Therapy for Amputees

Editors

Barbara Engstrom

Barbara has worked in a variety of settings (including acute hospitals, the community and prosthetic rehabilitation centres) in England and Canada in both general and amputee rehabilitation; she brings the generalist therapist's needs to this book. She worked at Roehampton for six years before pursuing a career in the clinical management of therapy services. She completed the certificate in lower limb prosthetics at Northwestern University, Chicago, ran wheelchair courses in her local health region, worked with the Chartered Society of Physiotherapy on their first standards booklet for people with amputations, has been a member of ISPO for over ten years and has lectured both nationally and internationally.

Catherine Van de Ven

Working in a centre of excellence at Roehampton for almost 30 years has given Catherine a specialist therapist's view of the need for this book; indeed it was started as a response to many telephone calls from physiotherapists and others requesting information and assistance. During her career she completed a Winston Churchill travelling fellowship to the USA to develop further knowledge about amputee rehabilitation, served on the McColl working party as the physiotherapy advisor for the Review of Artificial Limb and Appliance Services, was seconded to be the Physiotherapy Advisor to the Department of Health and was Chairman of the National Disablement Services Authority wheelchair training programme. She also gained the certificate in lower limb prosthetics from Northwestern University, Chicago, has been a member of ISPO for over 20 years (serving on the UK national committee) and was a member of the Council of the Chartered Society of Physiotherapy for five years.

For Churchill Livingstone:

Editorial director (Health Sciences): Mary Law
Project editor: Dinah Thom
Project controller: Derek Robertson

Therapy for Amputees

Edited by

Barbara Engstrom MCSP DipMgt(Open)
Formerly Therapy Services Manager, Nuffield Orthopaedic Centre NHS Trust, Headington, Oxford

Catherine Van de Ven MCSP
Formerly Physiotherapy Services Manager, Roehampton Rehabilitation Centre, Queen Mary's University Hospital, London

Illustrations by Jane Upton

THIRD EDITION

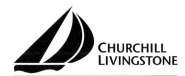

EDINBURGH LONDON NEW YORK PHILADELPHIA SYDNEY TORONTO 1999

CHURCHILL LIVINGSTONE
An imprint of Harcourt Brace and Company Limited

© Harcourt Brace and Company Limited 1999

◢ is a registered trademark of Harcourt Brace and
Company Limited

First published 1999

ISBN 0443 05975 6

British Library Cataloguing in Publication Data
A catalogue record for this book is available from the British
Library

Library of Congress Cataloging in Publication Data
A catalog record for this book is available from the Library
of Congress

Note
Medical knowledge is constantly changing. As new
information becomes available, changes in treatment,
procedures, equipment and the use of drugs become
necessary. The authors and the publishers have, as far as it is
possible, taken care to ensure that the information given in
this text is accurate and up-to-date. However, readers are
strongly advised to confirm that the information, especially
with regard to drug usage, complies with the latest
legislation and standards of practice.

The
publisher's
policy is to use
**paper manufactured
from sustainable forests**

Printed in China
NPCC/01

Contents

Contributors

Penny Buttenshaw MCSP
Clinical Specialist in Amputee Rehabilitation,
Roehampton Rehabilitation Centre,
Queen Mary's University Hospital, London

Fiona Carnegie DipCOT
Senior Occupational Therapist
Roehampton Rehabilitation Centre,
Queen Mary's University Hospital, London

Diana Dawes MCSP
Senior Physiotherapist,
Oxford Prosthetic Service,
Nuffield Orthopaedic Centre, Oxford

Barbara Engstrom MCSP DipMgt(Open)
Formerly Therapy Services Manager,
Nuffield Orthopaedic Centre, Oxford

Jane Greiller MCSP
Senior Physiotherapist,
Oxford Prosthetic Service,
Nuffield Orthopaedic Centre, Oxford

Clare Ireson DipCOT SROT
Head Occupational Therapist,
Nuffield Orthopaedic Centre, Oxford

Ann E Stead OBE DipCOT SROT
Clinical Director, Disability Services,
Nuffield Orthopaedic Centre, Oxford
(Born with a congenital lower limb deficiency, and a
prosthetic user since childhood, her role as an
occupational therapist has included work with users
in the development of services.)

Nicola Thompson MSc MCSP
Clinical Specialist in Gait Analysis,
Oxford Gait Laboratory,
Nuffield Orthopaedic Centre, Oxford

Maggie Uden MCSP
Senior Physiotherapist,
Roehampton Rehabilitation Centre,
Queen Mary's University Hospital, London

Catherine Van de Ven MCSP
Formerly Physiotherapy Services Director,
Roehampton Rehabilitation Centre,
Queen Mary's University Hospital, London

Brian Wade MBAPO
Director of Prosthetics,
Dorset Orthopaedic Co. Ltd,
Ringwood, Hampshire

Benna Waites BSc(Hons) DipClinPsych CPsychol
Chartered Clinical Psychologist,
Roehampton Rehabilitation Centre,
Queen Mary's University Hospital, London

Anne Zigmond DipCouns CQSW SRN
Accredited Counsellor,
Nuffield Orthopaedic Centre, Oxford

Preface to the third edition

This book is still intended as an introductory text for qualified and student physiotherapists as were the previous editions, but now it is also for qualified and student occupational therapists and for therapy assistants in the UK and overseas. It will also be of use to other members of the multidisciplinary team such as nurses, doctors, prosthetists, clinical psychologists, counsellors and amputees themselves.

Its purpose is to provide sufficient practical and theoretical information to enable therapy, relevant to the needs of the individual amputee, to be delivered by any therapist; the specialist therapist will find the wide range of ideas and avenues to pursue enables them to provide total integrated care for the amputee. It is hoped that the breadth of ideas will also help those working in more remote locations around the world to find rehabilitation solutions for amputees that are successful locally.

Since the second edition, many international changes have occurred resulting in an increase in the amputee population worldwide and consumer activism. Limited resources (both financial and human) and spiralling costs are pitted against increases in demand and advances in surgical and prosthetic technology.

Constant changes in the way healthcare is provided nationally have huge consequences and therapists have an increasingly difficult challenge to provide quality services to this group of people. Priority setting for such a specialised and small client group can be exceptionally difficult

when the demands of the whole of the physical disability client group (already poorly served) have to be met.

This third edition benefits from contributions from a wider range of healthcare professionals than previously and gives a broader, more flexible approach to rehabilitation due to greater awareness of the variety of different settings in which services are now delivered in the world. The contributors are a team of specialists in their field from the Roehampton Rehabilitation Centre at Queen Mary's University Hospital, London and the Prosthetic Service at the Nuffield Orthopaedic Centre, Oxford. New inclusions are chapters on the psychological impact of amputation, the user's point of view and therapy service quality. Considerable revision has been made throughout the text (using the latest international terminology), but with particular emphasis on prosthetic services and provision, wheelchairs, activities of daily living, pain management, multipathology and complex cases.

The authors have searched Medline, Cinahl, Recal and the Cochrane Collaboration databases; other references were found from these papers and authors in the field. It is recommended that therapists wishing to seek more in-depth information on any subject in the book make their own search using specific key words. For ease of reading, the authors have largely chosen to reference only at the end of each chapter and not in the text. The references, bibliography and appendix have been completely updated, although the reader must recognise that information is continually changing. For clarity throughout the book, the term 'therapist' is used to denote the healthcare professional delivering the treatment, and 'amputee' the person receiving it. It should be recognised that in practice the more correct term of 'person with an amputation' should be used to ensure that the person is recognised as an individual.

B. E.

Oxford & London, 1999

C. V. deV.

Preface to the second edition

Many changes have prompted us to revise the first edition.

Firstly, changes in the legislation and organisation of the National Health Service in the UK have resulted in the need for a more flexible and adaptable approach towards amputee management. These changes are ongoing and span across the acute episode in the hospital setting and care in the community setting.

Secondly, prosthetic and wheelchair supply and management have altered significantly following the McColl Report of 1986, allowing a more flexible service for the amputee's individual needs. Smaller companies are supplying a greater variety of prostheses: new designs and components are constantly being made available and will increase as the European Common Market and world markets expand. There is now a separation between prosthetic services companies and the manufacturers of components and hardware. There is no longer a national overview of the service, as it is now provided for either on a regional or local basis.

Thirdly, training, education, quality and standards issues are now also addressed at local level.

This second edition addresses some of these aspects and aims to help the clinical physiotherapist to cope with this constantly changing scene by paying attention to basic principles. It is still intended as a handbook for qualified and student physiotherapists and as such is still practically orientated. However, now more than ever physiotherapists must read more widely, paying attention to current literature including technical data concerning new prostheses, surgical techniques and rehabilitation research.

Many of our previous contributors have further assisted us; however, some no longer work in the amputee and prosthetic services but much of their original contribution remains in the text. The following people have supported us and contributed to this second edition:

For prosthetic rehabilitation services: Mrs P. Buttenshaw MSCP, Mrs J. Dolman MCSP, Mrs S. Smith MCSP, Mrs L. Robinson MCSP, Dr. S. Sooriakamaran MB BS LRCP MRCS FRCS (ENG EDIN & GLASG) Consultant in Rehabilitation, all from Richmond, Twickenham & Roehampton Health Authority; Ms P. Barsby MCSP and Dr L. Marks MRCP, Consultant in Rehabilitation, Royal National Orthopaedic Hospital Trust; Mr P. Lewis FBIST, Mr T. Morris FBIST, from C. A. Blatchford & Sons Ltd; Mr B. Fazackerely FBIST, Hugh Steepers Ltd. Mr P. Jamieson BSC, for photographic assistance from C. A. Blatchford & Sons Ltd.

Miss F. Carnegie DipCOT, who has revised Chapter 17 on upper limb amputation, and Miss B. Davis ONC MCSP, Kings Health Care, for suggestions on gait rehabilitation; Mrs V. Frampton MCSP, Canterbury and Thanet Health Authority, for further information on the aspects of pain and its control.

Miss S. Sharmin SRCh MChS DipPodM, for further information on chiropody, and Mrs S. Rigling RGN, for foot care advice and diabetes, both from Richmond, Twickenham & Roehampton Health Authority.

Ms H. Alper, Librarian, Queen Mary's University Hospital, for a literature search, the Medical Photography Department, Queen Mary's University Hospital, and S. Parapian, Medical Photography Department, University College and Middlesex School of Medicine, Mrs M. Lay, Physiotherapy Department Co-ordinator, Queen Mary's University Hospital, and Miss S. Skinner, University College Hospital, for secretarial support.

Dr M. F. R. Waters OBE FRCP FRCPath Consultant Leprologist, Hospital for Tropical Diseases; Mr A. Day OBE for assisting and coordinating much of the revised text; L. Crowder, Product specialist of Nomeq, for her technical help.

Lastly, but equally important, the voluntary organisations who have given so much assistance:

NALD
BLESMA
STEPS
BSAD
REACH

London, 1993

B.E.
C. V. deV.

Preface to the first edition

This is intended as a handbook for both qualified and student physiotherapists in the UK and abroad. Its purpose is to impart theoretical and practical knowledge, which can be used as a basic reference for those treating and caring for amputees during all stages of rehabilitation.

We have deliberately given a step-by-step approach because we feel this may simplify some of the complications encountered daily by patients and clinical staff. This may be criticised by those concerned with physiotherapy education, but we hope this book will provide advice for immediate and effective treatments in the clinical situation. This is particularly important during the prosthetic stages of rehabilitation, as it is essential to know how and where to obtain immediate assistance.

The majority of chapters are heavily illustrated to clarify procedures and activities. After each chapter there is a list of references, and there is also a general bibliography in the Appendix to permit the reader to deepen and widen existing knowledge. We have endeavoured to make these references as international and varied as possible. We have also included a list of useful addresses and a glossary of terms in the Appendix.

The contents of this book are our ideas and suggestions based on our experiences, which we have found successful over the years at Queen Mary's Hospital and the DHSS Limb Fitting Centre at Roehampton but, of course, each patient and situation must be approached individually.

We are most grateful to have been helped by many different professions in order to present an overall view of the Roehampton approach. Unfortunately, we cannot mention everybody by name, but we would like to thank the following, without whom this book would not have been possible:

Dr R. Redhead MB BS MRCS PhD, Senior Medical Officer, DHSS LFC, Roehampton, and Mrs F. Turner MCSP DipTP DipBioMech MPhil, who have read each chapter and given professional advice and assistance at all stages. Miss P. Langford MCSP and Mr J. Sim BA MCSP, who have commented on its clarity and understanding. Mr T. R. Frost FBIST, Chief Prosthetist, J. E. Hanger and Co. Ltd and Mrs D. Dixey MCSP, who have given specific advice on much of the contents.

Our main contributors: Miss A. Mendez OBE FCOT, former District Occupational Therapist, Richmond, Twickenham & Roehampton Health Authority, who has compiled and written Chapter 17; Miss A. Zigmond SRN CQSW, who has supplied written advice on social work and the psychological needs of the amputee; Mrs V. Long MChS SRCh, who has advised us on chiropody services.

Mrs J. Upton DipAD ATD, our illustrator, who has worked with us since the book's inception; much of the meaning of this book would be lost without her clear and accurate illustrations. Mr N. Babbage, consultant photographer, Bioengineering Centre, University College, London, for his excellent photographic work. Mrs W. Bevan, Librarian, Bioengineering Centre, who has helped us search the literature.

Other professional help and advice has been supplied by the following, from Queen Mary's Hospital, Roehampton: Dr I. H. M. Curwen MB ChB DPhysMed, former Consultant in Rheumatology and Rehabilitation, Mr B. G. Andrews FRCS, Consultant Orthopaedic Surgeon, Mr K. P. Robinson MS FRCSE FRCS, Consultant Surgeon, Dr P. Tidman MB BS FFARCS, Consultant Anaesthetist, Mr R. Ballard BSc FRCSEd MRCOG, Consultant Gynaecologist & Obstetrician, Mrs J. Hodder MCSP, Superintendent Physiotherapist, and Miss J. Jackson DipN, formerly ward sister, Limb Surgery Unit.

Dr N. Mustapha FRCS, Senior Medical Officer, Limb Fitting Service and Honorary Consultant to Queen Mary's Hospital, Dr D. J. Thornberry FRCS, and Mrs S. Riglin SRN, at DHSS LFC, Roehampton. Dr M. Dewer BSc PhD, Bioengineering Centre, University College, London, Dr J. Connolly MB MPhil FRCP FRCPsych, Consultant Psychiatrist, Maudsley Hospital, London, and Miss J. Guymer MCSP DipTP, Westminster Hospital, London. Mr M. Hammond supplied much of the information on sports for the amputee.

Mrs P. Ridgley, Manager, DHSS LFC, Roehampton, and many of her staff who have provided clerical assistance, in particular Mrs B. Spencer. Additional clerical help has been provided by Mrs C. O'Leary and Mrs M.

Pretty. Queen Mary's Roehampton Hospital Trust, and Mr J. Williams MBE, Clerk to the Trustees, for their financial help towards secretarial costs. Mrs G. Smith for her secretarial help in typing the final manuscript.

Miss S. M. Adams MCSP, District Physiotherapist, Richmond, Twickenham & Roehampton Health District, for her unfailing support and encouragement to us both during the production of this book and over the years. Also, the staff of the physiotherapy department, Queen Mary's Hospital, Roehampton, who have tried out the instructions for the functional activities and commented on them. The staff of Churchill Livingstone, for their help and advice.

We acknowledge permission to use photographs, illustrations and technical data of products of J. E. Hanger & Co. Ltd, C. A. Blatchford & Co., Vessa Ltd, Hugh Steeper (Roehampton) Ltd, and John Drew (London) Ltd. In particular, we would like to thank Mr B. O'Brien FBIST, and Mr R. Harrison LBIST, for prosthetic advice.

Lastly, but most importantly, we should like to thank all our patients, who, over the years, have taught us so much.

B. E.
London, 1985   C. V. deV.

Acknowledgements

The editors would like to acknowledge that without the support and encouragement of Penny Buttenshaw, Superintendent Physiotherapist at Roehampton Rehabilitation Centre, this third edition would not have come into being; also of Tod Frost, Emeritus Member ISPO, who not only has given a prosthetic overview while reading and re-reading the manuscript, but also has been a chef and wine waiter extraordinaire, without whom the editors would not have survived the last year. Our thanks are also due to many people who have contributed material, ideas and constructive criticism at various times throughout the project:

Prosthetists

Barry Fazackerely FBIST MBAPO Senior Prosthetic Manager, Hugh Steepers Ltd; Marie Kane MBAPO Prosthetic Manager, Orthopaedic Services Ltd; Joe McCarthy MBAPO Consultant Prosthetist, C. A. Blatchford and Sons Ltd; Anthony Millar MBAPO Clinical Services Director, Rehabilitation Services Ltd; John Mortimer MBAPO Prosthetist/ Orthotist, Otto Bock Ltd; Brian Wade MBAPO Director of Prosthetics, Dorset Orthopaedic Co Ltd

Prosthetic manufacturers

C. A. Blatchford and Sons Ltd: Suzanne Faulkener, PR / Sponsorship Coordinator; Gary Girling, Marketing Communications Manager; Paul Jameson, Regional Sales Manager

OrthoEurope: Michael O'Byrne MBAPO Chief Executive

Ossür UK: Toby Carlsson MBAPO

Otto Bock UK Ltd: Philip Yates, Managing Director

Hugh Steepers Ltd: Robin Cooper MBAPO Upper Limb Product Manager

Vessa Ltd: Keith Bell, Managing Director; James Parker, Technical Director; David Lindford, UK Sales Manager

Healthcare professionals

Queen Mary's University Hospital, Roehampton

Helen Ashton MCSP Superintendent Physiotherapist; P Burchell BSc SRD Dietetic Services Manager; Mary Jane Cole MCSP Senior Physiotherapist; Jane Duxbury BSc OT Senior Occupational Therapist; Carol Graves CQSW Social Worker; Neil Maffre LMPA RMIP Chief Medical Photographer; Dennis May BScHons PhD, CEng MIMechE Head of Clinical Science and Rehabilitation Engineering, QMUH Roehampton and Senior Fellow of the University of Surrey; Mary Pretty, Physiotherapy Assistant; Stuart Reeves RGN DMS Rehabilitation Service Manager; Professor K. P. Robinson, MSLond FRCSLond FRCSEd Consultant Surgeon in Rehabilitation, QMUH Roehampton and Visiting Professor Biomedical Engineering Group SMME University of Surrey; Sara Smith MCSP Senior Physiotherapist; S. Sooriakumaran MBBS LRCP FRCS(Eng) FRCS(Ed) FRCS(Glas) Consultant in Rehabilitation; Alison Swindells MCSP Superintendent Physiotherapist; Mandy Tottman MCSP Physiotherapy Services Manager

The Nuffield Orthopaedic Centre, Oxford

Bridget Burgess SSEN FAETC Manual Handling Advisor; Sarah Challacombe GradDip Phys Senior Physiotherapist; Adrian Dobson DTpADI DipDI DIAmond Driving Advisor, Mary Marlborough Centre; Barbara Edwards, Specialist Disability Services Manager; Jane Freebody GradDipPhys Senior Physiotherapist; Dr David Wilson MB BSc MRCP FRCR Consultant Radiologist and Medical Director NOC Senior Clinical Lecturer, University of Oxford

Other centres

Patsy Aldersea DipCOT Wheelchair Services Manager, Merton and Sutton Community NHS Trust; Professor Brånemark, Institute of Applied Biotechnology, Göteborg, Sweden; Dr A Bryceson MD FRCP Consultant Physician, Hospital for Tropical Diseases, London; David Condie, Rehabilitation Engineering Services Manager, Dundee Limb Fitting Centre; Elizabeth Condie FCSP Lecturer, National Centre for Training and Education in Prosthetics and Orthotics, University of Strathclyde; Dr Martin Dawes MD FRCGP Lecturer in Evidence-based Medicine, University of Oxford; Hilary Gooch BScOT BA(Hons) Lecturer, Brunel University; Ruth Hambrey DipCOT Manchester Disablement Services Centre; Rajiv Hanspal MBBS FRCS Consultant in Rehabilitation Medicine, Royal National Orthopaedic Hospital, Stanmore; Ann Hunter MA FCSP Practice Development Consultant; Amanda Lambert MCSP Superintendent Prosthetic Therapist, Castle

Hill Hospital, Cottingham; Wendy Matthias DipCOT Bristol Disablement Services Centre; Michelle McCreadie MCSP Deputy Director, Community Nursing, Community Health, Sheffield, NHS Trust; Judy Mead MCSP Head of Clinical Effectiveness, Research and Clinical Effectiveness Unit, Chartered Society of Physio-Therapy, London; Colin Stewart MD Associate Specialist in Rehabilitation, Dundee Limb Fitting Centre; Sue Stokes, National Coordinator, REACH; Grace Warren MD MS FRCS Previously Advisor in Leprosy and Reconstructive Surgery for the Leprosy Mission International in Asia (1975–1993), presently Associate in Infectious Diseases and Plastic Surgery at Royal Melbourne Hospital, Victoria and Consultant for Ortho-paedics (neuropathic limbs) Westmead Hospital, Sydney, Australia

Librarians

Helen Alper, MA MHSM ALA Library Service Manager, Queen Mary's University Hospital; Tina Craig BA Dip Lib Acting Librarian, Royal College of Surgeons of England; Eve Hollis, Library Services Manager, Girdlestone Memorial Library, Nuffield Orthopaedic Centre

Clerical help

Ellen Brewster, Secretary to the Roehampton Rehabilitation Centre; Gwyneth Follett, for assistance with the manuscript.

And last, our thanks to Dinah Thom and the staff of Churchill Livingstone, who have worked with us through all three editions and who have been most considerate of the difficulties faced by the editors during the last year.

1

Introduction

The purpose of this chapter is to introduce the subject to the reader in a general way; further details are to be found throughout the following chapters of the book. The authors have included a large and varied reference list and recommend that it be utilised by readers interested in specific details on any of the subjects covered in this chapter.

HISTORY OF AMPUTATIONS AND PROSTHESES

Archaeological evidence has shown that amputations were carried out as early as the Neolithic period with knives and bone saws, and skeletal remains with amputated bone stumps have been found.

In the latter half of the fifth century BC, Hippocrates wrote a treatise 'On Joints' in which amputation for vascular gangrene and cautery was described. In the first century AD, Celsus recommended that amputation should be between the healthy and the gangrenous tissues. There was an extremely high mortality rate brought about through shock and haemorrhage. The only forms of anaesthesia were wine and other alcoholic beverages and two assistants were needed to hold the patient down.

Ambroise Paré (1510–1590), the father of French surgery, improved ligation of large vessels during surgery and was vitally interested in the rehabilitation of the amputee, designing and manufacturing several prostheses for both upper and lower extremities. Ancient prostheses were very sophisticated by modern standards but were bulky and heavy. Many of the principles of modern prosthetics were developed and applied during this time.

The discovery of the circulation of the blood by Harvey in 1616 led to the invention of more efficient tourniquets, but speed of surgery was still essential. By the eighteenth century, better soft tissue coverage of bone ends with muscle flaps was achieved, but wound infection was frequent and often devastating. The modern concept of nursing was developed by Florence Nightingale during the Crimean War (1854–1856) in response to insanitary conditions in military hospitals. She replaced hospital chaos, filth and sorrow with scientific cleanliness, orderliness and increased well-being.

The development of anaesthesia in 1846 and Lister's aseptic technique in 1867 are the hallmarks of modern surgery. By the end of the nineteenth century the concept of allowing those muscles remaining to power the prosthesis was introduced. Prostheses at this time were fashioned out of wood. The Marquis of Anglesey, who lost his leg at the Battle of Waterloo, had a wooden prosthesis made for him by James Potts, and even today this type of prosthesis is still made and is called the Anglesey Leg.

HISTORY OF PROSTHETIC SERVICES IN THE UK

During the First World War, it became apparent that many men would survive their injuries and remain maimed by the loss of one or more limbs. In fact, by 1918, over 41 000 British ex-servicemen had become amputees.

The initiation of a service for amputees at Roehampton was followed by the setting up of services in other parts of the country, and in 1918, the first Director of Artificial Limb Supplies was appointed by the Minister of Pensions. During the Second World War there was a further influx of amputees but the service still existed predominantly for war injuries until the inception of the British National Health Service (NHS) in 1948. The system then expanded to take in civilian amputees as well as the ex-servicemen already under its care. This service model has been used as a framework for many nations who have adapted it to suit the specific needs of their populations. The supply of artificial limbs then became the responsibility of central government through the Department of Health and Social Security (DHSS) Artificial Limb Service.

The organisation of the Scottish prosthetic services became the responsibility of the NHS and is administered by the Scottish Home and Health Department. The local prosthetic services are operated by the health authority boards.

In May 1984, a group was set up 'to review and report on the adequacy, quality and management of the various services received by patients in Artificial Limb and Appliance Centres (ALACs) in England, on the respective roles of the staff of the centres and the NHS, and commercial manufacturers, having regard to the need to promote efficiency and cost effectiveness'. The group was chaired by Professor Ian McColl, now Lord McColl of Dulwich. The report recommended changes in:

- the organisation and management of the Artificial Limb and Wheelchair Service
- the provision of War Pensioners Appliances and the funding of Invalid Vehicle Services.

To enable these changes, a special health authority, the Disablement Services Authority (DSA) was created in 1987 and was integrated into the total service of the NHS in 1991. The McColl Report changed the overall service dramatically, enabling amputees to attend local prosthetic services rather than regional centres. Prosthetic supply also became more accessible giving both the prosthetist and amputee more choice and a greater variety of components. At the same time, the separation of prosthetic services from the manufacturing companies brought about changes in training and education for prosthetists (the profession is now for graduate entrants). For a description of the present day prosthetic services, see Chapter 8.

PRESENT DAY AMPUTEE POPULATION

Therapists and other healthcare professionals working in amputee rehabilitation need to know the characteristics of the population they serve. This will inform the professional training and education needed and the specific service components required by their clients, e.g. are the amputees mainly elderly people with a high incidence of concurrent disease or young people who have suffered trauma to either the upper or lower limb, or who have a congenital deficiency?

Data collection, evaluation and analysis varies depending on which country the therapist is working in. There may be national statistics (as in Denmark, Finland, Scotland and the Netherlands) or there may be smaller collections made in individual services or local regions, the latter giving a very fragmented view. Lack of a standardised approach to data presentation makes it difficult to draw conclusions and comparisons between regions and countries. The larger data collections are usually state funded and state driven to inform health care strategy. Innovative, small groups collect data for the benefit of their own units' research and audit. However, there are many studies available in the literature and the therapist must look for what is relevant to their specific service taking into account national characteristics, population age, amputation cause, and surgical and rehabilitation services.

National variables

When considering information from any country, the following background considerations must be taken into account:

- demographics of the population
- epidemiology of diseases that lead to amputation and the local management of these diseases
- amount of gross national product (GNP) available for social and healthcare provision
- economy of the country, as this will affect the type of workforce, degree of industrialisation, type of transportation used and how it is driven
- health and safety legislation and the degree to which it is adhered and monitored
- national social and healthcare policy, the availability and quality of medical and rehabilitation services and access to them

- timing of the periods of conflict that have occurred in that country, as this will determine the number of war wounded and people affected in the aftermath who commonly undergo amputation
- other local natural disasters, e.g. floods, earthquakes, etc.
- culture of the country, as this will affect the reporting of statistics and the attitude towards the rehabilitation provided.

Differences between developed and developing countries

More often, therapists treat amputees with major physical disability often made worse by concurrent disease. Therefore this chapter contains a small selection of the available information to help inform the need for rehabilitation locally, suggesting criteria for an approach to rehabilitation (always bearing in mind the quality of life) and aims of treatment intervention, suggesting reasons for the outcomes observed.

Cause of amputation

The cause of amputation in developing countries depends on the patient's stage of development; the country may be at war and in decline, or in post-war development and peace. In war zones, trauma results from fighting and landmines; in non-war zones, traffic and work-related accidents are the most common causes. Local disasters such as earthquakes also affect the numbers of amputees. The literature on amputee rehabilitation in developing countries reveals a constantly changing environment and progression of evolution. The total number of amputees in the developing world is not known, although efforts have been made to review areas of a particular country and the results are then extrapolated to predict national figures.

In the developed world, dysvascular conditions are the greatest cause of amputations; as these conditions are associated with ageing, concurrent pathology and ill-health, there is a direct relationship on the rehabilitation programme.

Table 1.1 Relative percentages of cause of lower-limb amputation

Developed world Cause	(%)	Developing world Cause	(%)
Peripheral vascular disease (approx. 25–50% have diabetes mellitus)	85–90	Trauma	55–95
Trauma	9	Disease	10–35
Tumour	4	Tumour	5
Congenital deficiency	3	Congenital deficiency	4
Infection	1	Infection	11–35

Differences in developed and developing world

Tables 1.1 and 1.2 contain a summation of information from the reference. In individual developing countries the percentages for tumour and trauma may be reversed.

Pathology

Peripheral vascular disease (PVD). PVD is referred to in some of the literature as a generic title encompassing disease of the blood vessels from a variety of presenting pathologies, and is subdivided by other authors into atherosclerosis, the effects of diabetes mellitus (DM), Buerger's disease, etc. This must be taken into account by the reader (See Ch. 2).

Over the past 2 decades, the incidence of amputation related to PVD in the western hemisphere has not changed and it is still the most common cause of lower limb amputation in the developed world. The incidence is increasing in the developing world as the economies of these countries and therefore lifestyle and diet alter, e.g. tobacco smoking lowers the mean amputation age in those with PVD by approximately 9 years.

It must be remembered that this is a disease

Table 1.2 Relative percentages of causes of upper limb amputation

Developed world Cause	(%)	Developing world Cause	(%)
Trauma	29	Trauma	86
Disease	30	Disease	6
Congenital deficiency	15	Congenital deficiency	6
Tumour	26	Tumour	1

of the older population, so concurrent pathology is likely to be present in 80% of those over the age of 65: these problems as well as the progression of the vascular disease may overwhelm older people. Half of the PVD-caused amputee population die of myocardial infarction or other cardiac disease; bronchopneumonia and carcinomatosis are other common causes of death.

In the developed world, it is estimated that one-third of dysvascular amputees die within 6 months of amputation, one-third have a major amputation of the contralateral leg within 2–3 years and one-third survive with one amputation beyond this time frame.

Risk factors for failed healing of amputation sites in the presence of vascular disease are pre-operative absence of gangrene in the ischaemic limb and pre-operative haemoglobin >120 g/L.

Renal disease. There is a high incidence of peripheral arterial occlusive disease in end-stage renal disease and in Tayside, Scotland, this subset of patients requiring limb amputation is now as large as those requiring amputation for tumour or trauma (Stewart, personal communication, 1997). The results of reconstructive procedures are generally poor, so lower extremity amputation may be the surgery of choice. It has been found that end-stage renal disease has a profound negative impact on morbidity.

Many of those on renal replacement therapy have diabetes (see later) and in the USA, the number of patients receiving dialysis has been increasing by 10% each year. The survival rate for those with diabetes and renal replacement therapy is, however, greater than for those without diabetes.

Buerger's disease. This occlusive disease affecting peripheral arteries occurs in young smokers (under 50 years of age), 98% of whom are male. There is a small major amputation rate that includes both upper and lower extremities.

Diabetes mellitus (DM). In 1991, the World Health Organisation (WHO) in Europe and the International Diabetes Federation (IDF, European region) accepted a programme for improved diabetes care known as The Saint Vincent Declaration. This set up certain goals to reduce the incidence of the most common diabetic complications. One of the goals was to achieve a reduction of 50% or more in major lower extremity amputations caused by diabetic gangrene. Preventative measures such as improved diabetic control, multidisciplinary teams looking after footcare and initiating optimal strategies to achieve healing, increased activity and better timing of vascular surgery and minor foot procedures, have helped achieve this goal in some localities.

Diabetic people have a 12–15-fold higher risk of an amputation compared to non-diabetic people but the absolute rate of amputation in DM appears to have been unchanged between 1981 and 1994. All diabetic amputees have a high postoperative mortality rate (8 times the expected rate during the first year following amputation) and a high rate of secondary amputation (30–50% at 3 years).

Trauma. There seems to be a positive correlation between population density and rate of traumatic amputation due to a heavy concentration of industry and mode of transport.

Natural environmental disasters can cause a substantial increase in amputation rates in a specific region. Conflict causes an increase in amputation in the military population as a result of the use of explosive devices. In the aftermath of conflict, indiscriminate use of landmines causes 80% of amputations in the civilian population. Landmines claim a new victim (either maimed or killed) every 22 minutes: for every 5000 mines cleared, one deminer is killed and two are injured. For every mine cleared, 20 new ones are planted.

However the injury is caused, the average age of traumatic amputees is significantly younger than that for PVD and diabetic conditions. It must be remembered that there are also borderline situations in which there is a sliding transition from trauma-related amputation to a vascular insufficiency amputation, e.g. a minor traumatic injury in a diabetic person can be one part of 'the causal pathway to amputation'.

In the UK, 63% of upper-limb amputations are due to trauma (1995 data), but the total number in the population is very small.

Frostbite. In some countries (e.g. Finland and Korea), frostbite is recorded as a separate statistic and in others as either a traumatic or vascular cause. The majority suffer cold injury either under alcoholic intoxication or as a result of being trapped in freezing conditions for too long, e.g. after motor vehicle breakdown.

Tumour. Tumours tend to require higher levels of amputation (approximately 80% are at hip disarticulation and trans-femoral levels) than other pathologies and are often carried out on younger people than people with PVD and DM (see Ch. 2). Approximately half of the total number are bone tumours, with soft tissue and skin tumours forming the majority of the rest.

Congenital limb deficiency. In most national studies, the incidence of congenital limb deficiency is 50 per 100 000 persons. One of the causes identified is an unexpected drug reaction, e.g. as in the thalidomide tragedy. Isolated limb deficiencies are usually sporadic occurrences. However, if they are associated with other abnormalities, or a family history, the risk to future pregnancies may be as high as 50%. The baby's anomalies may fit into a 'pattern' that constitute a syndrome. Recognition of a pattern of malformations may enable conclusions to be drawn about the mechanism and timing of the anomalies. The most common anomaly is transverse arrest at mid-forearm level, but there may be a variety of presentations from one absent limb to gross deficiency of all four limbs (see Chs 19 & 21).

Infection. Infections such as meningococcal septicaemia, may be the cause of amputation or infection following trauma, orthopaedic surgery (e.g. joint replacement), vascular surgery, etc. and may be recorded statistically as infection. Infection can be more common in developing countries because of the lack of medical facilities, antibiotics and hygiene. Leprosy (Hansen's disease) is an example of a successfully managed and treated infection with a supportive public education programme (see Ch. 21).

Age

In the developed world, the incidence of amputation of the lower limb is greater in people over 60 years of age and the average age of a patient requiring a first lower limb amputation is about 70 years.

The incidence of lower limb amputation in the over 65s is increasing dramatically with age, particularly in those over 80 years old; this can be linked to increased life expectancy in the developed world. The incidence of amputation in the under 65s is falling. However, in the developing world the picture is different, e.g. in Cambodia, where 80% of amputees are men between 18 and 40 years of age.

The incidence of common chronic disease in the over 65s is stated by Andrews (1996) as arthritis, 80%; impaired hearing/vision, 20–30%; diabetes mellitus, 10–15%; chronic heart disease, 15–20%; and cognitive disorders, 5% or more.

The average age of upper limb amputees is younger.

Gender

The male:female ratio varies slightly from country to country in the northern hemisphere – the further geographically north the country is, the more females undergo amputation.
Examples are:

Scotland: 3 males: 2 females
Denmark: 1.3 males: 1 female
London, UK: 2.4 males: 1 female (May, personal communication, 1998)
Korea: 4 males: 3 females
Saudi Arabia: 6.1 males: 1 female

Ratio of upper to lower limb amputations

Some examples are as follows:

- In the UK this was 1 upper limb: 5 lower limb in 1997.

- In Saudi Arabia this was 1 upper limb: 4 lower limb in 1977–1990.
- In Korea this was 1 upper limb: 2 lower limb in 1970–1994.

AMPUTATION SURGERY
Levels of amputation

There are certain levels of amputation that provide a residual limb suitable for prosthetic fitting, function and cosmesis. It is essential that one of these levels is selected rather than the boundary of the dead or diseased tissue with the viable tissue. Figures 1.1 and 1.2 illustrate these levels and further information can be found in the relevant chapters.

Statistics from all over the world indicate that the preservation of the knee joint in the lower limb amputee, and the elbow joint in the upper limb amputee, gives a far greater success with functional prosthetic use. Strenuous efforts are being made worldwide to increase the proportions of trans-tibial to trans-femoral amputations where possible, in order to keep more people ambulant.

Prevalence of amputation levels

Data is kept differently between centres and countries, however, Table 1.3 is a summation of information designed only to give the therapist an indication of the frequency with which treatment for each level will need to be provided.

Mortality

The operative mortality rate for lower extremity amputation is directly related to the level of amputation, the disease process, age and the presence of concurrent pathology: the higher the level of amputation, the higher the mortality rate. Data is kept in a variety of ways, i.e. in-hospital, postoperatively, within 3 months, and comparative. A range of 8–23% is the commonly reported mortality rate within 3 months.

Other mortality data from the developed world indicate 50–60% survival at 2 years and 30–40% at 5 years.

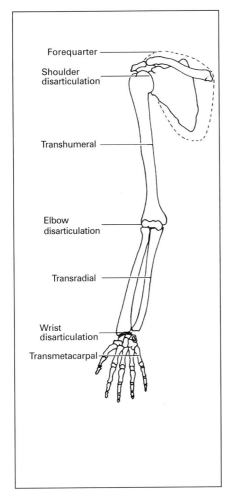

Figure 1.1 Levels of amputation in the upper limb.

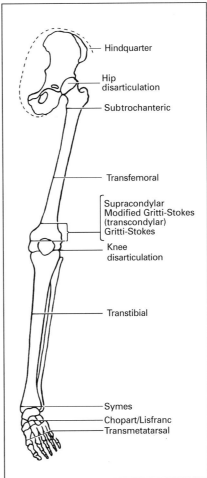

Figure 1.2 Levels of amputation in the lower limb.

Table 1.3 Levels of Amputation

Level	Developed world (%)	Developing world (%)
Lower limb		
Trans-tibial (including foot)	29–62	49–71
Trans-femoral (including knee disarticulation)	33–49	26–40
Upper limb		
Trans-radial (including wrist disarticulation)	32–66	21–33
Trans-humeral (including elbow disarticulation)	14–26	25–36

MODELS OF SERVICE DELIVERY

Every amputee is an individual and must always be considered within the context of their parti-cular abilities and wishes, and their medical and environmental status. Therefore no one model of care is right for all. Over the years, different models have emerged in different healthcare organisations and have been evaluated as to their outcomes (see Ch. 23) and now there is sometimes the flexibility of using different approaches for individuals starting from the same acute hospital setting. An ideal model, for example, is one in which the acute hospital team cares for the amputee at all stages from pre-operative assessment to discharge from outpatient services, with the amputee fully rehabilitated with prosthesis, wheelchair, home adaptations, etc.

Another model involves a transition from acute hospital to an inpatient rehabilitation unit with specialist prosthetic rehabilitation and all other forms of therapy needed by people with physical disabilities, and then follow-up as an outpatient at the same facility.

A community-based model transfers the amputee from the acute hospital either to their own home or to a community hospital at an early stage, and the community rehabilitation team provide the necessary care and therapy. If prosthetic services are required, they are provided on an outpatient basis at a specialist centre to which the team members may attend with their patient (see Fig. 1.3).

Therapists must know what models are available locally so that they can assess their patients in the relevant context. Prosthetic rehabilitation is not the goal for every amputee (see Chs 7 & 19) and even if it is, it may not be the most urgent priority in that individual's life at that moment. Indeed, surveys conducted in the developing world indicate that many amputees rank employment above the need for a prosthesis.

However, for any model to be successful, the following criteria must apply:

- good pre-operative assessment for the correct selection of amputation and performance of the operation by surgeons trained in amputation surgery

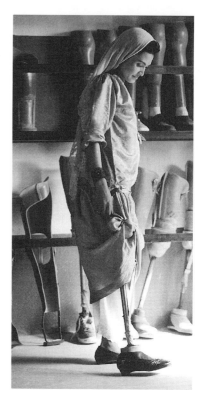

Figure 1.3 Victim of a landmine explosion in north west Afghanistan learns to walk. (Photograph by kind permission of Adrian Brooks and Times Newspapers Ltd.)

- an appreciation of the need for pre- and postoperative therapy and early mobilisation
- good integration of the prosthetic service with the acute or rehabilitation facility the individual is attending
- a team approach to amputee care (see Ch. 2).
- effective liaison between the rehabilitation team and the welfare services responsible for patient care in the community
- organised, regular follow-up of amputees by the specialist team in the prosthetic service and open access to this service by the amputee and/or their carers.

BIBLIOGRAPHY FOR PREVIOUS EDITIONS

Dallas Brodie I A O 1970 Lower limb amputation. British Medical Journal 4:596–604
Department of Health and Social Security Statistics and Research Division 1985 Amputation statistics for England, Wales and N. Ireland
English A W G, Gregory Dean A A 1980 The artificial limb service. Health Trends 12:77
Glattly H W 1964 Statistical study of 12 000 new amputees.

Southern Medical Journal 57:1373–1378
Glattly H W 1968 Preliminary report on amputee census. Artificial Limbs 7:5–10
Ham R, Thornberry D J, Regan J C et al 1985 Rehabilitation of the vascular amputee – one method evaluated. Physiotherapy Practice 1:6–13
Ham R, Van de Ven C 1986 The management of the lower limb amputee in England and Wales today. Physiotherapy Practice 2:94–100
Kay H W, Newman J D 1974 Amputee survey 1973–74; preliminary findings and comparisons. Orthotics and Prosthetics 28(2):27–32
Knight P, Urquhart J 1989 Outcomes of artificial lower limb fitting in Scotland. Information and Statistics Division, Common Services Agency for the Scottish Health Service, Edinburgh
McColl I 1986 Review of artificial limb and appliance centre services. DHSS, London, vols 1 & 2
Murdoch G 1977 Amputation surgery in the lower extremity. Prosthetics and Orthotics International 1:72–83
Murdoch G 1984 Amputation revisited. Prosthetics and Orthotics International 8:8–15
Narang I C, Jape V S 1982 Retrospective study of 14 400 civilian disabled (new) treated over 25 years at an Artificial Limb Centre. Prosthetics and Orthotics International 6:10–16
Orr J R, James W V, Bahrani A S 1982 The history and development of artificial limbs. Engineering in Medicine 11(4):155–161
Robins R 1984 An old Cornish hand. Journal of Hand Surgery 98:199–200
Robinson K P 1980 Limb ablation and limb replacement. Annals of the Royal College of Surgeons of England 62:87–105

BIBLIOGRAPHY FOR THE THIRD EDITION

Alaranta H, Alaranta R, Pohjolainen T, Kärkkäinen 1995 Lower limb amputees in Southern Finland. Prosthetics and Orthotics International 19(3):155–158
Al-Turaiki H S, Al-Falahi L A A 1993 Amputee population in the Kingdom of Saudi Arabia. Prosthetics and Orthotics International 17(3):147–156
Anderson S P 1995 Dysvascular amputees: what can we expect? Journal of Prosthetics and Orthotics 7(2):43–50
Andrews K L 1996 Rehabilitation in limb deficiency. 3. The geriatric amputee. Archives of Physical Medicine and Rehabilitation 77(3S): S14–17, S29–37, S81–82
Armstrong D G, van Houtum W H, Harkless L B, Lavery L A 1997a The impact of gender on amputation. The Journal of Foot and Ankle Surgery 36(1):66–69
Armstrong D G, van Houtum W H, Harkless L B, Lavery L A 1997b Seasonal variations in lower extremity amputation. The Journal of Foot and Ankle Surgery 36(2):146–150
Buttenshaw P, Dolman J 1992 The Roehampton approach to rehabilitation: a retrospective survey of prosthetic use in patients with primary unilateral lower-limb amputation. Topics in Geriatric Rehabilitation 8(1):72–78
Bottomley J M, Herman H 1992 Preventing amputation: Screening and conservative management. Topics in Geriatric Rehabilitation 8(1):13–21
Campbell W B, Kernick V F M, St Johnston J A, Rutter E A 1994 Lower limb amputation: striking the balance. Annals of the Royal College of Surgeons of England 76:205–209
Chappel P H 1992 Arm amputation statistics for England 1958–1998: an exploratory statistical analysis. International Journal of Rehabilitation Research 15:57–62
Chan K M, Cheung D, Sher A, Leung P C, Fu K T, Lee J 1984 A 24 year survey of amputees in Hong Kong. Prosthetics and Orthotics International 8(3):155–158
Condie E, Jones D, Treweek S, Scott H 1996 A one-year national survey of patients having a lower limb amputation. Physiotherapy 82(1):14–20
Cutson T M, Bongiorni D R 1996 Rehabilitation of the older lower limb amputee: a brief review. Journal of the American Geriatrics Society 44(11):1388–1393
Dossa C D, Shepard A D, Amos A M et al 1994 Results of lower extremity amputations in patients with end-stage renal disease. Journal of Vascular Surgery 20(1):14–19
Ebskov L B 1991a Epidemiology of lower limb amputations in diabetics in Denmark (1980 to 1989). International Orthopaedics 15:285–288
Ebskov L B 1991b Lower limb amputations for vascular insufficiency. International Journal of Rehabilitation Research 14:59–64
Ebskov L B 1993 Major amputation for malignant melanoma: an epidemiological study. Journal of Surgical Oncology 52:89–91
Ebskov L B 1994 Trauma-related major lower limb amputations: an epidemiologic study. The Journal of Trauma 36(6):778–783
Ebskov L B 1996 Relative mortality in lower limb amputees with diabetes mellitus. Prosthetics and Orthotics International 20:147–152
Editorial 1998 Aiding Landmine Survivors: the challenge awaits. Orthotics and Prosthetics Business World 1(1):22–34
Eneroth M, Persson B M 1993 Risk factors for failed healing in amputation for vascular disease. Acta Orthopaedica Scandinavica 64(3):369–372
Esquenazi A 1993 Geriatric amputee rehabilitation. Clinics in Geriatric Medicine 9(4):731–743
Fyfe N C M 1990 An audit of amputation levels in patients referred for prosthetic rehabilitation. Prosthetics and Orthotics International 14:67–70
Gailey R S, Nash M S, Atchley T A et al 1997 The effects of prosthesis mass on metabolic cost of ambulation in non-vascular trans-tibial amputees. Prosthetics and Orthotics International 21:9–16
Ham R, McCreadie M 1992 Rehabilitation of elderly patients in the United Kingdom following lower-limb amputation. Topics in Geriatric Rehabilitation 8(1):64–71
Hendry J A 1995 The utilization of physiotherapy services after lower-limb amputation in an academic hospital in South Africa. Proceedings of 12th International Conference of the World Confederation for Physical Therapy, Washington
Hettiaratchy S P, Stiles P J 1996 Rehabilitation of lower limb traumatic amputees: the Sandy Gall Afghanistan Appeal's experience. Injury 27(7):499–501

Jackson-Wyatt O 1992 Age-related changes in amputee rehabilitation. Topics in Geriatric Rehabilitation 8(1):1–12

Joss D M 1997 Global health issue. Anti-personnel landmine injuries: a global epidemic. Work 8(3):299–304

Kim Y C, Park C I, Kim D Y, Kim T S, Shin J C 1996 Statistical analysis of amputations and trends in Korea. Prosthetics and Orthotics International 20(2):88–95

Kulkarni J R 1995 Mobility after amputation of a lower limb. British Medical Journal 311:1643–1644

Lääperi T, Pohjolainen T, Alaranta H, Kärkkäinen M 1993 Lower limb amputations. Annales Chirurgiae et Gynaecologiae 82:183–187

Larsson J, Apelqvist J 1995 Towards less amputations in diabetic patients. Acta Orthopaedia Scandinavica 66(2):181–192

Lindholt J S, Bøvling S, Fasting H, Henneberg E W 1994 Vascular surgery reduces the frequency of lower limb major amputations. European Journal of Vascular Surgery 8:31–35

Loro A, Franceschi F, Mosha E C P, Samwell J 1990 A survey of amputations at Dodoma Regional Hospital, Tanzania. Prosthetics and Orthotics International 14(2):71–74

Nagashima H, Inoue H, Takechi H 1993 Incidence and prognosis of dysvascular amputations in Okayama Prefecture (Japan). Prosthetics and Orthotics International 17(1):9–13

O'Brien T S, Gray D R, Lamont P M, Collin J, Crow A, Morris P J 1993 Lower limb ischaemia in the octogenarian: is limb salvage surgery worthwhile? Annals of the Royal College of Surgeons of England 75:445–447

Pedersen A E, Bornefeldt O, Krasnik et al 1994 Halving the number of leg amputations: the influence of infrapopliteal bypass. European Journal of Vascular Surgery 8:26–30

Pell J P, Fowkes F G R, Ruckley C V, Clarke J, Kendrick S, Boyd J H 1994 Declining incidence of amputation for arterial disease in Scotland. European Journal of Vascular Surgery 8:602–606

Pernot H F M, de Witte L P, Lindeman E, Cluitmans J 1997 Daily functioning of the lower extremity amputee: an overview of the literature. Clinical Rehabilitation 11:93–106

Pohjolainen T, Alaranta H, Wikstrom J 1989 Primary survival and prosthetic fitting of lower limb amputees. Prosthetics and Orthotics International 13:63–69

Poonekar P 1992 Prosthetics and orthotics in India. In: Report of a research planning conference – prosthetic and orthotic research for the twenty-first century, Bethesda, Maryland, National Institute of Child Health and Human Development 23–25 July:233–239

Rommers G M, Vos L D W, Groothoff J W, Schuiling C H, Eisma W H 1997 Epidemiology of lower limb amputees in the north of the Netherlands: aetiology, discharge destination and prosthetic use. Prosthetics and Orthotics International 21(2):92–99

Sioson E R, Kerfoot S, Ziat L M 1993 Rehabilitation outcome of older patients with end-stage renal disease and lower extremity amputation. Journal of the American Geriatrics Society 41:667–668

Stewart C P U, Jain A S, Ogston S A 1992 Lower limb amputee survival. Prosthetics and Orthotics International 16:11–18

Stewart C P U, Jain A S 1992 Cause of death of lower limb amputees. Prosthetics and Orthotics International 16(2):129–132

Stewart C P U, Jain A S 1993 Dundee revisited – 25 years of a total amputee service. Prosthetics and Orthotics International 17(1):14–20

Takechi H 1992 History of prostheses and orthoses in Japan. Prosthetics and Orthotics International 16(2):98–103

Van Ross E R E 1997 After amputation: rehabilitation of the diabetic amputee. Journal of the American Podiatric Medical Association 87(7):332–335

Wainapel S F 1997 Rehabilitation of the older amputee. Journal of the American Geriatrics Society 45(8):1033

2

Assessment

The therapist's pre-operative assessment is concerned with the physical and psychological status of the patient, the social situation, home environment and available help. Following a diagnosis by the doctor, the therapist will relate the assessment of the patient to the implications of that diagnosis in order to:

- evaluate the patient's physical and psychological status
- evaluate the affected limb
- formulate a programme of action required to initiate immediate treatment, ensure safe discharge from the acute hospital and facilitate future rehabilitation.

CONDITIONS PREDISPOSING TO AMPUTATION

Each of the following conditions has important aspects that need to be considered by the therapist:

1. Vascular disease—atherosclerosis
2. Vascular disease—diabetes mellitus
3. Trauma
4. Tumour
5. Congenital limb deficiency.

Vascular disease: atherosclerosis

Atherosclerosis is a disease of the arterial system. Plaques of atheroma can be deposited in any artery of the body, for example:

- Cerebral atheroma can cause cerebrovascular accidents.

- Myocardial atheroma can cause myocardial infarction.
- Mesenteric atheroma can cause infarction of the gut.
- Peripheral vascular disease can cause limb ischaemia.

Therefore, it must be remembered that, although the presenting problem may be one of a gangrenous foot, the patient can also be suffering from vascular disease elsewhere in the body. Patients can complain of intermittent claudication and there may be open sore areas around the toes or heel. The appearance of the skin is hairless and shiny, and the colour can be white, red or blue and it will feel cold to the touch. Vascular reconstructive surgery may relieve these symptoms, but if the disease has progressed too far or surgery has failed, the symptoms that then bring the patient to amputation are:

1. *Gangrene.* Particularly if septicaemia is present.
2. *Rest pain.* This is intolerable ischaemic pain at rest, particularly at night. The patient does not sleep and may obtain relief by hanging the affected limb over the edge of the bed. This dependent position encourages blood flow to the extremity.

These two positive indications for amputation also apply to venous ulcers and Buerger's disease (this may also affect the upper limb). It is possible that the patient may have already had one leg amputated and requires further surgery to the residual limb or the remaining leg as the atherosclerosis progresses.

Investigations for vascular disease

Clinical examination of the limb. The general appearance and temperature of the limb is noted, together with the condition, colour and texture of the skin. The femoral, popliteal, posterior tibial and dorsalis pedis pulses are palpated.

Chest X-ray

Blood tests. Biochemical and haematological studies are carried out to detect factors that are known to affect the viscosity and hence reduce the flow of blood. The tests included are mea-surements of fasting serum cholesterol, platelet abnormalities and clotting changes.

Electrocardiogram

Doppler studies. A noninvasive technique that involves the application of an ultrasonic wave over the artery using a hand-held, battery-operated instrument. This wave is beamed over a moving stream of blood, producing a frequency shift, which is a function of the rate of blood flow. A pressure index can be ascertained by obtaining the ratio between systolic arterial pressure at the ankle and that in the brachial artery. Ankle pressure divided by brachial pressure is called the 'brachial index'. A value of 1 or more exludes significant vascular disease in the lower limb. Claudication indices are 0.4–0.8 and critical ischaemia indices are as low as 0.2–0.4. Advanced forms of this investigation are laser Doppler and duplex scanning. The latter provides an image of the vessels as well as a measure of the flow in them.

Arteriography. An invasive technique in which radio-opaque fluid known as 'contrast' is injected into the arterial system. X-rays are then taken, which indicate the patency of both the main and collateral vessels. This indicates whether reconstructive surgery is possible or if the lumen of the artery can be opened by the radiologist using a balloon catheter (balloon angioplasty) or using an expanding wire liner deployed by the balloon (intra-arterial stenting). Any recent occluding clot may be melted away by thrombolysis using streptokinase, urokinase or tissue plasminogen activator.

Venogram. An X-ray of the venous system – this can be avoided if venous duplex (colour flow Doppler ultrasound) can be carried out.

Thermography. A measurement of skin temperature in the whole limb, reflecting, among other factors, the level of cutaneous tissue viability, blood flow and hence the degree of ischaemia. A particular area cannot be considered in isolation but only in comparison with other areas.

Transcutaneous PO2 readings. A measurement of skin oxygen pressure that reflects the level of cutaneous blood flow, hence the degree of ischaemia.

Other tests may be carried out in specialist

centres with vascular laboratories, e.g. treadmill exercises, strain gauge plethysmography, echo and duplex imaging, digital subtraction angiography, radionuclide-distraction studies, nuclear magnetic resonance, isotope clearance structure of the skin and muscle.

Advanced technology is enabling more detailed clinical investigation and will become increasingly available in acute general hospitals in time.

Vascular disease: diabetes mellitus

Diabetes mellitus is a systemic disorder in which blood glucose may be intermittently raised above the normal range. The complications of diabetes may cause small blood vessel damage, which can affect different parts of the body in the following ways:

- Retinopathy can lead to impairment of vision and occasionally blindness.
- Glomerulosclerosis can lead to renal failure and death (see Ch. 1).
- Neuropathy of the peripheral nerves can lead to impaired sensation in the hands and feet; the distal portion of all digits is more severely affected.
- Small artery disease can lead to peripheral or coronary ischaemia.

Healing is often poor in these patients and even minor trauma can be a major problem. Non-healing ulceration of the feet can result from impaired circulation and poor sensation. The high glucose levels in the wound encourage bacterial growth, resulting in infection that may also extend to the bone. This can lead to gangrene, and while local amputation of parts of the foot can be attempted, these may not heal and a more proximal level must then be selected.

Because of a chemical reaction, people with diabetes are also more prone to vascular disease in large vessels, which could lead to cerebral and coronary ischaemia and peripheral vascular disease. Many of these patients therefore have both large and small artery disease. Reconstructive vascular surgery is not always successful in people with diabetes because they are prone to poor healing.

Each patient must seek individual advice from their dietician. Therapists need to be aware of the diet regime for each patient so they can attend to dietary needs appropriately if the patient attends the therapy facility for an extensive amount of time each day.

Investigations in diabetes

Blood tests. To estimate the blood sugar level. The normal range after 8 hours of starvation is 3.3–5.5 mmol/l. Haemoglobin A_{1C} gives an indication of the accuracy of control.

Urine tests. To estimate the sugar and ketone levels.

Trauma

Amputation of a limb can take place immediately at the site of an accident or the extensive trauma can cause sufficient damage or death of tissue to require subsequent ablation.

The aim in trauma management is to restore the limb to the best possible length with a good soft tissue covering. To achieve this, the expertise, cooperation and rational decision making of orthopaedic, plastic and vascular surgeons is necessary, with the consultant in prosthetic rehabilitation. This team must bear in mind priorities of surgical management from injury to successful prosthetic outcome. In an emergency setting, life may be saved by sacrificing the limb, but once the patient has stabilised, the decision concerning limb salvage and optimum level of amputation can be made. The psychological make-up of the patient and their goals and employment must be considered. The basic surgical techniques to achieve wound healing are appropriate, such as handling of soft tissue, wound debridement, secondary wound closure and control of sepsis, but these will inevitably delay rehabilitation.

The amputation can therefore take place immediately, or months or even years following the trauma, and this final decision should only be taken after extensive assessment and discussion between the patient, the surgeon and the rehabilitation team. Years of pain and lack of independence can possibly be avoided by seeking referral to the local prosthetic service for a pre-amputation consultation by members of the multi-disciplinary team. This will allow the patient to be given a realistic view of their future lifestyle as an amputee.

Additionally, a small number of elective ortho-paedic procedures, such as joint replacement, occasionally suffer overwhelming infection and, although two-stage revision with interim intra-venous antibiotics is the treatment of choice, amputation has to be considered in severe cases.

Examples of trauma

Various types of trauma can lead to amputation, including:

- Compound fractures, particularly those involving skin and soft tissue loss – often in association with multiple injuries
- Blood vessel rupture
- Severe burns
- Stab, gunshot or blast injuries
- Compression injuries
- Cold trauma, i.e. frostbite.

The factors listed above may occur in combina-tion; reimplantation and tissue transfer with microsurgery may often be necessary. Reimplan-tation is rarely successful in cases of adult proxi-mal upper limb or lower limb trauma. In young children, this technique may be successful and is valuable for treating forearm and hand trauma in adults.

Investigations in trauma

X-rays. Skeletal, arteriography, computerised axial tomography (CAT) scan, venography, (rarely magnetic resonance imaging [MRI] scan).

Estimation of skin loss. Wallace's Rule of Nines is used for burn patients. A visual assessment of the depth and area of soft tissue loss is noted in the non-burnt patient.

Clinical examination of the limb.
Assessment:

- physical
- psychological.

It may be necessary to explore both aspects by speaking to the relatives and friends of the acutely injured person where the patient is unable to provide an account of their situation.

Tumour

Patients with tumour usually present with pain or a history of trivial trauma, as a result of which an X-ray is taken and the tumour is discovered almost by chance. Sometimes there is a swelling present, but otherwise there is no other physical sign. Primary malignant tumours in bone are rare. The most common types of tumour are: osteo-sarcoma, chondrosarcoma, Ewing's tumour, fibro-sarcoma and giant cell tumour. The majority of patients with these tumours are under 20 years of age. Occasionally secondary deposits cause pa-tients to attend hospital with a pathological frac-ture. In the UK, there are specialist cancer centres for bone tumour investigation and treatment.

Following diagnosis of the tumour, the treat-ment may involve chemotherapy or radiotherapy, massive excision and endoprosthetic replacement, or amputation. However, it should always be remembered that even if massive replacement is the treatment of choice, the patient may eventually have to undergo amputation, either for recurrence of the tumour or infection in the replacement.

The therapist must communicate with the medical oncologist, surgeon and radiologist monitoring each case, in order to set appropriate and realistic goals of treatment. Whatever the choice of treatment, the psychological prepa-ration of both the patient and their parents or carers is of the utmost importance. In addition, the clinical psychologist or counsellor and thera-pists are involved to ensure that emotional and psychological problems are identified quickly and addressed effectively.

The physical rehabilitation programme must be flexible to accommodate the issues posed by concurrent treatments. As these patients are usually young, they can cope with extensive activity for the periods between chemotherapy. However, there are other times when no form of therapy is possible.

In adult life, metastatic tumours in the skeleton are much more common than primary malignant tumours. The primary lesions are usually found in the breast, prostate gland, kidney or lung. These patients more commonly present with pain or a pathological fracture. The treatment given is usually conservative, with internal fixation of the fracture.

Investigations for tumours

X-ray (mainly skeletal). Bone scintigraphy, angiography and CAT scans are very occasionally carried out.

MRI scan – to find the extent of soft tissue and bone involvement.

Biopsy. This is the most reliable means of diagnosis and is performed after the images have determined the site of the lesion. Needle biopsy is preferable to open biopsy to reduce the risk of spread, in many cases but not all. Blood tests may be performed for tumour marker substances.

Congenital limb deficiency

A child can be born with partial or complete absence of one limb, up to a total absence of all four limbs, or any combination between these two extremes. There may be absence of bone or another deformity present.

The classification of congenital limb deficiencies is complicated and the International Society for Prosthetics and Orthotics (ISPO) system is used, which is constructed on an anatomical basis. Deficiences are identified as being either transverse or longitudinal.

Transverse. The limb has developed normally to a particular level beyond which no skeletal elements exist, although there may be digital buds. Some children may have several of their limbs affected, but most commonly the child presents with a single deformity at mid-forearm level.

Longitudinal. There is a reduction or absence of a bone within the long axis of the limb; this will affect the development of structures distal to that bone. For example, a child with a short femur and absent tibia is likely to have absence of the lateral side of the foot as in the child in Figure 2.1, who is able to walk with the aid of extension prostheses.

Further details can be found on upper limb

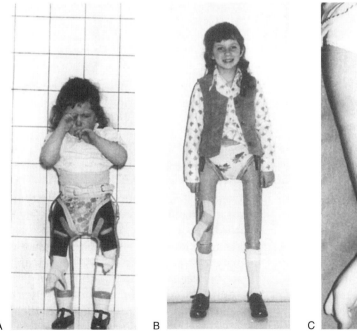
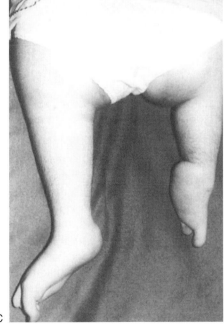

Figure 2.1 Extension prostheses: (A) child at 3 years; (B) Same child at 9 years; (C) this child's congenital deformities at 13 years.

congenital deficiency (see Ch. 19) and lower limb and multiple deficiency (see Ch. 21).

PRE-OPERATIVE THERAPY ASSESSMENT

Physical assessment

If the status of the limb appears critical, the therapist should ideally start the pre-amputation assessment before the actual decision to amputate has been made. The patient should be receiving treatment in a general surgical, medical, orthopaedic, plastic surgery or elder care ward (or even the intensive therapy unit), and should be observed closely during this time. The possibility of amputation must not be divulged to the patient – this is solely the surgeon's responsibility. However, in many cases there will be no time for a pre-operative therapy assessment due to the degree of medical urgency.

The therapist should tailor their assessment to the circumstances of the patient, for example:

- the option to amputate is being considered by the surgeon and the patient has been made aware of this possibility – in this case the multidisciplinary team are able to explain the full implications of the rehabilitation programme to them
- a patient requires an amputation within the next few hours or days
- a patient has just undergone an emergency amputation, sometimes during the previous night.

In all cases, the therapist must read the patient's medical notes, medication chart and nursing records before planning the order of the initial assessment. The information to be recorded by the therapist is as shown in Figure 2.2.

Muscle strength, range of joint movement and functional mobility must be recorded so that future comparison is possible. When measuring a joint, a goniometer must be used. The hip should be measured in Thomas' position (see Fig. 2.3). A number of positions can be used to measure the knee, but whatever method is chosen it is essential that subsequent readings are taken in

the same position. The size and position of fragile pressure areas should also be recorded accurately and functional activity levels assessed and recorded. The sequelae of other pathologies present must be recognised and assessed (e.g., musculoskeletal and neurological conditions). Furthermore, the general frailty associated with ageing, such as cognition, memory, etc. must be appraised, but it must be acknowledged that confusion may be the result of the acute medical condition and not a pre-morbid problem.

It must be noted that assessment is ongoing and never a one-off exercise. The patient may frequently be so systemically ill that accurate and detailed assessment is not possible. The therapist and patient must build up a relationship gradually so that communication is free and detailed subjective information can be gathered. Many patients are confused, in pain and anxious at this time, and subjective information may be inaccurate at this stage. For this reason, the relatives or carers should be approached whenever possible. The physical assessment and pre-operative exercise programme merge into one and the same activity. The aims and goals of treatment are planned at this stage and a care pathway and discharge plan are discussed by the hospital team. Legislation in the UK such as the NHS and Community Care Act, the Patient's Charter and the NHS Continuing Healthcare Guidance require that all hospitals ensure that all arrangements for care and ongoing rehabilitation have been organised before the patient leaves hospital. All care and discharge plans should be collaborative with the patient, their carer and any members of the primary healthcare team involved.

Treating the patient in this situation will require a tactful approach and care with the wording of questions is needed. The process of assessment must never cause the patient undue pain or distress – this will not build up confidence between the patient and therapist. Timing therapy sessions around analgesia is often essential to obtain the best possible response. To avoid repetition, it may be possible for the therapist to be present at the surgeon's initial examination. It may be appropriate to contact the local prosthetic

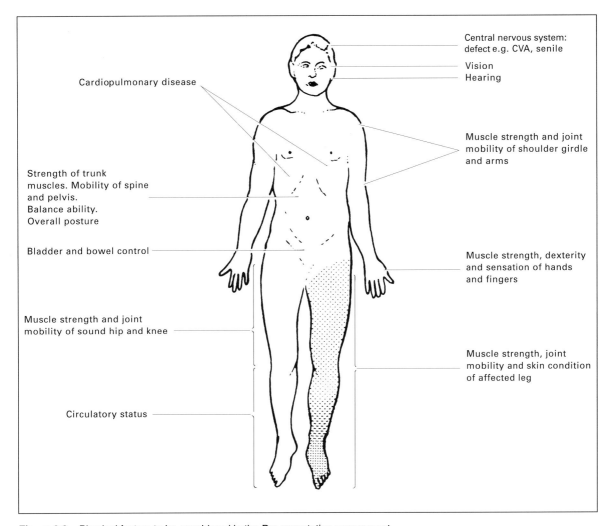

Figure 2.2 Physical factors to be considered in the Pre-amputation assessment.

service or one of the self-help organisations, e.g. the Limbless Association, the British Limbless Ex-Servicemen's Association or the Association of Carers Groups, if the patient and/or their carers wish to discuss the situation with another amputee.

Social assessment

Although the social assessment is not separate from the physical assessment, specific facts must be ascertained concerning the patient's home environment, support from relatives or friends, community support, place and type of work, leisure activities and any financial worries. Each patient's lifestyle will be affected by their medical condition to some extent.

Psychological assessment

Ideally a psychological assessment should run in parallel with the physical assessment, starting as early as possible. Access to psychological assessment should ideally be available for all patients (and partners/families where appropriate). However, ongoing psychological input will depend on the needs of the patient and will not be necessary for every amputee. In cases where memory

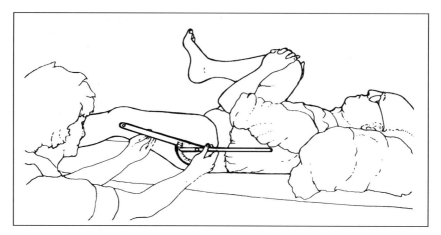

Figure 2.3 Thomas' test for measurement of hip flexion contracture.

or other cognitive problems are suspected or known, a neuropsychological assessment can be performed. This enables advance planning for rehabilitation and discharge (see Ch. 3).

DISCUSSION OF CHOICE OF AMPUTATION LEVEL

It is the responsibility of each team member to communicate their thoughts to the surgeon in charge regarding the most desirable amputation level. In making this decision, the clinical, physical, social and psychological assessments will be taken into account, along with consideration of the prosthetic possibilities.

As amputation is a final decision and so many healthcare professionals are involved, a case conference may be the best setting for discussion to take place. However, in an emergency situation, each team member should try to convey their recommendations (however brief) to the surgeon by telephone or fax. A unified team approach to the individual patient should always be the goal.

PRE-OPERATIVE PREPARATION

When the decision to amputate has been taken, the patient should be approached with the following information:

- an explanation of why the operation is necessary

- an explanation of what the operation entails
- a prediction of how the patient can expect to feel after the operation, including a description of phantom reactions and residual limb pain
- instructions concerning what to do about the pain (e.g. telling staff and relaxation)
- reassurance that the pain will pass
- introduction to, and explanation of, the local prosthetic service (provided the pre-operative assessment indicates a likelihood of prosthetic rehabilitation, see Ch. 7)
- realistic information regarding the possible effect of the operation on the patient's lifestyle
- an opportunity to talk over the patient's feelings about loss of the limb.

Pre-operative treatment

An active programme of pre-operative treatment may not be possible because of the medical condition of the patient, but the items listed in the treatment plan following should be attempted. Although the patient should ideally be brought to the therapy facility, this may not be possible if infection is present, drips are in situ, confusion is observed or the patient is reluctant to be moved.

There will be many pre-operative investigations and assessments carried out by other team members and the relative importance of all aspects of pre-operative care must be recognised.

Therapy treatment plan

Pre-anaesthetic chest physiotherapy. Many patients are smokers; any postural drainage position can be used as necessary, providing that care is taken with the affected limb.

Preparation for postoperative appearance. The therapist should reinforce the expected level of amputation by touching the patient's limb at the relevant point. The therapist can also discuss the appearance of the residual limb and warn the patient to expect i.v. drips, a drain in the residual limb and, in some cases, a urinary catheter.

Information about phantom sensation. The patient should be warned that it is completely normal to feel the sensation of the whole limb after amputation. This sensation usually diminishes as active rehabilitation, including handling the residual limb, resisted exercises and weight-bearing progresses (see Ch. 20). The therapist should be aware that the patient may not only describe feeling the phantom limb but also a wide variety of sensations, some of which can be distressing to the patient.

Instruction on bed mobility. The patient with an upper limb amputation should be shown how to move up and down the bed, and climb in and out of bed using one arm for support. The postoperative problems of balance should be explained to the patient.

A suitable high/low bed should be provided for the lower limb amputee so that the patient can transfer safely onto a wheelchair or commode. A firm base is necessary for balance. It must be explained to the patient that a bed rail may be necessary to aid mobility when moving from side to side in the first few postoperative days and not there because the staff expect the patient to be confused.

Instruction on use of a monkey pole to lift themselves onto a bedpan and relieve pressure areas may be needed while patients are relatively immobile. As the patients become stronger post-operatively, they will be taught to do push-ups and the monkey pole will be taken away as soon as the patient can manage without it.

Observation of all areas of the skin is important, particularly with Negroid and Asian skin tones, as erythema or ischaemic changes are harder to detect in these patients. Suitable care of pressure areas, particularly toes, heels, sacrum, trochanters and elbows, must be provided by the whole team. Special pressure relief mattresses can be supplied for elderly, dysvascular and other very immobile patients to reduce the risk of bedsores, but this may impair independent bed mobility.

Teaching transfers. A standing pivot transfer using the unaffected leg should be taught, but if the patient is unable to do this, a sliding board may be used, or a backwards transfer if neither leg can bear weight (see Ch. 4 & Figs 4.11, 4.12, 4.13).

Preserving joint mobility. All joints must be treated and active exercise is the ideal method of treatment. Passive stretching and positioning may be used. If there is a slight contracture present with a soft end feel in either a hip or a knee joint, pre-operative treatment gives the best chance of regaining a full range of movement. This becomes much harder postoperatively because handling the limb produces more pain and the leverage is shorter. The prone position should only be used if the patient can tolerate it without respiratory distress or undue discomfort (see Ch. 4).

If there is a gross contracture present, which after a week's treatment has shown no sign of improvement, this must be reported to the surgeon as it may have a direct bearing on the choice of amputation level. A severely contracted residual limb interferes with transfers and may prevent future prosthetic rehabilitation. Full mobility of both shoulder joints and the shoulder girdle is essential for any level of upper limb amputation.

Strengthening all muscles. Upper limb, trunk and lower limb muscles must all be treated within the limits of the patient's tolerance and cardiovascular status; this may only be a few gentle bed exercises in the ward or it may be an extensive programme in the treatment area.

Teaching wheelchair mobility. The therapist should loan a suitable wheelchair to the patient before the operation. All bilateral lower limb amputees and some unilateral trans-femoral amputees will require a wheelchair with the rear wheels set back 7.5 cm. This is so that the chair will not tip over backwards due to the altered weight distribution of the patient in the chair (see Ch. 6).

Correct use of the brakes and footplates is emphasised to ensure that damage does not occur to the skin of the lower legs, and chair mobility around obstacles in the ward is taught.

Walking. Where possible, this is the best active exercise for preservation of muscle strength, joint mobility and function of the lower limbs. Memory of the gait pattern is maintained, even if only a few lengths of the parallel bars are managed. However, it has been shown in one study that only 15% of patients can walk immediately prior to amputation of a lower limb. Temporary shoes can be supplied to fit over dressings on the affected foot, thus relieving pressure (see Fig. 2.4). If there is a hip and/or knee flexion contracture, a heel raise will be necessary to obtain a positive heel strike, thus facilitating the extensor muscles.

Treatment for co-existing conditions. Fractures, burns, arthritis, backache, soft tissue lesions, etc. may also need specific treatment.

Both the patient and their carers should be made aware of the reasons, stages and timing involved in the rehabilitation process to ensure their informed consent and maximal cooperation. The amount of detailed information given and the language or terminology used must be within every person's level of understanding and their comprehension should be checked regularly. The information may be given by the therapist or another member of the team. As many relatives only visit at evenings and weekends, the nurse or doctor must be available then for discussion. The therapist must be very sensitive to the reactions of the patient at this stage as some denial of the situation may be present. However, practical queries may be better clarified, either for the patient, relatives or carers, by another amputee of similar age and with the same level of amputation. The opportunity to discuss social, economic, personal, domestic and mobility issues may allay fears more effectively than by lengthy discussion with hospital staff.

Care must be taken if the patient wishes to see the type of prosthesis that they may use in

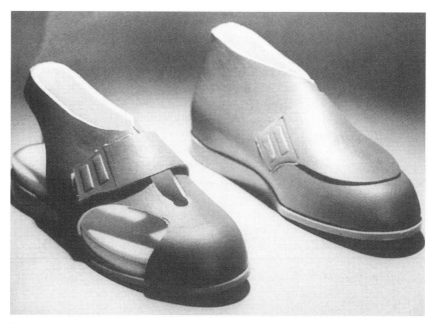

Figure 2.4 Drushoes. The shoe on the left has been cut out for a patient. (Photograph by kind permission of John Dew (London) Ltd.)

the future. This is because the level of amputation may not have been decided at that time and the hospital may not have up-to-date examples to show. If time permits, a visit to the local prosthetic service would provide more relevant information.

REHABILITATION TEAM

The need for effective communication during all stages between all members of the therapeutic team is paramount. Good communication and liaison ensures that a coordinated approach is achieved and therefore rehabilitation is likely to be more successful. It must also be remembered that the patient may relate different information to different team members and an accurate and composite picture must be obtained by all.

Therapists

Physiotherapist. The physiotherapist has expertise in manual therapy, electrotherapy, the facilitation of movement, exercise prescription and gait re-education and therefore sees the patient throughout all stages of the rehabilitation programme, although more than one individual may be involved. Physiotherapists are link members of the team overseeing and treating from pre- to postoperative stages and in pre- and postprosthetic mobility education. They will be involved in coordinating discharge planning procedures together with the nurse, occupational therapist and social worker. This will involve communication with the acute hospital, various outpatient clinics, prosthetic services, other hospitals, the community units and local authorities. Advice and support are also given regarding employment, sports and leisure activities.

Occupational therapist. The hospital occupational therapist (OT) will be involved in the assessment and management of the amputee from the pre-operative stage to resettlement at home. The focus is on helping the amputee achieve their optimum level of independence and quality of life following surgery. By facilitating the patient to identify their own goals and

by exploring their expectations, the occupational therapist helps the patient to re-establish their roles within the family and community. All aspects of daily living are assessed (including bathing, dressing, moving around the domestic environment and meal preparation) plus work, education and leisure activities. The treatment programme will consider physical, social, psychological and environmental factors that relate to the individual patient. Assessment of the home is carried out with the local social worker and community OTs so that assistive equipment, housing adaptations and homecare services can be promptly set up for the patient's safe return to the home.

Therapy assistant. The therapy assistant provides personal care, therapeutic exercise and activity with supervision from a qualified therapist, who prescribes the programme. Early in the rehabilitation, bed mobility, transfers, wheelchair practice, bed exercises and activities of daily living are commonly carried out with the assistant. Later on, gait re-education, home visits and early practice of leisure pursuits will be covered. The assistant often spends more time with the patient on a one-to-one basis and through this close relationship, may hear many issues raised by the patient that may not have been mentioned to the qualified therapist. The assistant will ensure that the right member of the team is alerted to any significant issue and should be present at team meetings.

Surgeon

The surgeon's role is to diagnose, order medical investigations, prescribe medication and ultimately inform the patient and relatives/carers of the severity of the condition and necessity for amputation. Wherever possible, amputations should be carried out in special units where consultant expertise is supported by the multidisciplinary team. Selection of amputation level should be determined by team discussion and all should understand the implications of wearing a prosthesis. The rehabilitation consultant and prosthetist may be consulted prior to surgery regarding the ideal level of amputation and future prosthetic potential. Postoperative medical treatment will be directed by the surgeon.

Nurse

The 24-hour observation of the patient is undertaken by the nurse who inevitably will take on a coordinating role. On admission an assessment is made of the patient's physical, psychological and social background, and an individual care plan is devised to take account of the following:

- fluid balance and nutritional state
- infection, pain, toxicity secondary to pain or infection
- preservation of skin – especially sacrum, heels and elbows
- spiritual and emotional needs
- general mobility.

Following surgery, the care plan will include monitoring and relief of pain, daily observation and treatment of the residual limb and remaining leg, and emotional support regarding altered body image, lifestyle and reduced mobility. Supervision of other activities, e.g. transfers, exercises, etc. is carried out as a continuation of the treatment plans of other members of the multidisciplinary team, so communication between everyone involved is vital.

Involvement of the relatives/carers is vital from admission in order to promote an understanding of the aims of the many facets of care and rehabilitation. Liaison with other nursing colleagues already involved in the patient's care is maintained; this may include the health visitor, diabetic nurse specialist, district nurse, practice nurse, community psychiatric nurse and continence advisor. The hospital stay is only a transient phase of the patient's life and it is important that links with existing professional resources and those of the family and friends are maintained in order to prevent the development of prolonged dependency.

The nurse is often the member of the team who explains and reassures both patients and carers, and offers counselling and emotional support. Where appropriate, the nurse will also encourage and supervise the patient in exercises and other techniques during evenings and at weekends.

Social worker/care manager

The role of the social worker/care manager is to give practical and emotional support to the patient, their family and carers, and to help them find realistic solutions to any social or economic problems related to hospitalisation and loss of a limb. They assist in providing assessment for care needs and for the arrangement and funding of community services such as homecare, provision of a daily meal, special transport schemes, daycare, respite care, etc. Where it is not possible for the patient to return to their previous accommodation, the social worker organises wheelchair accessible accommodation, sheltered housing or care in a residential or nursing home. The availability of such accommodation can be limited and early application is essential with full details and appropriate reasons for need proided. Social workers advise patients and their carers on their rights under legislation concerning disability discrimination and retraining for work. Financial worries may arise for all amputees due to loss of work or from their altered social and physical capabilities and the social worker can advise on any financial benefits to which they are entitled according to local and national policy.

Consultant in rehabilitation

The rehabilitation consultant's role is to provide long-term, committed medical care for the needs of the amputee throughout his or her life. In the pre-operative assessment phase, the rehabilitation consultant will help to advise the surgeon on the optimal level of amputation in difficult cases.

In the immediate postoperative phase, a disability-orientated, holistic assessment is carried out by the consultant, considering co-existing pathologies, psychological and social issues. A realistic appraisal of the future outcome of rehabilitation is discussed with the multidisciplinary team, patients and carers, and a proposed plan is made. Not all amputees will proceed to prosthetic replacement, so independent wheelchair mobility for the lower-limb amputee and uni-lateral manual dexterity for the upper limb amputee must be planned, trained and monitored. If prescription for the first prosthesis is made, the rehabilitation consultant will ensure early monitoring of both the residual limb and the prognosis of the general condition of the patient. In the follow-up phase, reappraisal of the patient's progress is made and refinement of the prosthetic prescription carried out as functional ability changes. Maintenance of the prosthesis and updating are carried out as monitoring of the changing needs of the patient and advancement in prosthetic technology indicate. It is often later, i.e. about 1 year following discharge from hospital, that the leisure needs and sports activities of the patient need careful prosthetic reassessment to optimise performance. The rehabilitation consultant will also identify and treat problems such as residual limb skin complications, phantom and residual limb pain, and will consult with other specialists as necessary. Links with staff in the community are made, e.g. family doctor, physiotherapist, occupational therapist, nurse, etc. to ensure the coordinated and specialised care of the amputee.

A research role is expected by means of clinical audit, evaluation of resource use and original clinical research; the rehabilitation consultant will also have a teaching role with junior medical staff and students, as well as with other members of the multidisciplinary team.

Prosthetist

The prosthetist's role is to provide care to patients with partial or total absence of a limb by designing, fabricating and fitting a prosthesis. The prosthetist is responsible for specifying the limb design, selecting materials and components, making all necessary casts, measurements and model modifications, including static and dynamic alignments. The prosthetist will evaluate the prosthesis on the patient, give instruction in its use and provide the rehabilitating therapists with any technical information required. In consultation with the referring doctor, the prosthetist may formulate the prescription for the prosthesis following examination and evaluation of the patient's prosthetic needs.

Additionally, the prosthetist is expected to keep abreast of technical developments worldwide and to supervise the functions of support personnel and laboratory activities related to the production and development of the prostheses. The prosthetist will remain the contact point for all the prosthetic needs of the amputee throughout their limb-wearing life. Advice can be given on new prostheses and designs and amputees can be put in touch with each other through the prosthetist regarding leisure and sports activities.

Clinical psychologist or counsellor

To enhance the process of physical therapy, it is helpful to have either a clinical psychologist or a counsellor on the team to work with the patient in order to understand the psychological processes that the patient experiences and to contribute to team assessment and decision making. Specific time is allocated by these team members for this work, particularly if they are required on an ongoing basis either by the patient or their partners or families.

The training undertaken by a clinical psychologist and counsellor is different: the clinical psychologist first completes a degree in psychology, then postgraduate training in clinical psychology, usually for 3 years, while the counsellor will undertake a recognised course of the British Association of Counsellors for 2–3 years. With their experience, both will fulfil the same aim of helping the patient explore the impact that an amputation has on their life and working towards making the necessary adjustments to ensure a fulfilled life in the future (see Ch. 3). Those patients with severe depression or other mental illness either before or following amputation will need the additional help of a psychiatrist – a medical doctor specialising in mental illness.

Carer

The role of the carer is complex: they provide information, act as a go between with the many healthcare professionals involved, give emotional support, motivation, instruction and practical help to the patient. Not all carers are able to fulfil this role and the carer's needs must be assessed by the rest of the team.

The makeup of the overall care team giving clinical support to the patient, surgeon and prosthetist will vary in different locations within a country and in different countries throughout the world. Remote locations, developing countries and different levels of healthcare budgets can be influential in the range of healthcare professions available. However, the above roles are essential to the optimal rehabilitation of the amputee and the skills required should be developed in the variety of healthcare professionals present in any team, however small.

BIBLIOGRAPHY FOR PREVIOUS EDITIONS

Barsby P, Lumley J S P 1987 Check-list for the management of the lower limb amputee. Surgery 41:985–986

Bradway J K, Malone J M, Racy J, Leal J M, Poole J 1984 Psychological adaptation to amputation: an overview. Orthotics and Prosthetics 38(3):46–50

Bruce J 1991 The function and operation of a parent support association. Prosthetics and Orthotics International 15:160–161

Clifford P C, Davies P W, Hayne J A, Baird R N 1980 Intermittent claudication: is a supervised exercise class worthwhile? British Medical Journal 21 June:1503–1505

Crowther H 1982 New perspectives on nursing lower limb amputees. Journal of Advanced Nursing 7:453–460

Day H J B 1979 Congenital lower limb deformities and extension prostheses. Physiotherapy 65(1):3

Day H J B 1991 The ISO/ISPO classification of congenital limb deficiency. Prosthetics and Orthotics International 15:67–69

Dean E 1987 Assessment of the peripheral circulation: an update for practitioners. The Australian Journal of Physiotherapy 33(3):164–171

Dowd G S E, Linge K, Bentley G 1983 Measurement of transcutaneous oxygen pressure in normal and ischaemic skin. Journal of Bone and Joint Surgery 65-B(1):79–83

Earl H M, Souhami R L 1990 Adolescent bone tumours: osteosarcomas and Ewing's sarcomas. The Practitioner 234:816–818

English A W G 1989 Psychology of limb loss. British Medical Journal 299:1287

Evans D G R, Thakker Y, Donnai D 1991 Heredity and dysmorphic syndromes in congenital limb deficiencies. Prosthetics and Orthotics International 15:70–77

Falkel J E 1983 Amputation as a consequence of diabetes mellitus. Physical Therapy 63(6):960–964

Fyfe N C M 1990 An audit of amputation levels in patients referred for prosthetic rehabilitation. Prosthetics and Orthotics International 14:67–70

Ham R O, Van de Ven C 1991 Patterns of recovery for lower limb amputation in the UK. WCPT 11th International Congress Proceedings Book II, pp. 658–660

Holstein P 1982 Level selection in leg amputation for arterial occlusive disease. Acta Orthopaedica Scandinavica 53:821–831

Hunter J, Middleton F R I 1984 Cold injury amputees – a psychosocial problem? Prosthetics and Orthotics International 8:143–146

Jackson J 1989 The role of the counsellor with amputees. Step Forward 16 (Autumn)

Jacobs P A 1984 Limb salvage and rotationplasty for osteosarcoma in children. Clinical Orthopaedics and Related Research 188:217–222

Jamieson C W, Hill D 1976 Amputation for vascular disease. British Journal of Surgery 63:683–690

Kasabian A K, Colen S R, Shaw W W, Pachter H L 1991 The role of microvascular free flaps in salvaging below-knee amputation stumps: a review of 22 cases. Journal of Trauma 31(4):495–501

Krebs D E, Edelstein J E, Thornby M A 1991 Prosthetic management of children with limb deficiencies. Physical Therapy 71(12):920–934

Lange L R 1982 Prosthetic implications with the diabetic patient. Orthotics and Prosthetics 36(2):96–102

Lempberg R, Ahlgren O 1982 Prosthetic replacement of tumour-destroyed diaphyseal bone in the lower extremity. Acta Orthopaedica Scandinavica 53:541–545

Liedberg E, Persson B M 1983 Age, diabetes and smoking in lower limb amputation for arterial occlusive disease. Acta Orthopaedica Scandinavica 54:383–388

Lind J, Kramhoft M, Bodtker 1991 The influence of smoking on complications after amputations of the lower extremity. Clinical Orthopaedics and Related Research 267 (June 91):211–217

Murray Parkes C 1972 Components of the reaction to loss of a limb, spouse or home. Journal of Psychosomatic Research 16:343–349

Murray Parkes C, Napier M M 1970 Psychiatric sequelae of amputation. British Journal of Hospital Medicine 4(5):610–614

O'Riordain D S, O'Donnell J A 1991 Realistic expectations for the patient with intermittent claudication. British Journal of Surgery 78:861–863

Reardon J A, Curwen I H M, Jarman P, Dewar M, Chodera J 1982 Thermography and leg ulceration. Acta Thermographica 7(1):18–23

Redhead R G 1984 The place of amputation in the management of the ischaemic lower limb in the dysvascular geriatric patient. International Rehabilitation Medicine 6:68–71

Roberts A 1988 Systems of life No. 160. Senior systems – 25. Peripheral vascular disease – 1. Nursing Times 84(18):49–52

Rose C A H, McIntosh C S 1991 Diabetes in the limb fitting centre. Practical Diabetes 8(4):146–147

Scales J T 1983 Bone and joint replacement for the

preservation of limbs. British Journal of Hospital Medicine 30:220–232

Setoguchi Y 1991 The management of the limb deficient child and its family. Prosthetics and Orthotics International 15:78–81

Simon M A, Aschliman M A, Thomas N 1986 Limb-salvage treatment versus amputation for osteosarcoma of the distal end of the femur. Journal of Bone and Joint Surgery 68A(9):1331–1337

Spence V A, Walker W F, Troup I M, Murdoch G 1981 Amputation of the ischaemic limb: selection of the optimum site by thermography. Angiology 32:155–169

Spence V A, McCollum P T, Walker W F, Murdoch G 1984 Assessment of tissue viability in relation to the selection of amputation level. Prosthetics and Orthotics International 8:67–75

Sweetman R 1980 Tumours of bone and their treatment today. British Journal of Hospital Medicine 24(5):452–463

Torode I P, Gillespie R 1991 The classification and treatment of proximal femoral deficiencies. Prosthetics and Orthotics International 15:117–126

Wake P, Mansfield A O 1980 Vascular surgery of the lower limb. British Journal of Hospital Medicine Aug:120–129

Williams L R et al 1991 Vascular rehabilitation: benefits of a structured exercise/risk modification programme. Journal of Vascular Surgery 14:320–326

BIBLIOGRAPHY FOR THE THIRD EDITION

Anderson S P 1995 Dysvascular amputees: what can we expect? Journal of Prosthetics and Orthotics 7(2):43–50

Apelqvist J, Ragnarson-Tennvall G, Persson U, Larsson J 1994 Diabetic foot ulcers in a multidisciplinary setting: an economic analysis of primary healing and healing with amputation. Journal of Internal Medicine 235:463–471

Armstrong D G, Lavery L A, Harkless L B, van Houtum W H 1997 Amputation and reamputation of the diabetic foot. Journal of the American Podiatric Medical Association 87(6):255–259

Armstrong D G, Lavery L A, Quebedeaux T L, Walker S C 1997 Surgical morbidity and the risk of amputation due to infected puncture wounds in diabetic versus nondiabetic adults. Southern Medical Journal 90(4):384–389

Berlin O, Stener B, Angervall L, Kindblom L-G, Markhede G, Odén A 1990 Surgery for soft tissue sarcoma in the extremities. A multivariate analysis of the 6–26-year prognosis in 137 patients. Acta Orthopaedica Scandinavica 61(6):475–486

Boulton A J M 1995 Why bother educating the multi-disciplinary team and the patient – the example of prevention of lower extremity amputation in diabetes. Patient Education and Counseling 26:183–188

Bunt T J 1995 Revascularization versus amputation for elderly patients. Association of Operating Room Nurses Journal 62(3):433–435

Bunt T J, Malone J M 1994 Amputation or revascularization in the >70 year old. The American Surgeon 60(5):349–352

Choong P F M, Sim F H 1997 Limb-sparing surgery for bone tumours: new developments. Seminars in Surgical Oncology 13:64–49

Clarke P, Mollan R A B 1994 The criteria for amputation in severe lower limb injury. Injury 25(3):139–143

Czyrny J J, Merrill A 1994 Rehabilitation of amputees with end-stage renal disease. American Journal of Physical Medicine and Rehabilitation 73(5):353–357

Eneroth M, Persson B M 1993 Risk factors for failed healing in amputation for vascular disease. A prospective, consecutive study of 177 cases. Acta Orthopaedica Scandinavica 64(3):369–372

Esquenazi A, Meier R H III 1996 Rehabilitation in limb deficiency. 4. Limb amputation. Archives of Physical Medicine and Rehabilitation 77:S18–S28

Fairhurst M J 1994 The function of below-knee amputee versus the patient with salvaged grade III tibial fracture. Clinical Orthopaedics and Related Research 301:227–232

Fletcher J P, Batiste P 1997 Incidence of deep vein thrombosis following vascular surgery. International Angiology 16(1):65–68

Frykberg R G 1997 Team approach toward lower extremity amputation prevention in diabetes. Journal of the American Podiatric Medical Association 87(7):305–312

Georgiadis G M, Behrens F F, Joyce M J, Earle A S, Simmons A L 1993 Open tibial fractures with severe soft-tissue loss. Limb salvage compared with below-the-knee amputation. The Journal of Bone and Joint Surgery 75A(10):1431–1441

Grimer R J, Carter S R, Pynsent P B 1997 The cost effectiveness of limb salvage for bone tumours. The Journal of Bone and Joint Surgery 79B(4):558–561

Gupta A, Rubin J 1994 Carotid brachial bypass for treating proximal upper-extremity arterial occlusive disease. The American Journal of Surgery 168:210–213

Gujral J S, McNally P G, O'Malley B P, Burden A C 1993 Ethnic differences in the incidence of lower extremity amputation secondary to diabetes mellitus. Diabetic Medicine 10:271–274

Harrington P 1994 Correspondence to the editor. The Journal of Bone and Joint Surgery 76A(10):1594–1595

Hierner R, Betz A M, Comtet J-J, Berger A C 1995 Decision making and results in subtotal and total lower leg amputations: reconstruction versus amputation. Microsurgery 16:830–839

Jain A S, Stewart C P U 1989 Tumour related lower limb amputation: a 23 year experience. Prosthetics and Orthotics International 13(2):82–85

Jeans W D, Cole S E A, Horrocks M, Baird R N 1994 Angioplasty gives good results in critical lower limb ischaemia. A five-year follow-up in patients with known ankle pressure and diabetic status having femoropopliteal dilatations. The British Journal of Radiology 67(794):123–128

Kennedy M J 1997 Am I better off without it?: a case study of a patient having a trans-tibial amputation after 52 years of chronic lower limb ulceration and pain. Prosthetics and Orthotics International 21(3):187–188

Larsson J, Apelqvist J, Agardh C-D, Stenström A 1995 Decreasing incidence of major amputation in diabetic patients: a consequence of a mutidisciplinary foot care team approach? Diabetic Medicine 12:770–776

Levin M E 1995 Preventing amputation in the patient with diabetes. Diabetes Care 18(10):1383–1393

Livingston D H, Keenan D, Kim D, Elcavage J, Malangoni

M A 1994 Extent of disability following traumatic extremity amputation. The Journal of Trauma 37(3):495–499

Lumley J S P 1993 Vascular management of the diabetic foot – a British view. Annals of the Academy of Medicine 22(6):912–916

Melchiorre P J, Findley T, Boda W 1996 Functional outcome and comorbidity indexes in the rehabilitation of the traumatic versus the vascular unilateral lower limb amputee. American Journal of Physical Medicine and Rehabilitation 75(1):9–20

Merimsky O, Kollender Y, Inbar M, Chaitchik S, Meller I 1997 Palliative major amputation and quality of life in cancer patients. Acta Oncologica 36(2):151–157

Mueller M J 1997 Therapeutic footwear helps protect the diabetic foot. Journal of the American Podiatric Medical Association 87(8):360–364

Novakovic B, Fears T R, Horowitz M E, Tucker M A, Wexler L H 1997 Late effects of therapy in survivors of Ewing's sarcoma family tumors. Journal of Pediatric Hematology/Oncology 19(3):220–225

Pell J P, Fowkes F G R, Lee A J 1997 Indications for arterial reconstruction and major amputation in the management of chronic critical lower limb ischaemia. European Journal of Vascular and Endovascular Surgery 13:315–321

Perler B A 1995 Cost-efficiency issues in the treatment of peripheral vascular disease: primary amputation or revascularization for limb-threatening ischaemia. Journal of Vascular and Interventional Radiology 6(6):111S–115S

Pinzur M S 1997 Current concepts: amputation surgery in peripheral vascular disease. Instructional Course Lectures American Academy of Orthopedics 46:501–509

Rougraff B T, Simon M A, Kneisl J S, Greenberg D B, Mankin H J 1994 Limb salvage compared with amputation for osteosarcoma of the distal end of the femur. The Journal of Bone and Joint Surgery 76A(5):649–656

Robicsek F 1997 Regarding 'Impact of arterial surgery and balloon angioplasty on amputation: a population-based study of 1155 procedures between 1973 and 1992'. Journal of Vascular Surgery 26(2):353

Sanders L J 1994 Diabetes Mellitus: prevention of amputation. Journal of the American Podiatric Medical Association 84(7):322–328

Sayers R D, Thompson M M, Varty K, Jagger C, Bell P R F 1993 Effects of the development of modern vascular services on amputation rates in Leicester, UK: a preliminary report. Annals of Vascular Surgery 7(1):102–105

Selby J V, Zhang D 1995 Risk factors for lower extremity amputation in persons with diabetes. Diabetes Care 18(4):509–516

Shenaq S M, Klebuc M J A, Vargo D 1994 How to help diabetic patients avoid amputation. Prevention and management of foot ulcers. Postgraduate Medicine 96(5):177–192

Shinoya S 1993 Buerger's disease: diagnosis and management. Cardiovascular Surgery 1(3):207–214

Simmonds T D, Stern S H 1996 Diagnosis and management of the infected total knee arthroplasty. American Journal of Knee Surgery 9(2):99–106

Simsir S A, Cabellon A, Kohlman-Trigoboff D, Smith B M 1995 Factors influencing limb salvage and survival after amputation and revascularization in patients with end-stage renal disease. The American Journal of Surgery 170:113–117

Tornetta III P, Olson S A 1997 Amputation versus limb salvage. Instructional Course Lectures American Academy of Orthopedics 46:511–518

Tseng C-H, Tai T-Y, Chen C-J, Lin B J 1994 Ten-year clinical analysis of diabetic leg amputees. Journal of Formosan Medical Association 93(5):388–392

Walker S C, Helm P A, Pullium G 1995 Total-contact casting, sandals, and insoles. Construction and applications in a total foot-care program. Clinics in Podiatric Medicine and Surgery 12(1):63–73

Williams J B, Watts P W, Nguyen V A, Peterson C 1994 Balloon angioplasty with intraluminal stenting as the initial treatment modality in aorto-iliac occlusive disease. The American Journal of Surgery 168:202–204

Williams M O 1994 Long-term cost comparison of major limb salvage using the Ilizarov method versus amputation. Clinical Orthopaedics and Related Research 301:156–158

Wütschert R, Bounameaux H 1997 Determination of amputation level in ischemic limbs. Diabetes Care 20(8):1315–1318

3

Psychological impact of amputation

Benna Waites
Anne Zigmond

Research on psychological reactions to amputation tends to show that while the majority of amputees recover from the experience without any lasting serious depression, a significant minority of patients are troubled by depression in the longer term. One study found that 30% of amputees showed signs of clinical depression following amputation (Kashani et al 1983); another found just under half their sample showed significant levels of psychological morbidity and significant levels of social isolation, both soon after amputation and at 1–2 year follow-up (Thompson & Haven 1983). Lerner et al (1983) reported that 85% of their amputees felt 'significantly mentally scarred'. Other studies, however have found much lower levels of morbidity (Stephen 1982) or have found that initially high levels of psychiatric morbidity resolve almost entirely by the time of discharge (Shukla et al 1982).

While this literature gives an idea of the overall levels of psychological morbidity, it gives little idea of the actual experiences of amputation. This chapter will seek to help the reader to understand how an amputee may be feeling, outline some models to place emotional responses in context, describe the work of clinical psychologists and counsellors in this field, and raise issues for therapists working with amputees in distress. Just as the physical health of the individual can have a powerful effect on their psychological state, so their psychological adjustment to amputation can have a significant influence on their involvement with and performance during rehabilitation and on their adjustment in the longer term.

PSYCHOLOGICAL RESPONSES TO AMPUTATION

Box 3.1 illustrates the vast range of emotional responses to amputation. In short, amputees and staff need to be prepared for anything. Many of these reactions may be transient, some are helpful and constructive, others less so, and a few may require further action (e.g. psychiatric assessment in the case of psychosis).

Many of the reactions listed in Box 3.1 can be found in other disabling conditions, and researchers comparing amputation to other conditions such as Parkinson's disease and stroke found that levels of depression were similar across these groups (Langer 1994, Schubert et al 1992). However, there are aspects of the psychological impact of amputation that are specifically related to the loss of a limb. Body image, which Henker (1979) defines as 'the individual's psychological picture of himself' is disrupted when a limb is amputated. Henker described a number of body image-related problems frequently experienced following amputation. These include anxiety, due to 'the discrepancy between the perceived disturbed physical state and the previously established body image' and depression, occurring when the person feels they have lost their previous image of themselves. Furst and Humphrey found that in their study of 19 amputees, 6 of the 8 women and 3 of the 11 men 'considered the change in body image as a more intrusive handicap than the impairment of function'. This indicates the significance of body image changes to many amputees. A conference held in 1997 at Roehampton Rehabilitation Centre indicated that amputees were keen for

further advances in the cosmetic appearance of artificial limbs to be actively pursued.

Studies have also documented changes in sexual function, which may in part be related to changes in body image. Reinstein et al (1978) found that 77% of their group of male amputees and 38% of female amputees reported a substantial decrease in the frequency of sexual intercourse following amputation. Reasons given for the decrease included impaired sexual function, decreased interest and mobility, an unwilling partner, and fear of poor performance or injury.

In most cases, the predominant experience of the amputee is one of loss: not only the obvious loss of the limb, but also resulting losses in function, self-image, career and relationships. These multiple loss issues most clearly affect younger trauma patients, for whom amputation is often the result of a sudden unforeseen event, and whose level of function following amputation normally compares unfavourably with their pre-amputation abilities. Frank et al (1986) found that younger amputees appeared to deteriorate in their psychological function over time compared to older amputees who improved. However, powerful feelings of loss are also frequently experienced by older dysvascular and diabetic patients. Their reactions can be particularly acute when they have not fully understood the need for amputation, or have had little time to prepare for the operation. A small black spot on the toe or an ulcer on the side of the leg can seem no justification for a trans-tibial amputation. The medical team should take time to prepare the patient as fully as possible before amputation (see Ch. 2). Even when this has been done and the patient may appear to understand the need for amputation at an intellectual or rational level, they may sometimes still struggle to adjust emotionally.

Box 3.1 Some possible emotional reactions to amputation

Grief	Anxiety
Anger	Hope/optimism
Relief	Tearfulness/distress
Sadness	Uncertainty
Denial	Vulnerability ('neediness')
Feelings of mutilation/	Depression
body image changes	Euphoria
Sexual difficulties	Mania
Regret	Psychosis

MODELS FOR UNDERSTANDING REACTIONS TO AMPUTATION

Bereavement models have been used to provide a framework for understanding the various emotional responses to amputation. The models presented in Boxes 3.2 and 3.3 are normally used

Box 3.2 Stages of grief and tasks of mourning based on work by Dr Colin Murray Parkes

Grief
1. Shock, numbness, disbelief
2. Yearning and searching for lost person; pangs of grief (deep sense of pain)
3. Disorganisation; discharging old patterns of living and becoming a new person
4. Re-organisation; accepting the loss (letting go and adjusting to new life)

Mourning
1. To accept the reality of loss
2. To experience the pain of loss
3. To adjust to the new environment without the person (or limb); finding new skills
4. Re-investment in life; finding new emotional energy in new life, relationships activities, etc.

Source: Murray Parkes C 1996 Bereavement. In: Doyle D, Hanks G W C, Macdonald N (eds) Oxford textbook of palliative medicine. Oxford University Press, Oxford, ch 14, p 665 (reproduced with kind permission).

Box 3.3 Stages of bereavement

lst STAGE: DENIAL ISOLATION
Pushing away. Limited communication
Shutting away. Disbelief. Unable to be in 'here and now' – stays in 'there and then'
Can be very proactive and angry
Denial can be helpful giving time to adjust, heal and prepare though not if it goes on for too long and becomes dysfunctional

2nd STAGE: ANGER
(Rage, envy, resentment). Releasing for patient but staff can find it more difficult to cope with. 'Why me' – 'if only the doctor' – blame others/world

3rd STAGE: BARGAINING
Less commonly experienced but equally relevant to patients
Bargaining is usually an attempt to postpone the reality of the loss

4th STAGE: DEPRESSION
Patient may feel numbness, stoicism, muted anger and rage; sleeplessness, lack of eating, self care and self worth
Anger / rage replaced by sense of deep loss
Preparatory } Depressions are very different
Reactive
Depression is often associated with result of past loss. Sharing this helps, and antidepressent therapy maybe required

5th STAGE: ACCEPTANCE AND HOPE

Adapted from: Kubler-Ross E 1970 On death and dying. Routledge, chs 3–8, pp 34–122

in relation to the death of a person, though Murray-Parkes has also applied this to the loss of a limb. It can often be helpful to the patient to point out some of the similarities in the grieving process between losing a loved one and losing a limb and can sometimes help them to understand some of the intense emotional reactions they may experience. It is important to note that for some patients who have experienced a previous bereavement (particularly the loss of a spouse), renewed feelings of loss may be triggered by the amputation. Kubler Ross' model is more detailed and encompasses a wider range of emotional expression.

Although a useful framework for some, grief models have key weaknesses that limit their usefulness and application to all patients. There is no objective evidence, to our knowledge, that supports stage models of grief. Thus while many of the reactions described in Boxes 3.2 & 3.3 may be familiar to most of us, there is no basis to expect that, for example, someone who is in denial will later move to being angry (rather than depressed). As Box 3.1 illustrated, the reaction to amputation may not always be negative, and grief models do not allow for this. When amputations occur after a long period of illness and loss of function, the patient may already have gone through a period of grieving and have no need to grieve again for the amputation. Therefore, there is a danger that the models could be used too prescriptively.

For this chapter, Anne Zigmond has developed 'The difference and adjustment model' (Fig. 3.1), which encompasses the amputee's experiences more fully. It has a therapeutic value in helping address issues that are important to them, without being prescriptive. It is also less threatening to those who may not relate well to concepts of grief or may be uncomfortable with a therapist who is expecting them to express emotion.

According to this model, the first task for the amputee is to acknowledge the difference the amputation has made to their life. There are various levels of difference that need to be acknowledged and in this context, it may be helpful to consider the World Health Organisation's

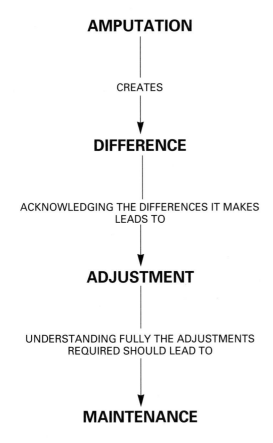

AMPUTATION

|
CREATES
|
↓

DIFFERENCE

|
ACKNOWLEDGING THE DIFFERENCES IT MAKES
LEADS TO
|
↓

ADJUSTMENT

|
UNDERSTANDING FULLY THE ADJUSTMENTS
REQUIRED SHOULD LEAD TO
|
↓

MAINTENANCE

Figure 3.1 Difference and adjustment in amputation (Anne Zigmond 1996).

(WHO) categorisation of impairment, disability and handicap (Fig. 3.2).

Physical *impairment* describes deficits in the structure or function of a part of the body resulting from underlying disease or disorder. *Disability* is defined as 'deficits in the performance of activities, arising directly from physical impairment' and *handicap* as 'deficits in social functioning'. Criticisms of this model will be considered later in this chapter, but it will be used for the time being to structure this discussion of difference and adjustment.

A minority of amputees experience denial in relation to accepting their impairment (i.e. the reality that their limb is missing). Where this occurs, it can be an attempt to return to what is known and familiar, perhaps in the face of unbearable levels of anxiety. In such cases, phantom sensation may play a role in reinforcing the denial. This degree of denial may lead to serious problems. Such a disconnection with reality may indicate some underlying psychosis and if this state persists for more than a few days and the amputee is not responding to counselling, a psychiatric assessment should be requested. A distinction should be made between the persistent denial of limb loss suggesting severe adjustment problems and occasional memory lapse, which may lead to minor accidents. It is not uncommon for individuals to forget about their amputation, particularly on awakening in the middle of the night, and attempt to get up out of bed as if their limb were present.

It is more common to experience denial in relation to *disability*, that is, accepting the 'difference' in physical function. This can be manifested in amputees who persistently 'overdo it' in relation to physical activity and can lead to problems with blistering or trauma to the skin on the residual limb. Some amputees may only understand the difference amputation is going to make to their lives when they start learning to walk again and realise the extent to which their function is compromised. Any amputee who has been assured pre-operatively that their 'new leg' will be 'as good as new' may have great difficulty adjusting to the reality of a prosthesis. *Handicap* is affected by many factors and is not an inevitable consequence of amputation. Many amputees may only become aware of possible handicaps (for example, jobs or hobbies they are no longer able to do) following discharge from hospital or from rehabilitation services. Amputees may also notice social issues living as a person with a disability, such as some friends treating them differently. These issues can be difficult to adjust to when individuals have spent most of their lives with the identity of an able-bodied person.

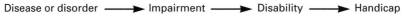

Disease or disorder ⟶ Impairment ⟶ Disability ⟶ Handicap

Figure 3.2 WHO model of impairment, disability and handicap.

There are therefore many levels at which the difference an amputation creates needs to be acknowledged and adjusted to. When adjustment has occurred, the amputee is able to meet the demands and challenges of amputation and a state of maintenance is achieved.

Another way of thinking about individuals' adjustment is to think about the meaning of the amputation in terms of losses and gains or pros and cons to the amputee. This partially explains why some people appear to cope easily with amputation, while others grieve to a greater extent or become depressed. Expressed in terms of the difference model just described, the differences some people face may be less significant or easier to adjust to than others. Losses can be functional, occupational or interpersonal (e.g. impact on relationship), but can also be less tangible, such as losses to identity or body image.

The advantage of Zigmond's and the losses and gains models is that they are not prescriptive and both allow for considerable individual variance. They allow for the amputee who comes to amputation of a limb that has caused them a great deal of difficulty over many years and reacts to the operation with relief and rapid acceptance. Such a person has experienced considerable gains to outweigh the loss of the limb, and the differences that must be adjusted to are not difficult to acknowledge and accept. However, if an amputee in the position just described experiences a profound sense of their own mortality, is troubled by others' view of them as disabled or is disturbed by their new body image, these losses may then outweigh the functional gains (or may present challenges in accepting the differences) and depression may result.

Both the Zigmond and the WHO models give us some explanation for why younger traumatic amputees may experience more difficulties in adjusting to their new impairment than older dysvascular amputees because of the greater extent of difference before and after amputation, and the greater losses relative to gains (see Frank et al 1986). However, as suggested before, difference or losses and gains can not always be observed externally and assumptions should not be made on the basis of a cursory analysis of someone's social or functional situation. Just as a dysvascular amputee may experience amputation as the first sign of ageing or future dependency and become depressed, a younger amputee whose injury was caused by trauma may be able to offset the inevitable functional losses against enhanced relationships or a greater sense of direction in life.

The processes that lead to an amputee's understanding of their amputation and the adjustment required, or losses and gains resulting from it, are complex and idiosyncratic. Thus, there is no clear linear relationship, nor a high correlation between level of impairment, disability and handicap when the WHO model is applied to clinical cases. In amputation, there is no clear relationship between the level of amputation (e.g., trans-tibial or trans-femoral) and psychological outcome (Langer 1994). Outcomes are determined by a complex interplay of factors, including the amputee's perception and appraisal of what has happened, their beliefs about it and their resources for coping with the situation. Figure 3.3 illustrates in simplified form the role of psychosocial factors in affecting psychological, social and functional outcomes.

The discussion above has shown some of the complex factors involved in individual reactions to amputation and provides some framework for thinking about and understanding them. By way of summary, and also to include factors

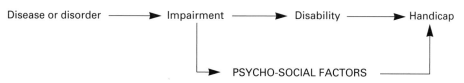

Figure 3.3 Adaptation of the WHO model.

not contained in the discussion so far, the various issues requiring consideration when assessing an individual's psychological reaction are listed as follows. This list is not fully inclusive as unique individual's situations always present new issues. It is also anticipated that the therapist may not always be in possession of all this information. However, it is hoped that it will encourage a breadth and depth of thinking about the patient and their situation.

FACTORS AFFECTING AN INDIVIDUAL'S REACTION TO AMPUTATION

Degree of difference/losses and gains pre- and postamputation.

See discussion of these issues above

Previous medical history

The circumstances surrounding amputation, the amputee's understanding of these, degree of control and role in the decision making are important, as well as previous experiences of the medical system, adjustment to the patient role and medical prognosis.

Cause of the amputation

Whether the cause is due to illness or trauma may be relevant to subsequent adjustment.

Post-traumatic stress disorder

This can hinder adjustment in amputees who have suffered trauma.

Expectations of rehabilitation

Effort should be made by the team to ensure these are as realistic as possible.

Previous experience of loss

Previous losses experienced by an individual may be triggered by amputation, giving the person additional difficulties to deal with.

Family history, reactions and attitudes

The amputee's current family reactions and their childhood family's attitudes (e.g. towards illness or disability) can have a powerful effect on adjustment.

Coping strategies

These strategies are sometimes learned in childhood and sometimes developed during adult life and have a critical impact on the way an individual adjusts.

Social support

The quality, rather than simply quantity seems to be important.

Cultural issues

It is important to recognise language, family dynamics, perceptions of illness and healthcare, compliance issues, religion, role and status, beliefs, etc.

Compensation claims

These can delay the adjustment process, though not always due to secondary gain.

Role changes

Family, relationships, social situation, employment and how the amputee views their role change are important.

Employment prospects

This has a powerful affect on individuals, both at the level of their sense of identity and their social and financial situation.

ROLE OF THE CLINICAL PSYCHOLOGIST/COUNSELLOR

Why refer to a psychologist/ counsellor?

Many people cope with the process of amputation by effectively utilising their own resources and those around them. They may find their own way of acknowledging difference and making the required adjustments successfully. However, there are those who find the process of adjustment overwhelming and may benefit from professional help.

Physiotherapists, occupational therapists, nurses and prosthetists often deal with many of the amputee's emotional concerns. However, there may be times when it is helpful for the team and the amputee to have a specialist to address more complex issues. For example, staff may feel overwhelmed and deskilled by an individual's distress. The dual role of task-focused therapeutic activities and counselling can also lead to patient confusion.

Box 3.4 lists reasons for considering referral to a psychologist/counsellor. However, many of these reactions may occur in a mild or transient form only: ultimately referral is a matter of the team's clinical judgement.

What does a psychologist/counsellor do?

Ultimately, all professionals working with the amputee's emotional well-being are aiming for adjustment to the amputation and current life situation. However, they may use different means to help the amputee achieve this, depending on their training and theoretical orientation.

Box 3.4 Why and when to refer to a psychologist/
counsellor

Expression of a need to talk
Depressive symptoms, e.g. insomnia, loss of appetite,
  hopelessness
Withdrawal
Irritability
Anger
Unrealistic expectations
Denial
Suspected residual limb abuse (see Ch. 21)
Self-neglect (personal hygiene, diabetic
  management, etc.)
Risk taking (e.g. trying to do too much too quickly)
Anxiety limiting progress in rehabilitation (e.g. can't or
  won't move)
Regression or excessive dependence
Sabotaging rehabilitation programme or discharge plans

For ease of expression, the term 'psychological therapist' will be used instead of counsellor/psychologist in this section. Two of the most common ways of working are described in turn as follows.

Counselling and the therapeutic relationship

All forms of therapeutic work have as their basis the relationship between the psychological therapist and client, and it is often the quality of this that determines how successful the work is. From the initial meeting, the psychological therapist attempts to establish a rapport with the client, which is the foundation for their working alliance, based on trust, respect and empathy. Many psychological therapists would also rate warmth, genuineness and unconditional positive regard for the client as key elements of this relationship. Listening actively and attentively and providing feedback (which can range from reflecting back and summarising to the client their view of the situation as they understood it, to more active questioning, interpreting or suggesting) are the main processes through which the therapy operates. Although the subject matter of therapy is often determined by what the client brings, there may be certain issues that benefit from the psychological therapist's specific enquiry or invitation. The most common issue is sexuality as clients often feel inhibited about sharing their concerns in this area.

When the process works well, the client feels they are able to be open and honest through good times and bad, and can share feelings without feeling guilty for burdening the psychological therapist. Many clients will report being able to talk through issues in therapy that they may not have discussed with even their closest friends and relatives for fear of upsetting them. It is common, particularly with amputees who have suffered trauma, for friends and relatives to insist on how lucky the amputee is in having avoided a worse outcome. This can be particularly acute when the amputee has been in intensive care and relatives have been told that they may not survive. The amputee, who has often had little awareness of this acute stage and emerges from this medical crisis facing the loss of a limb (or worse), may well be feeling far from lucky and can often feel very isolated with feelings of loss, anger or frustration. In such cases, the therapeutic relationship may be the one outlet for these emotions. Amputees may often feel frustrated with the restrictions and passivity of the patient role. They may have fears that expressing this to members of the core rehabilitation team may compromise their care or affect the team's view of them. The psychological therapist is often perceived as being one step removed from the team and the amputee feels able to 'let off steam' without fear of negative consequences.

In many cases, this therapeutic relationship may be sufficient to enable the amputee to make the necessary adjustments to amputation and its consequences and move on with their lives. Particularly in the early stages following (or preparing for) amputation, when distress can be high, establishing a relationship which the amputee finds supportive and which facilitates emotional expression may be all that is needed. However, later on in the process, particularly when the amputee appears to have become 'stuck' or when depression or anxiety have become chronic, a more structured approach can be helpful.

Cognitive-behavioural therapy

Cognitive-behavioural therapy (CBT) is an approach that offers many strategies applicable to the process of adjustment to amputation, and is also used in the psychological management of pain (described in more detail in Ch. 20). The following is a brief account of some CBT strategies that can be helpful in dealing with amputees. As in Chapter 20, what follows should be taken only as a summary of some of the techniques, and not a 'how to do it' guide.

Goal setting can be a valuable way of helping people to 'get moving' again if they have become very depressed or fearful. It is essential that goals are negotiated with the client so that they are attainable and provide an opportunity to succeed. Goals may be whole tasks or smaller components of a single activity, broken down

into smaller steps. They may be organised into a 'graded hierarchy' in which a series of tasks or steps are arranged in order of difficulty, so that the client can work up the hierarchy, building on the progress they have already made to face increasing levels of challenge. This more formal, systematic approach is most helpful when anxiety has become a severe problem. Figure 3.4 gives an example of a graded hierarchy for an amputee who has developed a phobia of leaving the house after being knocked down by a car. The hierarchy should be drawn up in collaboration with the amputee and moved through at their pace, using each stage to build confidence for the next one. The amputee is encouraged to stay on each level until they feel their anxiety reduce. Anxiety management strategies can be taught (such as relaxation, breathing, distraction and cognitive techniques (see later)) to facilitate this process of gradual exposure to the feared situation.

Goals may include specific rehabilitation tasks, looking at the residual limb, social activity, developing hobbies and interests, or finding work. Goals attempt to overcome avoidance, which can often arise as an attempt to avoid distress in the short term. Avoidance reinforces itself over time causing individuals to become trapped in vicious circles, which they often require structured help to overcome.

Helping clients to challenge their negative thinking can also be an important part of psychological therapy. CBT is not about blanket positive thinking; it is important to be aware of this for the amputee, who faces many losses and changes

Low anxiety

Going to the front gate

Standing on the pavement in front of the house

Going to the corner

Walking a short distance down the road

Walking round the block

Walking to the high street in the middle of the day

Walking to the high street in rush hour

High anxiety

Figure 3.4 Example of a graded hierarchy.

to their life that they have every right to perceive negatively. For example, an amputee who states 'walking will never feel the same again' is making an accurate statement that cannot be refuted. However, amputees who become deeply depressed by their belief that, for example, now that they have an amputation, they will never be attractive to the opposite sex again, or who become highly anxious because they believe that if another person learnt about their amputation they would be rejected, have beliefs that are open to more reality-based alternatives. This type of belief and others indicating high levels of social discomfort have been shown to be related to depression (Rybarczyk et al 1992) and are therefore particularly important to identify and challenge. The client should be encouraged to look at the effect the belief has on their mood and behaviour and consider alternative ways of thinking. They may be asked to consider how they would react if they talked to a close friend who expressed the same belief and what arguments they might use to illustrate the un-helpfulness of the belief. Clients are often more harsh in their judgement of themselves than of others and this can be a useful way of helping them to gain a more objective perspective on their thinking. Clients may also be taught typical thinking errors (such as all or nothing thinking, over-generalising and catastrophising, where events are predicted to have catastrophic consequences) to help them to identify negative, un-realistic beliefs. Challenging negative thinking often forms the basis for work directed towards building self-esteem.

Problem-solving techniques can often be helpful in assisting the amputee to make the many decisions that may face them following an amputation in a more structured and clear way. This approach takes the client through a series of stages, starting with problem definition and option generation, and moving on to weighing up the pros and cons of the various possibilities, enabling an option to be selected, and action planned, carried out and reviewed.

CBT is always carried out as part of a collaborative relationship in which the psychological therapist works alongside the client to help them

to apply the strategies at their own pace and in their own way. By the end of psychological therapy, the client should feel equipped with coping strategies that they can apply to a range of situations that may help them to prevent problems developing in the future.

Therapeutic setting

Traditionally, counselling and most forms of psychological therapy work within time boundaries of a 50-minute session: normally once a week, held on an individual basis in a quiet and confidential place. However, both authors have found that when practising psychological therapy in an applied hospital setting, there are benefits from a degree of flexibility in some cases. For example, both frequency and length of the sessions may be varied according to the amputee's needs. It may be helpful to involve a relative in a session or to see the relative separately (see section on friends and relatives), although bringing another person into the session should only be done with the agreement of the amputee. There may be times when it is helpful to observe the amputee in some of their rehabilitation settings, such as the therapy facility. This can enable a greater understanding of a particular problem an amputee may be having and can also facilitate liaison with staff.

Liaison with the team

Liaison with the rehabilitation team is an important part of the psychological therapist's role. Some counsellors prefer to work with strict confidentiality boundaries, which means they are unable to provide specific feedback to the rest of the team or to work with them closely in managing the amputee. While issues are sometimes covered in therapy which the amputee does not wish to be disclosed to the team (and it is almost always appropriate for this wish to be respected), many value their psychological therapist's close links with other staff as they feel it enables them to be better understood by staff who may not otherwise be able to get to know the amputee in the way that the psychological therapist can. This process sometimes promotes an advocacy role for the therapist, in which they may be the team member best placed to put forward the amputee's point of view.

Delayed presentation for psychological help

Many amputees benefit from psychological input in the early stages of adjusting to the amputation. However, it is important when providing psychological and counselling services for amputees to allow for longer-term follow-up, giving the option of contact months and years following their amputation. The reasons for these delayed presentations vary. Some amputees sail through their rehabilitation, buoyed up by the attention and structure this medical input provides. It is often only when faced by the challenges of returning home, that some issues (perhaps at the level of accepting difference at the handicap level as mentioned earlier) suddenly arise, which seem overwhelming. Some amputees present years later following the breakdown of a relationship or the loss of a job.

Working with family and friends

One study by Thompson and Haran (1985) addressed the psychological adjustment of relatives to amputation, and found significant levels of social isolation and risk of psychiatric illness in well over one-third of their sample of carers, in addition to impact on the ability to work, changes in sleep patterns and financial strain. Foort found that amputees' most commonly voiced concern was the need for psychological insight on the part of care givers. It is therefore important to recognise the impact of amputation on the system surrounding the amputee.

Friends and family may go through many of the same feelings that the amputee experiences, and when communication is clear and open between the amputee and their social support networks, there may be no need for the psychological therapist to become involved. However, it is very common, particularly in trauma cases, for con-

cern about the amputee's well-being to lead to family and friends becoming highly protective and trying to bottle up their concerns or distress. This desire to protect is similar to amputees' own protectiveness, and may lead to conversations that determinedly focus on the bright side. Significant others may therefore benefit from a confidential place in which to share their concerns. Confidentiality becomes critical when working with an amputee and their friend/ relative, and information should not be shared without consent.

The most important time for relatives' needs to be taken into account is when their adjustment difficulties appear to be hindering the amputee's progress. This may be remedied by involving them in the rehabilitation process to a greater extent, giving them the opportunity to ask questions of the rehabilitation team, but may be an indication that they are in need of psychological help in their own right. There are occasions when the psychologist/counsellor may see the relative on their own or when their intervention may be entirely on a couple or family basis.

Group interventions for amputees

Some studies have evaluated the effects of group interventions for amputees. Fischer and Samelson (1971) found that their group discussion programme facilitated adjustment and covered a diverse range of topics such as fears of falling and failing, and changes in body weight and health issues. Caine (1973) found similar benefits. More recently, Delehanty and Trachsel (1995) found that a preventive psycho-educational series of 2–3 groups aiming to provide information, anticipate and normalise future stressors and build coping strategies, resulted in significantly lower levels of distress at 8 months following discharge.

Useful points for physical therapists

Many physiotherapists, occupational therapists, nurses and prosthetists work in teams without psychologists or counsellors, and even where such a resource is available, many amputees will choose to talk to one of these professionals,

---

> **Box 3.5**   Useful points to note when an amputee wants to talk
>
> Observe non-verbal as well as verbal cues
> Listen actively, reflect back what the amputee is saying and be empathetic
> Be wary of making assumptions; verify understanding by asking the amputee
> Don't feel something has to be accomplished; sometimes just being with the amputee is enough
> Keep an open mind; bear in mind the vast range of individual reaction
> Have a good knowledge base of what might happen and how an amputee might feel
> Ensure that you feel comfortable, and are not getting 'out of your depth'
> Refer to a specialist when necessary
> Get to know the specialist where possible to facilitate liaison
> Be aware when the amputee's issues may trigger own personal issues
> Talk to a colleague, supervisor or manager about any of the above if concerned

and do not always wish to be referred on to a specialist. Box 3.5 offers some ideas for making this process less burdensome and de-skilling for the therapist, and more effective and helpful for the amputee.

There is no substitute for referring to a professional with expertise in psychological matters and where one does not exist, staff should be making a case to managers for the provision of such a service. All NHS trusts should employ clinical psychologists, most often within mental health resources, and alongside community psychiatric nurses who can also offer supportive counselling and sometimes CBT. Some general practitioners (GPs) now have psychologists and counsellors in their practices. Thus even where there is no dedicated service to amputation, there are other ways of accessing this input, though there can sometimes be a long wait for this. If the amputee is keen to find a private psychologist, they should be encouraged to consult the British Psychological Society's (BPS) *Directory of Chartered Psychologists* (available through public libraries or directly from the BPS). The British Association of Counsellors provides a list of registered counsellors across the country. Addresses for both of these organisations can be found in Appendix 1.

SUMMARY

Reactions to amputation are many and varied: amputees cannot be expected to follow a set pattern of adjustment that parallels the stages of the rehabilitation process. Although many amputees may experience significant distress, at least transiently, most will adjust and recover, and some may react very positively to their amputation. Models have been presented in this chapter that may make amputee's reactions more understandable, though care should be taken not to apply any one model too rigidly. The psychologist/counsellor works with those amputees who need help to adjust to the reality and consequences of their amputation using a range of different techniques. Physical therapists may work with a good deal of amputees' distress and suggestions are made for managing this side of their work, as well as ways of accessing a specialist when there is not one attached to the team.

CONCLUSION

One of the authors was recently visiting a therapy facility at another centre and witnessed an angry outburst by an amputee toward a physiotherapist. The amputee had made excellent progress in his rehabilitation and the physiotherapist had been working hard to successfully reduce his flexion contractures. The therapist was in the process of telling the amputee how well he was doing when he turned on her and started expressing his sense of futility about the work they had done together. He said that there seemed little point in being more mobile if every day when he returned home he had to face the trauma of what he had lost – the emptiness of his life since the accident and the hopelessness of his future. Although such feelings are not encountered frequently in such an extreme way (and even less frequently expressed), this case illustrates the enormity of psychological adjustment required by some amputees and the challenge for therapists' work with amputees who have been severely traumatised by their amputation.

It is important to try to find a balance while working with such amputees between acknowledgement of the trauma they are facing alongside a gentle persistence at the physical goals that they will ultimately benefit from achieving. Losing sight of the former can lead to a less than sensitive approach to the amputee; losing sight of the latter can lead to the therapist becoming demoralised and burnt-out. Progress can sometimes be slow with a distressed amputee, but taking the time to establish a good relationship can pay dividends in terms of their long-term outcome. Adjusting to life with an amputation is a psychological as well as a physical journey. By caring for the amputee in a multidisciplinary setting, which includes attention to psychological needs alongside physical rehabilitation, the team gives the amputee the best possible chance of long-term adjustment. Understanding the psychological impact of amputation, addressing this as part of the amputee's rehabilitation and referring to a specialist where appropriate are all an essential backdrop to the therapist's work with the amputee.

BIBLIOGRAPHY FOR THE THIRD EDITION

Akesode F A, Iyang U E 1981 Some social and sexual problems experienced by Nigerians with limb amputation. Tropical Geographical Medicine (33):71–74

Beattie G W 1979 On becoming an artificial arm user. New Society (31):510–512

Bradway J K, Malone J M, Racy J, Leal J M, Poole J 1984 Psychological adaptation to amputation: an overview. Orthotics and Prosthetics (38):46–50

Breakey J W 1997a Body image: the lower limb amputee. Journal of Prosthetics and Orthotics 9(2):58–66

Breakey J W 1997b Body image: the inner mirror. Journal of Prosthetics and Orthotics 9(3):107–112

Burger H, Marincek C 1997 The lifestyle of young persons after lower limb amputation caused by injury. Prosthetics and Orthotics International 21:35–39

Butler D J, Turkal N W, Seidl J J 1992 Amputation: pre-operative psychological preparation. Journal of the American Board of Family Practitioners 5:69–73

Caine D 1973 Psychological considerations affecting rehabilitation after amputation. Medical Journal of Australia 2:818–821

Caplan L M, Thomas M D 1963 Emotional effects of lower limb amputation in the aged. New England Journal of Medicine 269(22):1166–1171

Delehanty R D, Trachsel L 1995 Effects of short-term group treatment on rehabilitation of adults with amputations. International Journal of Rehabilitation and Health 1(2):61–73

Dembo T, Ladieu-Leviton C, Wright B A 1952 Acceptance of loss – amputation. In: Garrett J F (ed) Psychological aspects of physical disabilities. US Government Printing Office

English A W G 1989 Psychology of limb loss. British Medical Journal 299:1287

Fischer W G, Samelson C F 1971 Group psychotherapy for selected patients with lower extremity amputations. Archives of Physical Medicine 52:79

Foort J 1974 How amputees feel about amputation. Orthotics and Prosthetics 28: 21–27

Frank J L, Herndon J H 1974 Psychiatric – orthopaedic liaison in the hospital management of the amputee war casualty. International Journal of Psychiatry in Medicine 5:105–114

Frank R G, Kashani J H, Kashani S R, Wonderlich S A,

Umlauf R L, Ashkanazi G S 1986 Psychological response to amputation as a function of age and time since amputation. British Journal of Psychiatry 144:493–497

Frierson R L, Lipman S B 1987 Psychiatric consultation for acute amputees. Psychosomatics 28(4):183–189

Furst L, Humphrey M 1983 Coping with the loss of a leg. Prosthetics and Orthotics International 7:152–156

Gilder R 1988 Emotional reactions to the loss of a body part. Loss, Grief and Care 2(3–4):11–13

Gingrass G, Mongeau M, Susset V, Lemieux R, Chevrier J M, Voyer R 1956 Psychosocial and rehabilitative aspects of upper extremity amputees. Canadian Medical Association Journal 75:819–824

Goldberg R T 1984 New trends in the rehabilitation of lower limb extremity amputees. Rehabilitation Literature 45(1–2):2–11

Ham R, Cotton L 1991 Limb amputation: from aetiology to rehabilitation. Chapman and Hall, London, ch 10

Hansen S T, Jr 1987 Editorial: the type IIIC tibial fracture: salvage or amputation. American Journal of Bone Joint Surgery 69A:799

Hanspal R S, Fisher K 1991 Assessment of cognitive and psychomotor function and rehabilitation of elderly people with prostheses. British Medical Journal 302:940

Henker F O 1979 Body image conflict following trauma and surgery. Psychosomatics 20(12):812–820

Johnston M 1996 Models of disability. The Psychologist 9(5):205–211

Kashani J H, Frank R G, Kashani S R, Wonderlich S A, Reid J C 1983 Depression among amputees. Journal of Clinical Psychiatry 44:256–258

Katz J 1992 Psychophysiological contributions to phantom limbs. Canadian Journal of Psychiatry 37:811–821

Katz J, Melzack R 1990 Pain 'memories' in phantom limbs: review and clinical observations. Pain 43:319–336

Kegel B, Carpenter M L, Burgess E M 1977 A survey of lower limb amputees: prostheses, phantom sensations and psychological aspects. Bulletin of Prosthetics Research (Spring):43–60

Laatsch L, Rothke S, Burke W F 1993 Countertransference and the multiple amputee patient: pitfalls and opportunities in rehabilitation medicine. Archives of Physical and Rehabilitation Medicine 74:644–648

Langer K 1994 Depression in disabling illness: severity and patterns of self-reported symptoms in three groups. Journal of Geriatric Psychiatry and Neurology 7:121–128

Lerner R K, Esterhai J L, Polomano R C, Cheatle M D, Heppenstall R B 1993 Quality of life assessment of patients with post-traumatic fracture nonunion, chronic refractory osteomyelitis, and lower extremity amputation. Clinical Orthopaedics and Related Research 295:28–36

Macbride A, Rogers J, Whylie B, Freeman S J 1980 Psychosocial factors in the rehabilitation of elderly amputees. Psychosomatics 21:258–261

Monforton M, Helmes E, Deathe A B 1993 Type A personality and marital intimacy in amputees. British Journal of Medical Psychology 66:275–280

Murray-Parkes 1996 Bereavement. In: Doyle D, Hanks G W C, Macdonald N (eds) Oxford textbook of palliative medicine, Oxford University Press, Oxford

Nissen S J, Newman W P 1992 Factors influencing reintegration to normal living after amputation. Archives of Physical Medicine Rehabilitation 73:548–551

O'Toole D M, Goldberg R T, Ryan B 1982 Functional changes in vascular amputees. Proceedings of the American Congress of Rehabilitation Medicine Meeting, Houston, Texas

Parkes C M 1975 Psycho-social transitions: comparison between reactions to loss of limb and loss of a spouse. British Journal of Psychiatry 127:204–210

Pell J P, Donnan P T, Fowkes F G R, Ruckley C V 1993 Quality of life following lower limb amputation for peripheral arterial disease. European Journal of Vascular Surgery 7:448–451

Pinzur M S, Graham G, Osterman H 1988 Psychologic testing in amputation rehabilitation. Clinical Orthopaedics and Related Research 229:236–240

Randall G C, Ewalt J R, Harry H 1945 Psychiatric reaction to amputation. Journal of the American Medical Association 128(9):645–652

Reinstein L, Ashley J, Miller K H 1978 Sexual adjustment after lower extremity amputation. Archives of Physical Medicine Rehabilitation 59:501–504

Rybarczyk B D, Nyenhuis D L, Nicholas J L, Schulz R, Alioto R J, Blair C 1992 Social discomfort and depression in a sample of adults with leg amputations. Archives of Physical and Medical Rehabilitation 73:1169–1173

Schubert D S P 1992 Increase of medical hospital length of stay by depression in stroke and amputation patients: a pilot study. Psychotherapy and Psychosomatics 57:61–66

Schubert D S P, Burns R, Paras W, Sioson E 1992 Decrease of depression during stroke and amputation rehabilitation. General Hospital Psychiatry 14:135–141

Shukla G D, Sau S C, Tripathi R P, Gupta D K 1982 A psychiatric study of amputees. British Journal of Psychiatry 141:50–53

Stephen P J 1982 Psychiatric aspects of amputation. British Journal of Psychiatry 141:535–536

Thompson D M, Haran D 1983 Living with an amputation: the patient. International Rehabilitation Medicine 5:165–169

Thompson D M, Haran D 1985 Living with an amputation: the helper. Social Science and Medicine 20(4):319–323

Walker C R C, Ingram R R, Hullin M G, McCreath S W 1994 Lower limb amputation following injury: a survey of long-term functional outcome. Injury 25:387–392

Weinstein C L 1985 Assertiveness, anxiety and interpersonal discomfort among amputees: implications for assertiveness training. Archives of Physical Rehabilitation. Medicine in Rehabilitation 6:687–689

Wells L M, Schacher B, Little S, Whylie B, Balogh P A 1993 Enhancing rehabilitation through mutual aid: outreach to people with recent amputations. Health and Social Work 18(3):221–229

Wittkower E 1947 Rehabilitation of limbless: joint surgical and psychologic study. Occupational Medicine 3:20–44

4

Immediate postoperative treatment

The care and treatment given to the amputee at the early postoperative stage is concerned with mobility both in bed and about the immediate surroundings of the ward. It commences on the first postoperative day and is continued for as long as the amputee's condition indicates.

The prime consideration is healing of the wound. The wound drains may remain in situ for 24–48 hours and movement may therefore be restricted. Prevention of contractures and wound management are the most important factors at this time. It may be unnecessary to give general mobilising and strengthening exercises to younger amputees in the first 2–3 postoperative days.

However, those suffering from vascular disease and diabetes are generally older, unfit and possibly confused, and thus more at risk from the complications of bed rest, i.e. bronchopneumonia, pressure sores, urinary tract infection, etc. Therefore, immediate mobilisation on the first or second postoperative day is recommended.

Respiratory therapy is started immediately but other exercises are added as the individual recovers. Postoperatively, all amputees experience a certain amount of pain, and this must be controlled adequately, particularly during the very early stages. Therapy must be organised around analgesia; short but frequent treatments given daily achieve the best result.

The correct bed and accessories will have been already organised pre-operatively (see Ch. 2, p. 19). The type of mattress, sheets and other pressure care items must also be considered, particularly as in the first 2–3 postoperative days the amputee finds alternate side lying uncomfortable for long periods. A pressure risk assessment score (such as Waterlow, see Ch. 6) should be carried out to ensure that a correct mattress is supplied. This should be re-evaluated regularly to reduce the risk of developing pressure sores. However, if an amputee requires a pressure-relieving mattress, bed mobility and transfers are more difficult to perform. It may be necessary to add sheepskins, foam pads, sponge leg gutters, etc., to protect the remaining foot and leg. Bed cradles are necessary to relieve pressure of bed-clothes from the residual limb and toes of the remaining foot.

EARLY THERAPY

Following amputation, the amputee may have difficulty in coming to terms with the residual limb psychologically as it is sometimes very un-sightly during the initial stages of healing. Some may not look at the residual limb for some time and may deny to themselves that amputation has been performed. For others it may be a very gradual process of acceptance. It has been noted that if the entire therapeutic staff refer to and handle the residual limb normally, then the amputee can learn to accept this new concept of their body. If this fails, then there are a few who will present with the syndrome of distorted body image. Gentle acknowledgement of reality and reinforcement will help this type of individual make this major physical and psychological adjustment. However, there are a few who never fully achieve this. Observation of the amputee can be important in these early stages as acute transitional reactions (e.g. intense anxiety or distress) can occur. The most appropriate way to manage extreme distress at this time is probably to listen, acknowledge, reassure and contain the emotional reaction. The amputee is often engaged in a process of trying to make sense of what has happened to their body and accommodate new feelings and sensations. Some may have diffi-culty looking at their newly amputated limb. Support and encouragement may be offered but amputees should not be pressurised to look

before they are ready to do so. Concerns about family members and their reactions are often picked up at this time. It is helpful to offer family members support and specialist psychological/counselling input where necessary, particularly where the family's reaction appears to be hindering the amputee's adjustment.

Phantom sensations are frequently encoun-tered at this time. It is important for amputees to be given permission to describe their experi-ences, particularly as some find the feeling so bizarre they may begin to question their sanity. Until relatively recently, phantom sensation was considered by some to not exist, or to be evidence of psychiatric disorder and some may still labour under these misapprehensions. Care should be taken to distinguish phantom sensation from phantom pain, as many who experience phantom sensation will not necessarily find this painful (see Ch. 20).

It is important that the therapist, at the first postoperative treatment session, observes the amputee's ability to move the residual limb inde-pendently. Handling the residual limb should first be attempted by the amputee, before the therapist provides either assistance or resistance to movement. Sensitivity of approach is neces-sary at this first session, as it may be the first time the amputee touches the residual limb and fully realises that amputation has taken place (see Fig. 4.1).

Active movements

The active movements that are attempted first are hip flexion, extension, adduction and abduc-tion, static quadriceps and knee flexion exercises, and contractions of the muscles in the trans-tibial residual limb. To aid bed mobility, exercises such as bridging, rolling, moving up and down the bed, sitting forwards and pushing up using the arms, can be attempted on the first postoperative day and continued until the amputee is fully mobile in bed. Active exercise of the remaining limb can also lead to 'overflow' to the residual limb, thus encouraging active movement.

All these techniques, except push-ups, can be attempted with drips, drains or catheters in situ

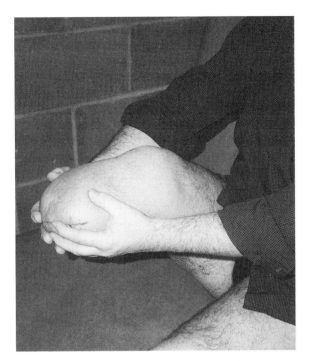

Figure 4.1 Handling the residual limb to aid with desensitising. (Note that there is no dressing as the wound is healed and sutures are removed.) (Photograph by kind permission of Richmond, Twickenham and Roehampton Healthcare NHS Trust).

(see Figs 4.2–4.4). The therapist should continue to encourage the amputee to gently touch the residual limb over the dressings, to assist movement, re-educate sensation and aid psychological acceptance. Vascular and diabetic amputees must always take great care when moving about so that neither the residual limb nor the remaining leg is knocked on the cot sides, wheelchair or the bed cradle. Even this minor trauma can cause a major complication; any team member who observes this must report to the nursing staff immediately. It is more difficult to observe minor damage to the skin of Negroid or Asian patients, so the team must be constantly vigilant.

Prevention of contractures

In preventing contractures, there are four important factors to note:

1. If the amputation is below the knee joint, the knee must rest in full extension immediately after the operation. Any dressing applied should not pull the residual limb into flexion. Pain frequently causes a flexor withdrawal pattern, involving both hip and knee, and must not be allowed to persist; sufficient analgesia must therefore be given.

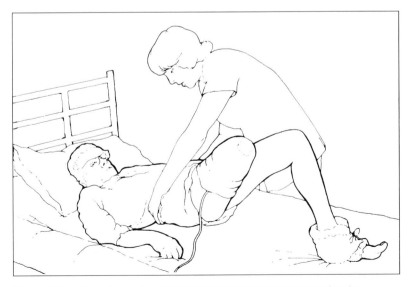

Figure 4.2 A trans-femoral amputee bridging on the first postoperative day.

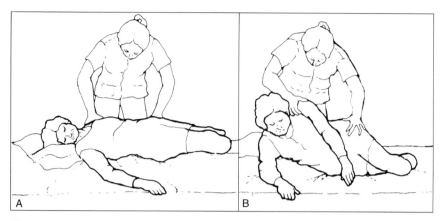

Figure 4.3 A bilateral trans-tibial amputee rolling. Note the hand positions of the therapist.

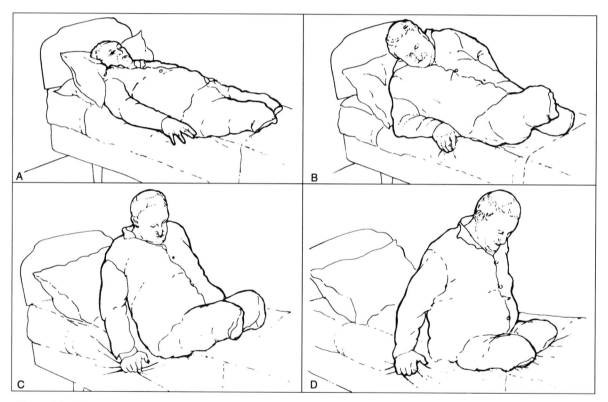

Figure 4.4 Four-stage movement for a bilateral trans-femoral amputee to sit up in bed. Note arm positions and trunk rotation.

The therapist can passively extend a transtibial residual limb, temporarily fixed in flexion, after a night's sleep or a midday rest, by placing both hands either side of the knee, pushing the patella proximally with the thumbs and sliding the tibia forwards with the fingers (Fig. 4.5). Once full extension has been achieved the amputee should perform static quadriceps exercises and be able to maintain the extended position independently. This extended position is maintained

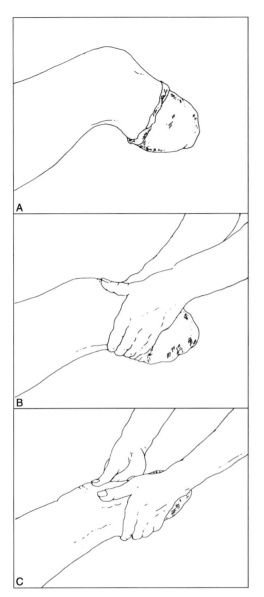

Figure 4.5   Passive extension of a trans-tibial residual limb.

by providing a stump board for the wheelchair (Figs 4.6 and 4.7).

The use of weights, sandbags and pillows to maintain this position is inadvisable. The weight of these objects can occlude circulation in the residual limb which causes pain and in turn causes increased flexor withdrawal.

2. If the amputation is through or above the knee joint the major concern is the development of a hip flexion contracture, but it must be remembered that the short trans-femoral residual limb can also become abducted as a result of the unopposed pull of the intact gluteus medius and gluteus minimus. Active hip extension and adduction exercises must be undertaken. However, the long trans-femoral and knee disarticulation residual limbs can become adducted because the strong pull of the long intact adductor longus and adductor brevis is greater than that of the hip abductors. Therefore, in these cases active hip extension and abduction exercises must be given.

3. The amputee will, of necessity, be sitting up in bed or in the wheelchair for long periods of time. Therefore, set periods of either supine or prone lying, to obtain neutral hip alignment, must become part of the daily routine. The prone position may be inappropriate for some amputees, e.g. those with cardio-respiratory problems, kyphotic spine, large abdomen or gross arthritis. For these patients, it is important to find a position in which they can achieve neutral alignment at the hip, e.g. high side lying with the residual limb supported.

The treatment programme must be gradually altered each day to attain the correct positioning, i.e. supine lying for only 10 minutes may be all that is possible for some amputees; others will progress to prone lying for 30 minutes, twice daily (see Fig. 4.8).

4. All joints in the upper and lower limbs and trunk must be actively treated, as contractures and loss of range of movement of any joint can occur while the amputee is relatively immobile.

Washing

Immediately after the operation, the amputee will usually have an assisted wash whilst remaining in bed. When sufficient sitting balance has been achieved, the therapist will progress the amputee to sitting on the edge of the bed, washing using a bowl on a table of a suitable height, and then encourage mobility and personal care tasks to be undertaken from the wheelchair in the ward bathroom facilities.

The amputee may remain seated in their

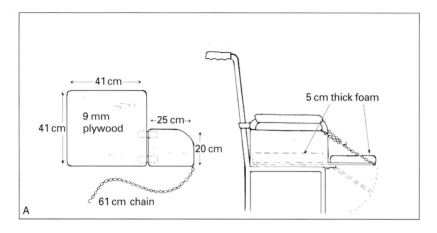

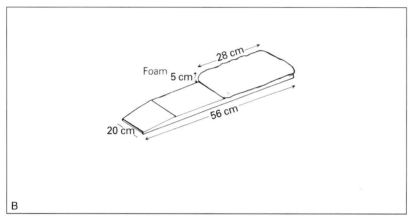

Figure 4.6   Two designs of stump board. (A) An adjustable stump board: the angle can be varied for comfort. (B) A fixed stump board: this slides underneath the wheelchair cushion.

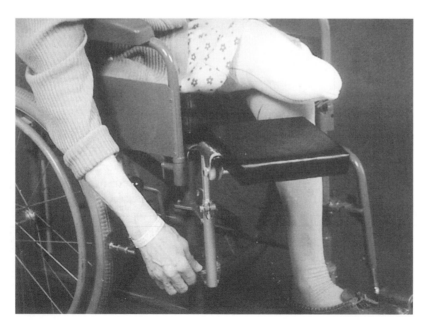

Figure 4.7   The King's stump support (made by Remploy Healthcare) is 29 cm long.

No pillows or *one* pillow

Arms positioned wherever comfortable for patient

Residual limb lying flat (with knee straight if t/t) *No pillow*

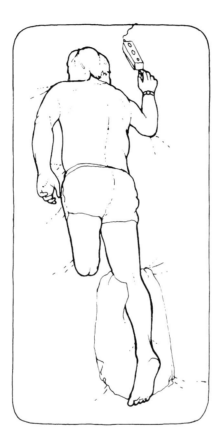

Nurse call bell placed within patient's reach

Head turned to sound side

Patient wearing a watch to time period prone

Both hips completely flat on bed

Remaining leg supported on a pillow to prevent toes from digging into bed

Footboard and bedclothes turned right back out of the way

Points to remember

1. To roll prone, the amputee must turn towards the sound side, the nurse ensuring that the residual limb is lowered gently.
2. Initially the amputee lies prone for about 10 minutes.
3. The amputee should then build up to lying prone for 30 minutes three times a day.

Figure 4.8   The correct position for prone lying (t/t denotes trans-tibial).

wheelchair or use a high stool at the wash basin. Washing aids with long handles may be needed to enable the amputee to reach their remaining limb.

Dressing

Getting dressed can be very tiring for the amputee in the early stages of rehabilitation, and it may be necessary to grade this activity carefully. The unilateral amputee should start dressing by lying on the bed using the bridging technique to pull their lower garments up, (see Fig. 4.9). Good sitting balance is required to put on upper garments. This is usually easiest while sitting on the edge of the bed. Bilateral amputees may find it easier to put on lower garments by rolling from side to side. When sitting balance permits, the unilateral amputee should progress to sitting on the edge of the bed, leaning forward to pull on lower garments, and then standing on the remaining limb. Abducting the residual limb can help to prevent garments from falling down.

Some amputees (e.g. those with hemiplegia, arthritis, bilateral lower limb amputation and some with upper limb amputation) may require assistive equipment to achieve independence in dressing. Those with limited hip flexion, back pain or breathing problems may need to use a reaching aid, long shoehorn and sock/stocking aid to reach the remaining limb. A reaching aid is also useful for the amputee to reach items or clothes that they have dropped and are out of their safe reach.

The amputee should be encouraged to wear comfortable, loose clothes that are easy to put on and take off, which will not hinder movement or rub on the wound. The therapist and therapy assistant may need to practice this activity several times with the amputee before they feel totally confident to manage unsupervised.

Some very frail amputees may need ongoing assistance from a carer. It is important to involve the family and carers at all stages so they are aware of where the amputee needs assistance and how they can achieve independence.

Clothing should not be adapted permanently until it is known whether the amputee will progress to prosthetic rehabilitation or not. Trouser legs can be taped or pinned temporarily so that the garment does not impede movement.

It is important to regain the individual's daily routine as soon as possible in preparation for their return home from hospital. The amputee

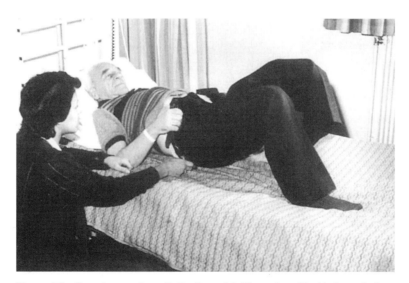

Figure 4.9 Dressing practice with the therapist. (Reproduced by kind permission of Faber & Faber, from Downie P A (ed) 1990 Cash's textbook of general medical and surgical conditions for physiotherapists.)

will often report that they feel much better having got dressed and are resuming a normal and familiar routine. It is important to note that if it is still impossible for an amputee to put on underpants or trousers independently after daily dressing practice, it is very unlikely that the independent donning of a prosthesis will be possible (see Ch. 7).

Using the toilet

The amputee may require assistive equipment such as a raised toilet seat, rails on the wall or fixed floor-mounted rails (Fig. 4.10).

Transfers

The stage at which amputees are able to sit out of bed in a wheelchair will be governed by their medical condition. The general rule for starting to learn independent transfers, as opposed to

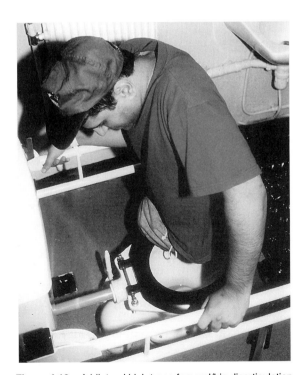

Figure 4.10 A bilateral high trans-femoral/hip disarticulation amputee transferring forwards onto a toilet using fixed hand rails (photograph by kind permission of Richmond, Twickenham and Roehampton Healthcare NHS Trust).

using a hoist, is that the amputee must be alert and capable of responding to instruction. The therapist will decide which transfer method is most suitable, taking account of risk factors to the amputee and the therapist, and give instruction and help with the transfer. It is possible for the amputee to sit out of bed in a wheelchair while the drip, wound drain and catheter are still in situ if suitable care is taken, which is frequently as early as the first or second postoperative day.

A suitable wheelchair should have been loaned pre-operatively and must be self-propelling (see Ch. 2); the amputee should not sit in a static armchair. The use of the wheelchair greatly improves both the physical and psychological state of the amputee. The assessment for a suitable and safe loaned wheelchair must be carried out by a qualified therapist, who will also decide on the need for, and prescription of, a permanent wheelchair (see Ch. 6).

Methods of transfer

The amputee must have a well-fitting shoe on the remaining foot before attempting a transfer. There are three methods of transfer for the amputee:

1. Standing pivot transfer (Fig 4.11)
2. Backwards/forwards transfer (Fig. 4.12)
3. Sliding board transfer (Fig. 4.13).

Once a safe method of transfer for both the amputee and the staff has been decided, it must be recorded so that the same method is always used and the amputee is encouraged to gain independence.

Manual handling policy

It is essential that all staff are aware of their employer's policy. Every employee has a responsibility to ensure that any task that involves the handling of patients or loads will not present a risk to the health and safety of themselves or others. Training in manual handling is mandatory for all staff in Europe under EEC regulations.

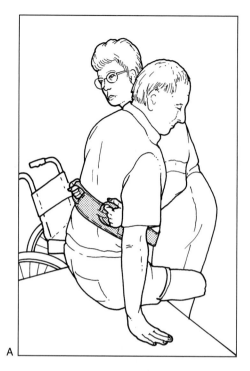

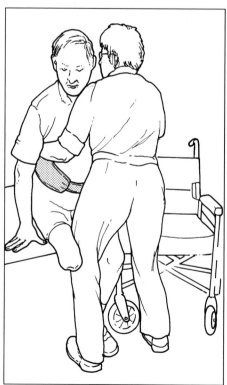

B

Figure 4.11 The standing pivot transfer using a lifting belt.

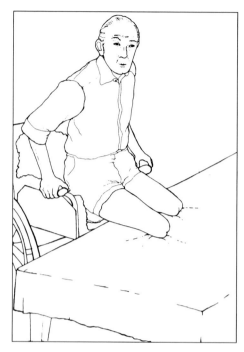

Figure 4.12 The backwards/forwards transfer. Note that the wheelchair and bed are level. While this transfer is more often used by bilateral amputees, it is also suitable for other patients unable to bear weight on either leg.

Use of the wheelchair (see Ch. 6)

After the method of transfer has been established, the amputee must be taught how to manoeuvre the wheelchair safely. A stump board must be provided for knee disarticulation and trans-tibial levels. This will protect the residual limb from knocks, prevent knee joint contracture and control oedema (Fig. 4.6). Some amputees with poor sitting balance, e.g. hemiplegics and bilateral amputees, may need a seat belt.

Those with poor eyesight, hearing, weak hands or arms, and poor sensation, require lengthy instruction and practice in wheelchair management. The confused amputee also requires constant supervision.

Young, fit and agile amputees may be unwilling to use a wheelchair. The therapist must explain the dangers of the dependent position of the residual limb while using crutches in these very early postoperative days. The problems of pain, oedema and the possibility of delayed

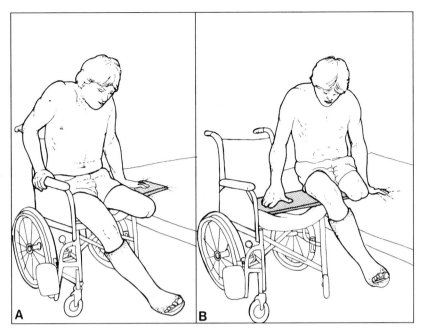

Figure 4.13   The sliding board transfer. Note that the wheelchair and bed are level and that the sliding board is sufficiently long to allow the patient to slide smoothly over the gap between the bed and chair. This method is also ideal for transferring from wheelchair to car seat.

wound healing must be understood by the younger amputee.

RESIDUAL LIMB OEDEMA

Residual limb oedema occurs immediately after the operation as a result of surgical trauma and may also recur at any future time in the amputee's life from a variety of other causes (see Fig. 4.14). It is important that the therapist recognises the total problem and all aspects of its management, so that the amputees can be taught to recognise it and thus cope with their own future management.

Methods of treatment of residual limb oedema

Elevation

The foot of the bed can be elevated, providing the blood pressure is stable and the vascularity of the residual limb and the remaining leg is adequate.

The trans-tibial residual limb should be elevated on a stump board when using the wheelchair (see Fig. 4.7, p. 46).

Trans-tibial amputees who are not wearing prostheses all day at home should be provided with a stump board for use with their own wheelchair. Those who occasionally remove their prosthesis should elevate the residual limb on a stool or chair.

Exercise

Active contraction of the residual limb muscles is the best method of reducing oedema. A regular pumping action by the opposing muscle groups is needed.

- The trans-tibial amputee must imagine the performance of alternate dorsiflexion and plantar flexion in order to achieve this muscle contraction.
- The knee disarticulation and trans-femoral amputee must perform alternate hip flexion

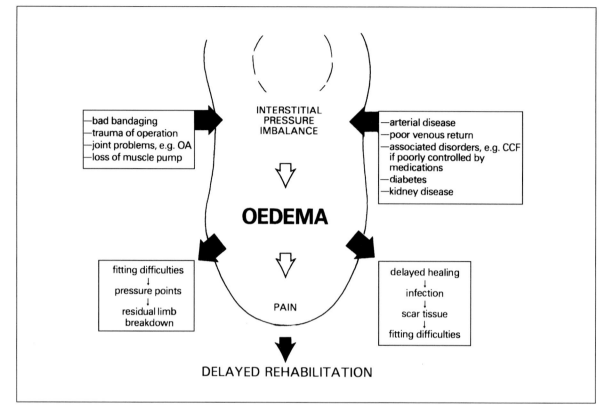

Figure 4.14 Causes of residual limb oedema.

and extension and hip abduction and adduction, encouraging strong contractions in the residual limb.

These active exercises must be performed at regular intervals throughout the day; 10 repetitions performed hourly is a useful guideline. Bilateral activities often achieve a more vigorous contraction in the amputated side. Any amputee who has strong and well-coordinated residual limb muscles can look forward to a better prosthetic future, e.g. a strong and muscular transfemoral residual limb is suitable for retaining and controlling a self-suspending knee component (see Ch. 13).

Bandaging

It is a misconception to think that bandaging will shape the residual limb. Bandaging is a technique that has been used from the early 1900s. In those days the main reason for amputation was trauma and the majority of patients had normal residual limb vascularity. The prostheses then had simple conical-shaped sockets fashioned out of wood, and bandaging was important to enable the residual limb to fit into the socket. Today the considerations are very different:

- In the developed world, over 80% of new amputees now suffer from peripheral vascular disease and/or diabetes. The pressure exerted by a bandage can frequently exceed the arterial pressure in the blood vessels of the residual limb, causing pressure necrosis, which in turn can lead to a higher level of amputation. This is particularly true in the trans-tibial amputation when it is safer to dress the residual limb with just a light supportive covering, e.g. Tubifast.

- Surgeons are now fashioning the muscle

flaps of the residual limb with greater expertise as they liaise with both the rehabilitation consultants and prosthetists and are more aware of prosthetic socket shape and manufacture. This factor alone will determine the final shape of the residual limb: bandaging can never change residual limb shape without the danger of interference with the local circulation. Incorrect bandaging can distort the tissues.

• Prosthetists now have many more techniques and materials available for making the socket of the artificial limb fit the individual residual limb. It should be remembered that a uniformly oedematous residual limb is more readily fitted than one that has become misshapen with bandaging (see Fig. 4.15).

Bandaging may be required for tissue support early in the postoperative period, before a shrinker sock can be used, or instead of a shrinker sock, depending on the availability of suitably skilled application and of stock available in any facility. In many countries around the world, a bandage is all that there is available (see Fig. 4.16).

Shrinker socks (e.g. Juzo)

These elasticated stump socks are available in various sizes from the prosthetic centre. They are only to be used for the healed residual limb with oedema (see Fig. 4.17). They are less likely to wrinkle and cause a tourniquet effect than other elasticated materials, as the correct size can be supplied. It is advisable that when the elasticated sock is first tried, it is worn for at least half an hour under the supervision of the therapist. The residual limb must be observed carefully

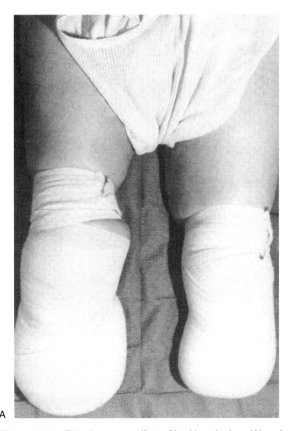
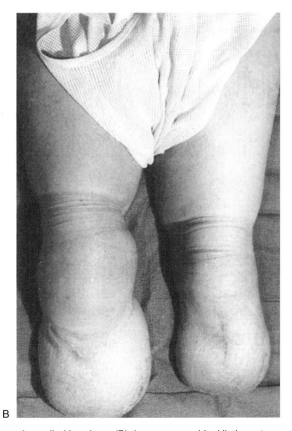

A   B

Figure 4.15   The disastrous effect of bad bandaging: (A) an incorrectly applied bandage; (B) the uneven residual limb contour produced by the incorrectly applied bandage.

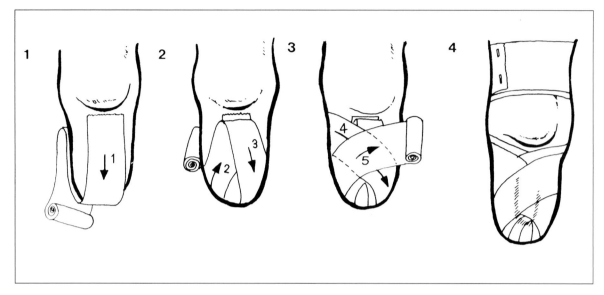

Figure 4.16   The method of bandaging a trans-tibial residual limb. From an original leaflet produced by Seton Ltd.

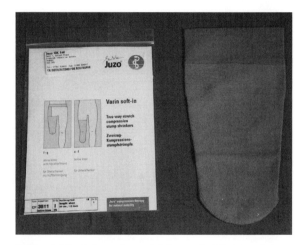

Figure 4.17   A Juzo stump shrinker sock. (Photograph by kind permission of Richmond, Twickenham and Roehampton Healthcare NHS Trust).

during this time for colour change and indentation, which may indicate that the sock is not the correct size. The sock should only be used when the amputee is awake but not wearing the prosthesis. It is inadvisable for the amputee to sleep wearing the elasticated sock, as damage to the residual limb may occur should a tourniquet effect develop. The amputee should apply the

sock by rolling it down on itself before applying it to the limb, and then proceed by gradually unrolling it up the residual limb. It is easy to overstretch the sock by pulling it from the top.

Rigid dressing

Some young traumatic trans-tibial amputees may have a plaster-of-Paris dressing applied.

Plaster-of-Paris or other rigid material should not be used for any residual limb in which wound healing is doubtful. However, it can be very useful in specialised centres, where early postoperative temporary sockets made of either plaster-of-Paris or thermoplastic material are constructed. Early gait rehabilitation is then achieved.

Pneumatic mobility aids

This pneumatic postamputation mobility aid (Ppam aid) and the amputee mobility aid (AMA) can be used before prosthetic delivery, or for periods when the prosthesis no longer fits when oedema is present (for further description see Ch. 6).

Intermittent variable air pressure machines (e.g. Flowtron)

There are a variety of these machines available, but the general principle employed is that, by varying the air pressure around the residual limb in a predetermined cyclic fashion, the circulation of blood and lymph can be modified with beneficial results. The pressures imposed by these machines on the tissues are uniform throughout the length of the residual limb, regardless of size or shape, so a tourniquet effect is impossible.

BIBLIOGRAPHY FOR PREVIOUS EDITIONS

Ham R, Richardson P 1986 The King's amputee stump board Mark II. Physiotherapy 72(3):124

Hamilton A 1977 Device for supporting the stump of a below-knee amputee. Physiotherapy 63(10):318

Koerner I 1976 To bandage or not to bandage: that is the question. Physiotherapy Canada 28(2):75–78

Murdoch G 1983 The postoperative environment of the amputation stump. Prosthetics and Orthotics International 7:75–78

Redhead R G, Snowdon C 1978 A new approach to the management of wounds of the extremities. Controlled environment treatment and its derivatives. Prosthetics and Orthotics International 2:148–156

Sarmiento A 1972 Postoperative management. Orthopedic Clinics of North America 3(2):435–446

Tilbury B, Slack H N, Mancey C 1985 The Exeter amputee stump support board. Physiotherapy 71(11):477

BIBLIOGRAPHY FOR THE THIRD EDITION

Arksey H, Heaton J, Sloper P 1998 Tell it like it is. Health Service Journal 108(5588):32–33

Condie E, Jones D, Treweek S, Scott H 1996 A one-year national survey of patients having a lower limb amputation. Physiotherapy 82(1):14–20

Eneroth M, Apelqvist J, Larsson J, Persson B M 1997 Improved wound healing in trans-tibial amputees receiving supplementary nutrition. International

Orthopaedics 21:104–108

Lambert A, Johnson J 1995 Stump shrinkers: a survey of their use. Physiotherapy 81(4):234–236

Yeager R A, Moneta G L, Edwards J M, Taylor L M, McConnell D B, Porter J M 1995 Deep vein thrombosis associated with lower extremity amputation. Journal of Vascular Surgery 22(5):612–615

5

Exercise programme and pre-prosthetic activities of daily living

This chapter describes the general fitness programme that is required for all ages and levels of lower limb amputee. The treatment of the upper limb amputee is continued in Chapter 19. The exercises described may be carried out during all stages of progress, from about 1 week postoperatively.

Illustrated here are examples and ideas for treatment, but every individual must be assessed separately and an appropriate treatment plan devised. This is a programme of general exercise that may be carried out in any facility, large or small, or alternatively in the home.

PRIMARY AMPUTEE

Following removal of the wound drain, the amputee should be up and dressed during the day; the exercise programme can then continue in the therapy facility. For this programme to take place, it is necessary that the amputee is not confused, the pain is adequately controlled and the amputee's medical condition has stabilised (particularly important for diabetics). Incontinence should not prevent treatment, as catheters or tubing can be connected to a leg bag worn under the clothing, and special incontinence pads and pants are available. Exercises should be performed daily.

It is ideal for new amputees to remain in hospital until they are fully rehabilitated on their first prosthesis. However, it is likely that most who have undergone surgery at an acute hospital will be discharged early on in their recovery.

Ongoing treatment will be provided by specialist prosthetic rehabilitation units, community therapists, day hospitals or on an outpatient basis at the acute hospital.

Some amputees may never progress to using a prosthesis; in this case it is essential that the therapist ensures that the amputee is able to be as independent and safe as possible within their own environment without the use of a prosthesis. As high a level of physical fitness, stamina and independence as possible must be obtained before the patient is discharged home using a wheelchair.

Whatever the individual situation, the new amputee must exercise regularly under supervision and continue until either prosthetic rehabilitation is complete or all adaptations have been completed to ensure that they can manage at home mobilising in a wheelchair or with other mobility aids.

Contractures, weakness and loss of function are often the result of inadequate supervision during this time. It is the hospital therapist's responsibility to oversee the management of amputees until they are fully rehabilitated and are using the prosthesis. This is not easy and much time and energy is required to ensure that the amputee progresses smoothly through prosthetic fitting stages, and eventually achieves full prosthetic rehabilitation. Individuals may vary greatly in their tolerance of rehabilitation and their resulting fatigue. Being given encouragement and support to achieve attainable goals is important to minimise discouragement. Psychologically, the experience of preparing to learn to walk for the second time is a powerful one.

Some new amputees can feel deskilled and demoralised by the experience of rehabilitation, which prepares them to relearn to walk and may cause them to become anxious or angry. These early stages of rehabilitation can be a time when individuals are confronted, sometimes for the first time, by the extent of their loss, and once again, extreme emotional reactions can also be expected at this time.

Some, on the other hand, may become excited, even euphoric at times, at learning a new skill and contributing to their own progress in such a clear way. This can help them to deal with difficult feelings by keeping them busy and providing a distraction. Although concern is sometimes expressed by staff at this stage that more euphoric amputees are 'in denial' (see Ch. 3), this state of energetic enthusiasm can often be highly adaptive for making progress with the task in hand.

With any problems arising through this period (and indeed any other throughout rehabilitation), it is important to think psychologically as well as functionally.

ESTABLISHED AMPUTEE PRESENTING WITH A NEW PROBLEM

If for any reason an established limb wearer cannot wear the prosthesis, the same principle of exercise should be followed. Examples of problems these amputees may encounter are:

- Residual limb breakdown
- Surgical retrim of the residual limb
- Other surgery, fracture or acute episode
- Recurrence of tumour
- Other medical conditions, e.g. minor stroke, diabetic upset, cardiorespiratory problems
- Social difficulties.

If surgical revision to a higher level of amputation is carried out, the amputee must be regarded as a primary amputee. Balance, proprioception and muscle control are altered and the amputee must be made aware that using the new prosthesis will be very different. The full exercise programme must be given.

AIMS OF TREATMENT RELATED TO AGE

The aims of rehabilitation are basically the same for all age groups, namely personal, domestic, social and economic competence. There are, however, specific factors to be taken into account when planning treatment programmes, always bearing in mind each individual's needs.

Young people. The aims of the physical treatment for the young are perfection of movement, coordination and full muscle strength. These people become easily bored, so that constant variation and imagination in their exercise programme is necessary. Realistically hard exercises must be given with daily progression, with particular emphasis on the residual limb. The therapist must also be prepared to give time and find the opportunity to listen carefully to the younger amputee and maybe to prompt them, in a sensitive manner, into voicing their concerns. Often they are discharged home from hospital quickly and by the time they have found out what is involved in their changed circumstances, opportunities for receiving information and professional advice are lost. Young amputees generally have high expectations of themselves and their ability and are surprised at how difficult tasks are to achieve. It is important therefore that they do have an opportunity to try tasks within a secure environment before discharge, e.g. domestic tasks, use of public transport, visiting shops/ pubs, etc.

Elderly people. The aim of treatment for elderly people is safe function in the activities of daily living. A few relevant exercises must be repeated in the same way each day, ideally during short treatment sessions. Balance, transfers and upper limb strength are essential to the amputee so that they can be independent in their wheelchair. Those who proceed to prosthetic rehabilitation also require maximal lower limb strength. Both types of rehabilitation may challenge the individual's cardiovascular system. The therapist will need to be aware of any cardiovascular insufficiency that may affect rehabilitation. For the mentally alert, the same degree of stimulation needs to be given as for the younger amputee.

Elderly frail people may tire more easily, have sensory or perceptual impairments, and will undoubtedly have more than one medical condition. Vascular amputees in particular may lose the remaining leg within 2 years and have a short life expectancy. These amputees require practice in tasks of daily living to enable them to be safe in their home and local environment. They are likely to use a wheelchair for all or part of the time. The whole team must therefore work towards ensuring an acceptable quality of life in the remaining years of these amputees' lives.

IDEAS FOR THE EXERCISE PROGRAMME
Starting positions used

Sitting

The amputee should be seated on a large plinth that is at the same height as the wheelchair to ensure safe transfer. Sitting balance must be achieved before anything else. The proprioceptive neuromuscular facilitation (PNF) technique of rhythmic stabilisation can be used, with manual contacts on the scapulae and pelvis. This can be progressed to throwing and catching exercises and a balance board can be used (Fig. 5.1).

Arm exercises should be carried out by all amputees, particularly those with upper limb weakness. Exercises include push-up blocks (Fig. 5.2) with which rhythmic stabilisations can again be performed. Weight and pulley systems, restive exercise bands and other means of graded resistance can be used very effectively,

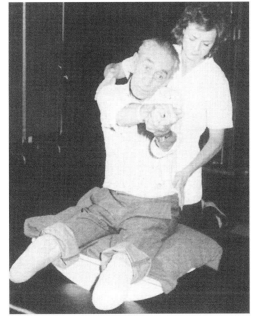

Figure 5.1 Sitting balance board exercise.

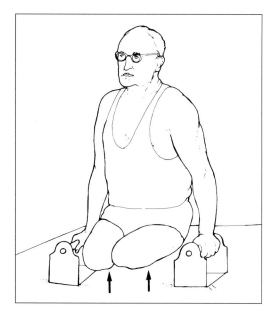

Figure 5.2 A bilateral trans-femoral amputee using push-up blocks.

particularly for graded bilateral resisted latissimus dorsi work. All amputees must be able to push up in order to lift their buttocks off the bed or chair to relieve pressure and therefore prevent the development of pressure areas.

Supine lying

In this position, the remaining leg, trunk and arms can be effectively treated in a variety of ways. PNF patterns to the remaining leg or upper limbs can be particularly useful to facilitate muscle work in order to increase strength and endurance. Also, using the principle of overflow, they can be used to facilitate muscle work on the amputated side. Once the most appropriate patterns have been selected, pulley and weight systems or other means of graded resistance can be set up to provide the appropriate resistance so that the amputee can perform contractions.

The weight and number of repetitions can be increased daily. This often gives the amputee, particularly the younger one, a measurable goal of achievement. Residual limb exercises can also be effectively performed in this position with manual assistance or resistance.

Side lying

Initially, many amputees require assistance to roll into this position. PNF patterns of the head, upper limb and trunk can be useful to facilitate the movement. With practice, many amputees will achieve this independently, although the very frail or those with other problems, e.g. neurological, might not. This position is particularly useful for facilitating hip extension. Again, PNF techniques of repeated contractions, plus hold, as well as advanced repeated contractions can be useful, especially to re-educate the hip extensors and/or abductors. If hip extension is limited, hold-relax of the flexors can be performed in order to increase the range of extension.

Prone lying

It must be emphasised that amputees with cardio-respiratory problems, kyphotic spines or gross arthritis will never be comfortable in this position, in which case, it is inappropriate to choose this position for exercises.

For those who are able to tolerate lying prone it is a particularly effective position for arm exercises, e.g. press-ups, trunk and hip extension exercises. McKenzie exercises can be used to mobilise the lumbar spine and maintain hip extension passively.

Kneeling

Providing wound healing is complete, the trans-tibial and knee disarticulation amputee, both unilateral and bilateral, can try to exercise in two-point or four-point kneeling or standing with the residual limb resting on a stool. The purpose is to improve balance reactions, weight transference and sensation in the residual limb to prepare for prosthetic use. It is hard exercise, and inappropriate for some elderly amputees (Figs 5.3 and 5.4).

It is necessary in the early stages, particularly for the knee disarticulation amputee, to place a soft covering over the residual limb, or to place a pillow under the residual limb to protect the skin while kneeling. Rhythmic stabilisations

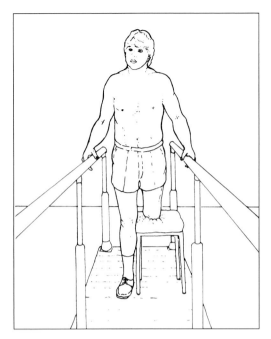

Figure 5.3   Supported standing applying graded pressure to a knee disarticulation residual limb.

with progressive speed and resistance can be used. Kneeling increases stability for those with transtibial and knee disarticulation levels whilst dressing.

Dynamic residual limb exercises

Dynamic residual limb exercises are simply multipurpose exercises combining the actions of the muscles of the residual limb with the rest of the body. They are used in the pre-prosthetic stage (and during any period when the prosthesis is not worn) to facilitate restoration of body symmetry. Some of these exercises are very hard and may not be suitable for very elderly or frail persons. However, they can be adapted to suit most individuals. Their advantage is that the amputee can carry out these exercises independently either in the hospital ward or at home.

The effects gained from dynamic residual limb exercises include:

1. The residual limb muscles are strengthened with emphasis on adductors, extensors and internal rotators.

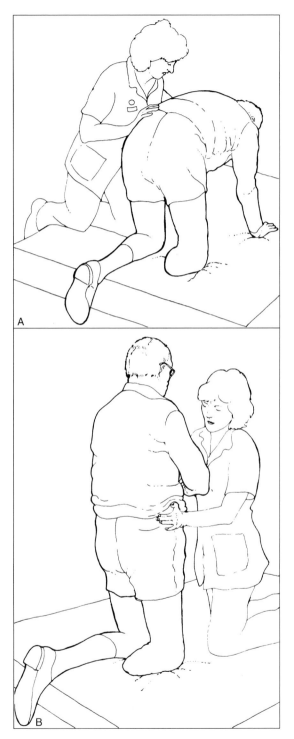

Figure 5.4   Kneeling exercise with manual resistance: (A) four-point kneeling; (B) two-point kneeling.

2. The residual limb becomes accustomed to taking pressure, in preparation for prosthetic use.
3. The circulation is increased.
4. The flexibility of joints is maintained.
5. The muscle tone is promoted.
6. The amputee's proprioceptive sense is re-educated in that the exercises at the same time involve movement of the rest of the body.
7. The amputee learns the muscle coordination required of the residual limb in preparation for using a prosthesis.

The following items are used for the exercises:

- Thick towels or pillows made into rolls of different sizes
- Stool 18 cm high with a soft padded top
- Firm wide plinth.

Exercise 1. Residual limb extension with anterior pelvic thrust

Position (Fig. 5.5). The amputee lies supine with a pillow under their head. The residual limb is placed on a 18 cm stool, with the opposite leg flexed (to reduce lumbar lordosis).

Movement. The amputee presses the residual limb forcibly against the stool so that their hips

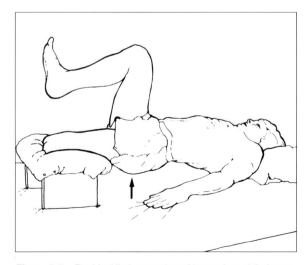

Figure 5.5 Residual limb extension with anterior pelvic thrust.

are lifted off the mat and held there momentarily. The therapist can either assist or resist the movement.

Purpose. The action is similar to that which occurs during the gait cycle as the prosthesis enters the support phase, and the remaining limb enters swing phase after the foot leaves the ground.

Exercise 2. Adduction of the internally rotated residual limb with lateral pelvic thrust

Position (Fig. 5.6). The amputee lies on the unaffected side with the residual limb resting on the stool; the opposite leg is flexed forwards and held up off the plinth. The trunk is stabilised by the arms. Some amputees need an extra pillow on top of the stool.

Movement. The internally rotated residual limb is pushed strongly downwards into adduction, and the pelvis is elevated. The therapist can either assist or resist the movement.

Some amputees tend to roll forwards, thus elevating the rear rather than the side of the pelvis; the therapist must then stabilise the upper shoulders and hips of the amputee. Shoulder, hip and residual limb must then remain in a straight line.

Purpose. In the prosthetic gait cycle of the trans-femoral amputee, there is a tendency to bend the trunk over the supporting side. The adductors and internal rotators should contract as weight is put on the prosthesis.

Exercise 3. Residual limb abduction with pelvic elevation

Position (Fig. 5.7). The amputee lies on the affected side. The residual limb is adducted with a stool, towelling roll or pillow placed under its abductor surface. The amputee stabilises the position by using the arms.

Movement. The amputee abducts the residual limb hard down on the stool or pillow until the pelvis is lifted. Extension must be maintained. Range can be increased by moving the stool or pillow distally if it is not too painful for the amputee.

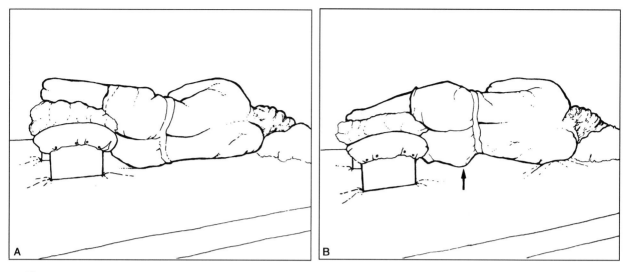

Figure 5.6   Adduction of the internally rotated residual limb with lateral pelvic thrust.

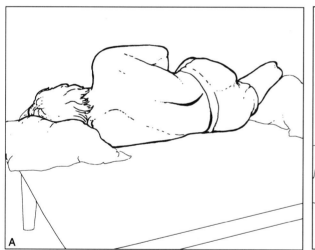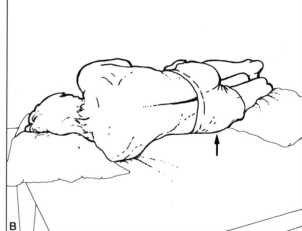

Figure 5.7   Residual limb abduction with pelvic elevation.

Purpose. This exercise should prevent the Trendelenburg gait. Any amputee who has not walked for a length of time will have weak hip abductors.

Exercise 4. Residual limb adduction with extension

Position (Fig. 5.8). The amputee lies prone, with the hips flat on the mat. A pillow or rolled towel is placed between the thighs.

Movement. The amputee presses the thighs together and squeezes the roll. This causes simultaneous back and hip extension.

Mechanically resisted exercises

Pulleys

A weight and pulley system can be used for arm or leg exercises, either to simulate the gait

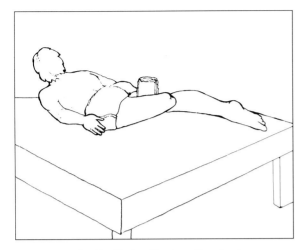

Figure 5.8 Residual limb adduction with extension.

pattern or as an isolated movement. Any starting position can be used. Repetitive exercises can be carried out, which help build up muscle endurance and general fitness. The weight and number of repetitions can be increased daily. This often gives the younger amputee, in particular, a measurable goal of achievement.

Isokinetic exercise

In this type of exercise the speed of the muscular performance is controlled rather than the amount of resistance or the distance moved. Equipment used may be pre-set to hold the speed of a body movement at a constant rate, irrespective of the magnitude of forces generated by the participating muscles. The resistance offered by the machine matches the amputee's immediate and specific muscular capacity of a body segment throughout a range of motion, but without permitting acceleration to occur. This type of exercise is also termed 'accommodating resistance exercise'.

The mounting of the isokinetic device is adjustable so that the lever arm can be positioned for movement in virtually any plane; a large variety of exercise patterns are thus possible.

The apparatus can be used in measurement of muscle performance with great accuracy and provides an objective measure of torque, total work and power rates for evaluation purposes.

Examples of these systems are the KinCom and Cybex.

This type of exercise is particularly useful for the fitter amputee, who needs to exercise all four limbs. The lever arms may not accommodate knee or elbow flexion/extension with a short residual limb; however, they can be used for full hip and shoulder movements (Fig. 5.9). Later in the amputee's rehabilitation, when the residual limb is healed and prosthetic tolerance has been built up, the isokinetic systems can be used wearing the prosthesis. The lever arm should be positioned proximal to the end of the residual limb in order to prevent a shear force between the socket and the skin of the residual limb.

Points to consider during the exercise programme

1. Amputees can be treated both individually and in groups. A period of individual work daily will enable the therapist and therapy assistant to observe progress and to increase the exercise programme where appropriate. Communication between amputee and therapist is ongoing. Group work with other amputees or patients with different conditions is fun and of great psychological value.

Exercise classes can be given in a gymnasium area for the fitter patients. The therapist must remain sensitive towards amputees' feelings when they are being viewed in a group or class situation.

2. A programme of home exercises must be taught. It should include the most relevant exercises for each individual and must not be complicated. Generally, a maximum of five exercises is recommended. They should be written down or illustrated in a form understandable to the amputee and presented in an appropriate format.

3. The therapist should always handle both the residual limb and remaining leg with care. The position of hand holds and mechanical resistance (of pulley harness, straps, restive exercise bands, sandbags, etc.) must be considered. Damage to the tissues of the residual limb or remaining leg, particularly in the dysvascular amputee, can easily occur if padding is inadequate.

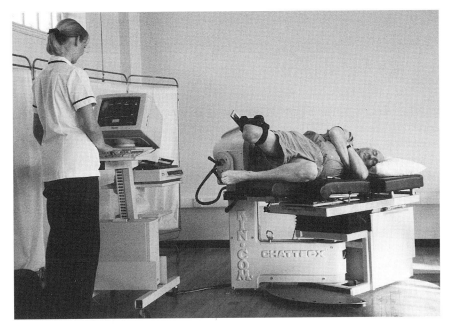

Figure 5.9   A transtibial amputee using the KinCom to strengthen hip abductors.
(Photograph by kind permission of the prosthetic physiotherapy service, Oxford, UK)

IDEAS FOR THE TREATMENT OF CONTRACTURES

Reasons for contractures

1. Contractures can occur pre-operatively as a result of pain and inactivity. The body's reaction to pain is to hold the limb in a flexed position. The contracture should be noted, measured and recorded pre-operatively by the therapist. However, following amputation, the amputee may maintain a flexed position through habit, muscle imbalance and immobility. If the amputee has an underlying neurological condition, altered tone may influence the position of the residual limb.

2. Vascular surgery, particularly if multiple operations were carried out, result in extensive scar tissue. This may initially limit full range of movement at the hip and knee.

3. Specific joint problems (such as osteoarthrosis and rheumatoid arthritis) may present with muscular, capsular and ligamentous tightness; the joint may be flared up in an acute phase. Furthermore, there may be permanent restriction of the joint caused by previous fractures or trauma.

4. If the amputee is an established limb wearer and has to stop using the prosthesis for any reason for a period of time (see p. 58), contractures both at the hip and knee joints can develop through sitting for prolonged periods.

5. Pain that persists after the amputation will cause the limb to be held in flexion; analgesia should be reviewed and the cause investigated. If there is ischaemic pain, the amputation may not have been performed sufficiently proximally to ablate the disease, or the disease may have progressed. Also, with increasing age the established non-vascular amputee can develop peripheral vascular disease. The whole team must be aware of this problem: it is often the night nurse who observes the amputee clasping the residual limb in flexion or dangling it over the edge of the bed to try to alleviate the pain (see Ch. 20).

Treatment

The techniques listed below are for both the prevention and treatment of contractures:

1. Active or resisted muscle work, either directly to the limb or to the rest of the body to gain over-

flow: proprioceptive neuromuscular facilitation techniques are particularly appropriate.

2. Diligent positioning of the residual limb or remaining limb to prevent contracture: the whole team must be aware of correct positions and constantly remind the amputee. The prone or supine positions and use of stump boards, etc., are mentioned in Chapter 4.

3. Passive stretching must be performed with great care and sensitivity, particularly with regard to the underlying pathology. The therapist should be experienced enough to 'feel' the end of the range, whether it is elastic or blocked.

To reduce existing contracture other modalities can be used depending on the pathology present:

a. Ice
b. Passive mobilisations
c. Ultrasound therapy
d. Plaster-of-Paris or thermoplastic materials for serial splints.

Amputees with contractures require frequent but short periods of daily treatment. Accurate measurement of the joint using a goniometer and noting the starting position used must be recorded at least weekly. It must be realised that treatment may only prevent the contracture getting worse, rather than improving it. These principles of treatment apply to contractures of joints in both the residual limb and the remaining limb, the difference being that there is inherent muscle imbalance in the residual limb.

IDEAS FOR THE TREATMENT OF ADHERENT SCARS

Adherent scars on the residual limb may result from slowly healing wounds or previous surgery to that limb. They can present problems with prosthetic fitting, especially when they immediately overlie a bony prominence. Treatment should commence when healing is complete and no open areas remain.

Treatment

1. Gentle thumb and finger massage, using a non-reactive cream, to mobilise the tissues.

This may be taught to the amputee and/or carer.

2. Ultrasound, using a high-frequency, low-intensity beam directly over the scar. (The usual contraindications to this treatment apply.)

CONTINUOUS ASSESSMENT

While the therapist is treating the amputee, ongoing assessment must take place. Observation of strength, movement, balance, perception, motivation and psychological state will enable an accurate assessment of function so that realistic goals of treatment can be planned with the amputee and their carers.

It is most important that there is free communication between therapists and amputees. The amputee's wishes must be known and understood so that individual identity is preserved. Not all amputees wish to achieve the goal the therapists has in mind. Weekly meetings with the other team members are important to communicate the amputee's achievements and to plan their future progress.

FUNCTIONAL TASKS

The amputee should be encouraged to regain their independence in activities of daily living as early as possible in the hospital ward. Having gained some early mobility through the use of a wheelchair, the amputee can begin to care for themselves. Achieving even small tasks helps to build confidence.

It is important that the physiotherapist and occupational therapist liaise frequently to discuss the amputee's progress. Treatment plans can be graded and modified appropriately according to the amputee's needs and should be complementary to each other.

Pre-prosthetic activities

Re-education for personal care, dressing and transfers will have been carried out while the amputee is on the hospital ward (see Ch. 4). Once they are able to attend the therapy facility, a wider range of functional tasks relevant to their individual needs can be addressed.

Bathing

Most amputees will require simple assistive equipment to bathe safely. A bathboard, seat, non-slip mat and rail on the wall are often recommended.

The more frail amputee may require an electro-mechanical bath lift, particularly where upper limb strength is poor. The bilateral amputee should be shown how to position the wheelchair next to the bath, remove the armrest of the wheelchair and slide across onto the bath board (see Fig. 5.10).

Some people will prefer to use a shower rather than attempting to climb into the bottom of the bath. A slatted shower board may be used with an over-bath shower. Cubicle showers often have a deep step into the tray. The unilateral amputee may manage this and sit on either a free-standing stool or wall-mounted seat. The therapist should advise on the position and fixing of wall-mounted rails for safety.

The bilateral amputee will require a level access shower tray and a self-propelling shower chair for use within the bathroom. Prosthetic users should be advised or remove their prosthesis and undress close to their bathing facilities.

Armchair

Not all amputees will wish to remain seated in their wheelchair all day. Armchairs should be adjusted to a suitable height for the amputee to transfer safely. The height may be altered by additional foam cushions or by chair raisers fitted onto the legs/castors of the chair.

Car

The amputee should practice getting in and out of a car. It is usually easier to transfer from the wheelchair into the front passenger seat of the car. The seat should be pushed backwards to give sufficient room for the amputee to avoid knocking the residual limb and to allow the carer to assist where necessary. If the amputee cannot manage a standing pivot transfer, a banana-shaped sliding transfer board can be tried. Bilateral amputees will need to use a transfer board to slide across to the car seat. This should always be attempted on level ground and away

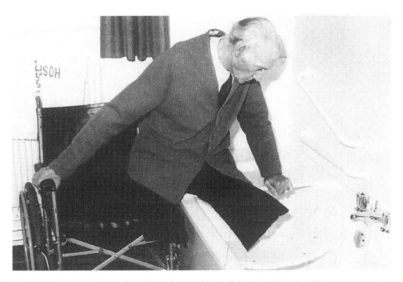

Figure 5.10   Bath transfer. Note the position of the wheelchair with one arm rest removed. Bath board, inner bath seat and two grab rails are in situ.

from the kerb. A seat swivel transfer disk may also assist the amputee to get into the car.

Wheelchair practice

All amputees will use a wheelchair in the pre-prosthetic stages of their rehabilitation. Wheelchair mobility is an excellent method for developing independence in the hospital ward and therapy facility (see Ch. 6 for details).

Arm strengthening exercises

Some activities are directed towards upper limb strengthening while others enable the amputee to gain skills and confidence in independent living. Activities such as woodworking and printing can be carried out in the workshop facility and domestic tasks such as cooking, washing and ironing personal clothing can be carried out in the rehabilitation facilities. Gardening and modified leisure activities, particularly in a group setting, can stimulate and motivate the amputee. All activities can be graded according to each individual's needs. The grading may be in length of time, complexity of the task, amount of strength

required or the amount of wheelchair mobility required.

Domestic activities

The therapist should encourage the amputee to regain independence in some domestic tasks. Beverages, simple snacks and meals can be prepared in the rehabilitation facility. (see Fig. 5.11). The amputee will need to practise reaching and carrying items from their wheelchair. On the home visit assessment, the therapist can help the amputee to plan how they will manage cooking, what items of equipment will need to be used and any changes required to the layout of the kitchen.

Self-expression

It is often when the patient is engaged in a familiar activity that personal feelings may begin to be expressed, either to the therapist or to another patient. The less rushed and less clinical atmosphere lends itself to quiet discussion that should be seen as an adjunct to specialist counselling help.

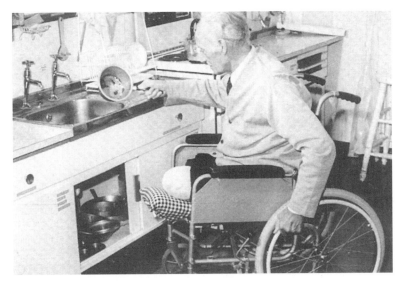

Figure 5.11   Cooking practice.

Discharge home from hospital

Owing to the short length of stay associated with acute care it is likely that the amputee will be discharged home from hospital prior to using a prosthesis. The multiprofessional team should liaise regularly to discuss progress and propose a discharge date for the amputee to return home.

From the initial therapy assessment (see Ch. 2), the therapist will have obtained information about the amputee's home and social situation. Early discharge planning involving the patient, carer and professionals both within the hospital and community is necessary. This will ensure that any equipment or care needs identified can be planned and organised in advance of the patient going home.

Once the amputee is medically stable, their wound is healing well and they are reaching their optimum level of mobility and independence, the therapist will start to coordinate the necessary arrangements for discharge home as safely and independently as possible. It is advisable to carry out an early home visit to obtain an accurate assessment of the environment that the amputee will be returning to. This visit will often be carried out without the amputee. This allows the therapist to identify any particular problems such as difficult access, inaccessible rooms and equipment requirements (such as bed raisers to make transfers easier, bathing aids, etc.), before taking the amputee home from hospital on a home visit assessment to plan the final arrangements. There will be time to obtain items or equipment or for the family/carers to move furniture around to make room for the wheelchair. In some cases it may be possible to carry out this early visit pre-operatively.

Home visit assessment

The therapist will coordinate the visit with the amputee, carer and any relevant community support agencies including the community therapists and nurse. The aims of the visit are to ensure that the amputee is able to function safely and independently with their wheelchair, to identify any hazards and risks, and any equipment

and care needs such as personal care, wound management, pressure area care and domestic tasks. The therapist should measure and assess for necessary equipment and minor adaptations and arrange to provide the equipment prior to the individual's return home. This may include altering furniture heights (see Fig. 5.12), providing toileting and bathing equipment including any temporary arrangements such as moving a bed downstairs, provision of a commode for night use or temporary ramps for wheelchair access.

The therapist should assess the home for both wheelchair and prosthetic use, e.g. where the amputee will put on and take off the prosthesis and whether a second stair rail is required. The community therapist will be responsible for the longer term needs of the amputee and for any major housing adaptations required for independent living. Home visits can be very emotional for the amputee, particularly if they have been in hospital for a long time and because of

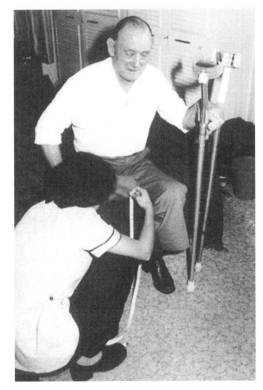

Figure 5.12 The home visit. All functional activities in the home are checked both with and without the prosthesis.

the change in their ability. Sometimes the home visit can be the deciding factor as to whether a person can actually go home and manage with support or whether alternative accommodation such as a nursing home or residential home is necessary. The therapist should be sensitive to the situation and provide support and reassurance to the amputee and/or carers.

BIBLIOGRAPHY FOR PREVIOUS EDITIONS

Alpert S H 1982 The psychological aspects of amputation surgery. Orthotics and Prosthetics 36(4):50–56
Baruch I M, Mossberg K A 1983 Heart-rate response of elderly women to nonweight-bearing ambulation with a walker. Physical Therapy 63(11):1782–1787
Chadwick S J D 1986 Restoring dignity and mobility in the amputee. Geriatric Medicine 16(7):43–46
Eisert O, Tester O W 1954 Dynamic exercises for lower extremity amputees. Archives of Physical Medicine and Rehabilitation 35:695–704
Furst L, Humphrey M 1983 Coping with the loss of a leg. Prosthetics and Orthotics International 7:152–156
Kavanagh T, Shephard R J 1973 The application of exercise testing to the elderly amputee. Canadian Medical Association Journal 108:314–317
Moncur S D 1969 The practical aspect of balance relating to amputees. Physiotherapy 55(2):409–410
Moverley L 1990 Discovering water's redeeming features. Therapy Weekly 17(7):4
Parkes C M 1972 Components of the reaction to loss of a limb, spouse or home. Journal of Psychosomatic Research 16:343–349
Thompson D M, Haran D 1984 Living with an amputation: the patient. International Rehabilitation Medicine 5(4):165–169
Tilbury B 1981 Some general thoughts on the rehabilitation of the elderly amputee. Newsletter of the Demonstration Centres in Rehabilitation 26:44–52

BIBLIOGRAPHY FOR THE THIRD EDITION

Bailey M J, MacWhannell C 1997 Clinical monitoring of dysvascular lower limb amputees during initial gait training. Physiotherapy 83(6):278–283
Edelstein J E 1992 Preprosthetic and nonprosthetic management of older patients. Topics in Geriatric Rehabilitation 8(1):22–29
Kulkarni J, Wright S, Toole C, Morris J, Hirons R 1996 Falls in patients with lower limb amputations: prevalence and contributing factors. Physiotherapy 82(2):130–136
Powers C M, Boyd L A, Fontaine C A, Perry J 1996 The influence of lower-extremity muscle force on gait characteristics in individuals with below-knee amputations secondary to vascular disease. Physical Therapy 76(4):369–377
Renström P A F H, Alaranta H, Pohjolainen T 1995 Review: leg strengthening of the lower limb amputee. Critical Reviews in Physical and Rehabilitation Medicine 7(1):11–32
Ward K H, Meyers M C 1995 Exercise performance of lower-extremity amputees. Sports Medicine 20(4):207–214

6

Wheelchair use and early walking aids

Achieving an independent means of moving around early in the rehabilitation programme has many obvious advantages for both elderly and young amputees and wheelchair mobility is advisable for all before a trial with an early walking aid (EWA). No longer having to rely on others for daily living activities (such as going to the toilet), being able to socialise out of the ward environment with relatives and friends and building upper limb power is of great psychological benefit and the amputee is reassured that greater mobility will soon be possible.

Amputees should carry out regular progressive exercise programmes in the therapy facility during this phase. Independent wheelchair activities and the use of EWAs should usually commence within the first 2 weeks postoperatively. Hopping is not encouraged until the residual limb is healed.

WHEELCHAIR MOBILITY

Individual needs regarding wheelchair use vary; some people will use a wheelchair in the early postoperative days and subsequently only if a major problem with other illness, the prosthesis or residual limb arises. Others will continue to use the wheelchair if their pathology overcomes their other mobility achievements using the prosthesis; others will use the wheelchair as their main means of functional independence.

Temporary wheelchair

Whatever the eventual outcome for wheelchair

use, all amputees will need a temporary wheelchair for mobility at an early stage in the acute hospital environment. This will help to prevent dependent oedema of the residual limb at this stage. Standing and hopping are not recommended and can be particularly difficult for elderly amputees. The remaining foot may have fragile tissue viability and be unable to take vertical and shear forces. The benefits of using a wheelchair at this stage include:

- upper limb strengthening
- increased cardiovascular output
- increased stamina and tolerance
- independence in activities of daily living.

The temporary wheelchair may not be the ideal solution for the individual as most hospitals have a limited range of loan wheelchairs, but providing basic safety features are correct, it will serve its purpose for independent mobility for a short time. Box 6.1 provides a checklist of details to ensure safety of temporary wheelchairs.

Whilst the amputee may associate the provision and use of a wheelchair with permanent disability, it is the therapist's responsibility to explain the benefits of using the wheelchair in these early stages (based on knowledge and reasoning) and encourage the user to gain maximum independence in function and mobility, and to develop upper limb strength. However, the amputee may be unwilling initially to use a wheelchair; the therapist and the rest of the team should give them time to adapt to realising the benefits it provides.

In the early stages of rehabilitation, a wheelchair will often be the only method of mobility. The only amputees who should attempt to hop with a frame or crutches are those in the youngest age group, who find it very frustrating to use a wheelchair all the time. However, support in the form of a stump bandage or shrinker sock should be used to prevent gravitational oedema, even for short hops. A few elderly amputees may have to hop to manage at home, e.g. in getting to the toilet as the home may not be adaptable for wheelchair use. Some amputees will only use a wheelchair in the early stages of their recovery but for others, a wheelchair will become their main means of achieving not just mobility but also greater independence.

Assessment for the provision of a permanent wheelchair

If a permanent wheelchair is required, the assessment for the type of chair and the specifications that will need to be considered should be carried out once the amputee's condition has stabilised and must include assessment of the main environment where the chair is to be used. The range and choice of wheelchairs available from local health services will vary from one area to another due to different funding levels and local requirements. The hospital therapist should identify the specifications and contact the local wheelchair service at an early stage. The specialist wheelchair therapist may also wish to carry out their own assessment for more complex or specialist cases together with the hospital therapist.

Assessment criteria

A wheelchair is not simply a mobility aid to get from one place to another – if well assessed and appropriately prescribed, the wheelchair can improve independence and enhance the user's quality of life. All aspects of the user, their lifestyle, level of ability and environment as well as the needs of their carer should be included.

Box 6.1 Checklist for temporary wheelchair safety

Ensure that:

- Brakes are safe
- Tyres are inflated to correct pressure
- Chair is stable and will not tip over backwards due to the alteration of the user's centre of gravity
- Cushion is suitable for pressure and posture requirements
- Footplate is correctly adjusted to provide stability and equal weight distribution under buttocks
- Stump board is supplied if necessary
- Chair features are suitable for ease of transfer by user and carer
- Size is appropriate for access to all necessary facilities, e.g. toilet

---

Box 6.2 Criteria for wheelchair assessment

Individual physical and clinical features
- Height and weight
- Skin condition
- Site of amputation, e.g. uni- or bilateral; level of amputation
- Postural ability; deformities of the spine/hip – fixed or correctable
- Weight distribution with regard to rearward stability
- Prosthetic prescription
- Care and supervision required

Functional ability
- Able to change position (for pressure relief)
- Method of transfer
- Manual dexterity and coordination
- Cognitive and perceptual ability
- Level of independence

Environment
- Home, work, school, leisure – frequency of use
- Access
- Floor surfaces
- Turning spaces
- Furniture or work surface heights
- Storage space for chair

Transport
- Car
- Converted van
- Minibus
- School bus
- Public transport

Other relevant factors in assessment
- Attitude
- Motivation
- Preferences of user
- Abilities and preferences of carer
- Pain
- Incontinence

The checklist provided in Box 6.2 will assist in the assessment process.

Type of chair required

There are a number of different chairs on the market today. The basic types are:

- Self-propelled
- Attendant pushed
- Powered model.

Maintenance and care of wheelchair

Routine maintenance and care of the wheelchair by the user or their carer will help to keep it in good working order. People should always follow the manufacturer's instructions in the handbook provided. The following is a list of items that should be checked regularly by the user/carer:

- Tyre pressures (pneumatic tyres)
- Brake function (contact repairer if these are not working properly)
- State of seat and back canvas
- Condition of cushion
- All surfaces and working parts for routine cleaning including:
  — clips on detachable arms
  — footrest mechanism
  — folding backrest
- Regular charging of battery (powered chairs).

The user or carer must be trained to perform these tasks and they must have the relevant telephone numbers of the local wheelchair provision centre and repairer. Any technical problems should be reported to the repairer and should not be dealt with by the user or carer.

Model of wheelchair

Self-propelling folding chairs

These are usually prescribed for amputees (see Fig. 6.1.)

Accessories. Detachable or swing back armrests and swing back detachable footrests may assist with transfers and transporting the wheelchair. If the amputee has a prosthesis with a rigid pelvic band and finds standing up out of the chair difficult due to the prosthesis getting caught on the front of the armrests, the front armrest slot can be outset approximately 2.5 cm on a self-propelling chair.

A stump board (see Ch. 4, p. 46) is essential for the trans-tibial amputee and advisable for knee disarticulation amputees.

The rear wheels of the wheelchair should be set back 7.5 cm for all bilateral amputees and for some unilateral amputees to provide rearward stability, particularly on an upward incline. This will increase the wheelbase and thus a larger turning space is required. This is important when

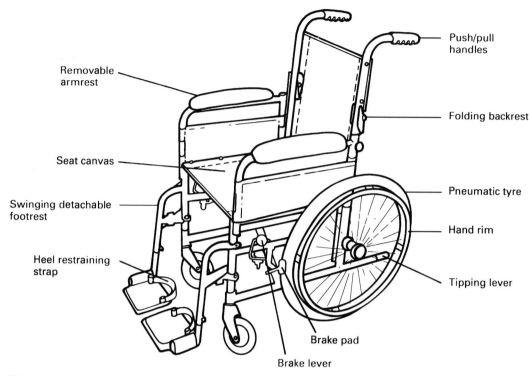

Removable armrest

Seat canvas

Swinging detachable footrest

Heel restraining strap

Push/pull handles

Folding backrest

Pneumatic tyre

Hand rim

Tipping lever

Brake pad

Brake lever

Figure 6.1 A basic self-propelling wheelchair.

considering how the chair will manoeuver in small areas such as lifts, small rooms and narrow passages.

Some wheelchair models are designed to allow adjustability in the position of the propelling wheel and/or castors. This alters the stability of the chair and will allow a more able user to achieve rear-wheel balance ('wheelies') and enable the user to mount low kerbs, steps or traverse more easily over rough ground. Unless the user is very experienced, altering the position of the wheels should only be carried out with agreement from the specialist wheelchair therapist or engineer.

Electrically Powered Indoor-Outdoor Wheelchairs (EPIOCs)

Amputees who are severely disabled (i.e. full-time wheelchair users who are unable to walk or self-propel indoors) may obtain increased independence and freedom when successfully using one of these models. In the UK they are classified as pavement vehicles. They use gel batteries, have a top speed of 4 m.p.h. and can travel some 10–12 miles on a full battery charge.

Assessment of the amputee and their environment for provision of a powered chair involves consideration of:

- suitable access within the home and immediate environment
- good general vision or an ability to adapt appropriately if visually impaired (e.g. for crossing roads and manoeuvring on a busy public pavement)
- ability to understand and anticipate possible hazards (e.g. children on bicycles)
- space at home and suitable floor coverings (a chair that is used for both outdoor and indoor use is likely to bring dirt into the home and heavy tread tyres may leave track marks on thicker carpets)
- ability of the amputee or their carer to recharge the battery

- ability of the amputee to access a breakdown service to rescue them away from home
- ability of the user to purchase insurance in case of an accident.

Selection of the most suitable features must be identified during the assessment period, e.g. central or side curb climbers; padded or canvas seat and back; folding mechanism for occasional travel; style and position of the controller.

Training is essential if the user is to obtain maximum benefit from a powered indoor-outdoor wheelchair.

Selection of cushion

Most amputees will use a 5 or 7.5 cm foam cushion with a wipeable cover. A plywood base or crescent-shaped insert can be used to reduce the sag in the canvas, improving weight distribution and stability. For users with fixed postural deformity or those at risk from skin breakdown due to pressure, an alternative cushion may be provided. A full assessment should be carried out taking into account the results of any risk assessment scale used, e.g. Waterlow, Norton, Gordon, etc.

The therapist should ensure that the cushion remains in place when the amputee transfers from the wheelchair (particularly bilateral amputees). Tie tapes stitched to the back of a cushion or the use of a non-slip mat under the cushion can prevent slipping or sliding. A range of pressure-relieving cushions, or others suitable to encourage a good sitting position, are generally available.

It is important to note that special cushions will not heal pressure sores once formed, but correct selection together with advice on caring for the cushion will reduce the risk of pressure sores developing.

Wheelchair supply

Government healthcare funding: each wheelchair service has an identified budget for their local population; the range of choice will depend on the level of funding and local requirements. Amputees with a high level of ability and good

upper trunk stability may benefit from provision of a lightweight, high-performance chair that may or may not be available from the local service.

Private supply: some amputees are able to purchase their own wheelchairs, but it is essential that appropriate advice regarding correct prescription features is obtained from an experienced therapist so that expensive mistakes are not made by purchasing an inappropriate model.

Voucher schemes: This was introduced in the UK in 1996 to offer a wider choice to users willing to contribute financially towards their wheelchair. As an alternative to accepting the model prescribed by the wheelchair service, the user may accept a voucher and either select a suitable chair from a larger specified range, but still receive free maintenance and repairs (partnership scheme), or an independent scheme where the user has a wide choice of chair, but will take responsibility for repairs and maintenance. Details of these schemes are available from the local wheelchair service.

Charitable organisations: a number of charities will consider providing finance towards purchasing a private wheelchair. Details can be obtained from the local wheelchair service, disability information centre or social worker.

Instruction to user and carer

Training in handling the wheelchair and regular practice is essential if the user is to gain maximum benefit from the equipment. The therapist should explain the importance of keeping the wheelchair clean and in good working order.

Independent wheelchair activities will be part of the rehabilitation programme in the therapy facilities (see Ch. 4). Suitable positioning for toilet and bed transfers should be identified and the patient should practise manoeuvring the wheelchair through doorways, into lifts, around corners, and on different floor surfaces and gradients. Further practice should take place on a visit to the environments in which it will be most used.

Written information with contact addresses and telephone numbers for maintenance and advice are essential for the amputee and their carer.

Both the amputee and their carer should be shown how to lift, fold and unfold the chair correctly, paying due attention to safe manual handling techniques and therefore the minimisation of injury. Negotiation of steps and kerbs must be practised to find the safest and least strenuous method that both feel comfortable using.

Review

Most wheelchair services in the UK accept self-referrals from registered users who can contact the service direct with any queries or requests.

People who have been supplied with a wheelchair may need review appointments to ensure ongoing needs are being met. Individual needs alter over time particularly for those with a chronic progressive disease such as peripheral vascular disease and diabetes. For the amputee, the general decline of strength and mobility with increasing age and possible accommodation change, can be compounded by weight change, more proximal amputation of the existing residual limb, loss of the remaining limb and the decline in cardiopulmonary function with consequent loss of exercise tolerance. A reassessment of the original prescription should always be carried out to ascertain the changes in needs. Particular care should be taken by the amputee not to increase their weight as this will not only limit the range of chairs available to them, but also put additional strain on any self-propelling user and attendants or carers carrying out transfers, etc.

The therapist based within the community is frequently the team member best placed to monitor changes and initiate the process whereby prescription review can be carried out. A complete checklist for assessment, prescription, provision and review of wheelchairs can be found in Appendix 2.

HOPPING

The purpose of achieving hopping with an aid is to offer the amputee an alternative method of mobility about the home. Going to the toilet and bathroom early in the morning and late in the evening is often easier without the prosthesis. Access to these areas in the wheelchair is not always possible so the ability to hop short distances is frequently essential. If there is mechanical breakdown of the prosthesis or tissue damage of the residual limb, the amputee must either hop or use the wheelchair.

However, too much hopping in the early stage of the rehabilitation programme is inadvisable because:

1. The residual limb is dependent, therefore oedema, discomfort and pain may result.
2. Those with vascular insufficiency may have an ischaemic and fragile foot through which the sudden force of full weightbearing during hopping is dangerous and inadvisable.
3. Prolonged hopping, especially in the younger amputee, may cause temporary postural defects such as pelvic tilt and spinal rotation. It can be dangerous when hopping at high speeds as the residual limb can be carelessly knocked.
4. Many elderly people are unwilling to stand and hop, not only because of physical problems, but because they feel unsafe and lack confidence.
5. A new bilateral amputee must not try to hop using the original prosthesis, even if they are fit and a trans-tibial amputee. This is unsafe and puts too great a stress through the soft tissues of the residual limb. However, standing transfers using the prosthesis may be possible, initially under the therapist's supervision.

An alternative to hopping is toe/heel swivelling. This has the advantages of requiring less arm strength and giving greater stability as the foot is always in contact with the floor. The great danger for the patient with vascular insufficiency is the large shear forces on the plantar soft tissues.

Individuals will often find their own solutions to mobility needs and those who feel unsafe hopping, or who cannot gain access using a wheelchair, may shuffle around on their bottom. This is inadvisable for anyone at risk of tissue breakdown. There are however strap-on bottom protectors, which are not easy to put on, but may help if this method of mobility has to be used. Stairs may be more accessible this way rather than by any other means. The therapist and amputee or carer should check the condition of the amputee's skin regularly.

EARLY WALKING AIDS (EWAs)

Pneumatic Post Amputation Mobility Aid (Ppam aid)

The Ppam aid is a partial weightbearing early walking aid that must only be used under clinical supervision in the therapy facility – it is not for ward or home use. This aid can be used from 5–7 days postoperatively while the sutures are still in the wound, provided the surgeon is satisfied that wound healing is progressing satisfactorily and has given permission for its use, and the therapist has observed the state of the wound. It consists of a basic frame (in three lengths), two inflatable airbags that surround the residual limb and a foot pump with a calibrated gauge protected for overpressure from 40 mmHg (Fig. 6.2). The Ppam aid is manufactured in the UK by Vessa Limited, who produce a leaflet that is free on request and describes the equipment and method of application for the trans-tibial amputee.

The therapist must ensure adherence to hygiene, including keeping one set of bags per patient, which are washed in appropriate cleaning solutions after use to prevent cross-infection.

Advantages

There are a number of advantages of the Ppam aid, including:

1. The great psychological boost gained by walking very soon after amputation.
2. The ability to assess the amputee in terms of prosthetic fitting and rehabilitation prospects. Particular examples of this are those with stroke or severe cardiorespiratory disease. Mild confusional states often improve once standing and walking commence.
3. The reduction of oedema. As weight is taken on the amputated side, the pressure in the bags is

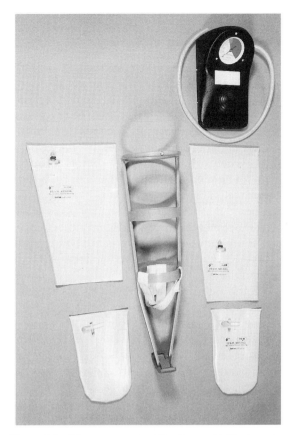

Figure 6.2 The components of the Ppam aid. The bags for trans-tibial and knee disarticulation amputees are on the right of the frame; the trans-femoral bag is on the left. (Photograph by kind permission of the prosthetic physiotherapy service, Oxford.)

increased and when weight is removed, pressure decreases. This pumping action reduces oedema and promotes wound healing. The support that the inflated air bags offer provides comfort for the dependent residual limb.

4. By encouraging partial weightbearing at an early stage, postural reactions are re-educated. This is important for those who have not stood up or walked for a long period of time prior to amputation. Muscle control of the trunk, remaining limb and hip on the amputated side is stimulated and balance is improved.

5. Preparation of the residual limb for the harder socket of a prosthesis is achieved by maintaining pressure around the residual limb. This may help in reducing phantom sensation.

Disadvantages

The disadvantages of the Ppam aid are:

1. If a fixed flexion contracture is present, the residual limb is more liable to break down. The anterior aspect of the knee may rub against the metal frame and there can be excessive pressures on the distal end of the residual limb.

2. Where there are fractures present in the femur (whether internally fixed or not) sufficient union or stability must be present to permit partial weightbearing. However, it must be remembered that rotational stress may occur while using the somewhat unstable Ppam aid; it may be safer to wait until the prosthesis can be supplied. If there is any doubt, the orthopaedic surgeon must advise.

3. If the amputee is very heavy or has a 'heavy footed gait,' excessive pistoning may occur and there will be insufficient support.

4. The experienced limb wearer who has further surgery to the residual limb finds partial weightbearing difficult and may try to use the Ppam aid as a normal prosthesis.

5. The amputee uses a stiff knee gait pattern, which is unnatural for those with a trans-tibial level of amputation.

6. The inflation pressure required to ensure stability in standing (approximately 40 mmHg) may be greater than the arterial pressure in the residual limb. This can lead to dysvascular changes if used for too long at any one session or too often in any one week.

Application of the Ppam aid

The method of application of the Ppam aid for trans-tibial and knee-disarticulation amputees

1. The fully dressed amputee sits on a chair inside the parallel bars. The wound dressing remains in place.

2. The therapist inflates the small bag to no more than one-quarter full, invaginates it and places it over the distal end of the amputee's residual limb and trousers, if worn (see Fig. 6.3A). The amputee is asked to hold this in place. If the residual limb is large or if bulky dressings are present, the small bag is folded in half, slightly inflated and held against the distal end of the residual limb.

3. The large bag (uninflated) is pulled over the residual limb and small bag, ensuring a smooth fit right up to the groin and buttock crease (see Fig. 6.3B).

4. The correctly sized frame is eased up over the two bags and residual limb until it is about 8 cm from the top of the large bag (see Fig. 6.3C).

6. The cruciate webbing straps are then fixed so that support is given to the distal end of the large bag.

7. The amputee is asked to straighten the knee of the remaining leg so that a check of the length of the frame can be made.

8. The large bag is then inflated using the foot pump to approximately 40 mmHg pressure (see Fig. 6.3D)

9. The amputee then stands in the parallel bars and the fit of the Ppam aid is checked before balance exercise and walking are attempted (see Fig. 6.3E).

The method of application of the Ppam aid for trans-femoral amputees

1. The amputee starts in the same position as for the previous method.

2. The large bag is pulled over the residual limb with the inflation tube on the lateral side (see Fig 6.4A).

3. The small bag (the same as for trans-tibial and knee-disarticulated amputees) is folded in half and is inflated slightly. This is then pushed up inside the larger bag so that it touches the distal end of the residual limb.

4. The frame is eased up over the large bag and the patient holds it in place; the length is checked with the remaining leg (see Fig 6.4B).

5. The large bag is semi-inflated just enough so that it is held in position by the frame.

6. The amputee then stands up on the remaining leg, but is instructed *not* to bear weight yet through the Ppam aid. At this stage the therapist pulls the large bag up as high as possible anteriorly and posteriorly and adjusts the length of the frame (see Fig. 6.4C). The cruciate webbing straps may or may not be in a position to support

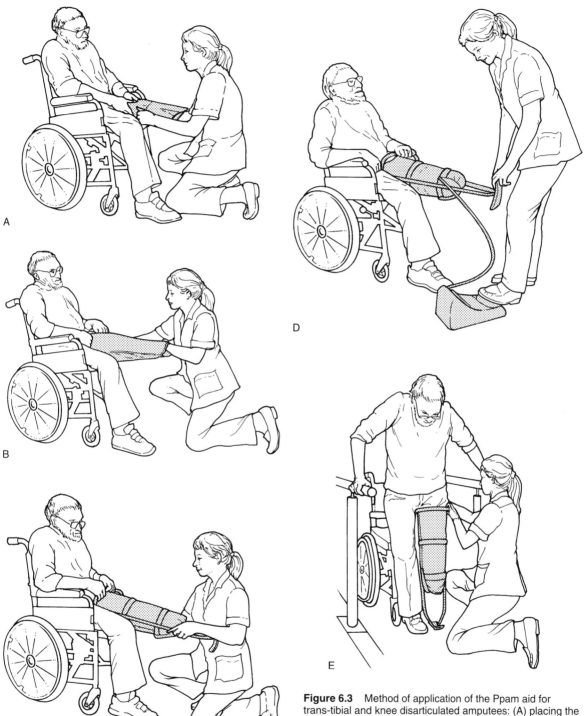

Figure 6.3 Method of application of the Ppam aid for trans-tibial and knee disarticulated amputees: (A) placing the small bag; (B) putting on the large bag (C) putting frame on; (D) inflating the bag; (E) Checking the fit.

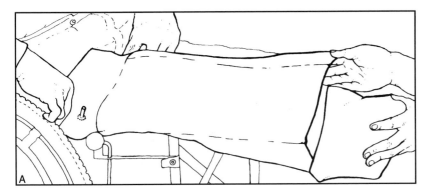

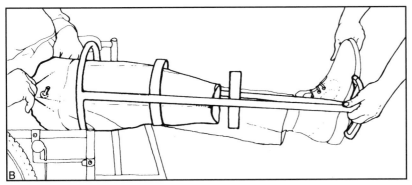

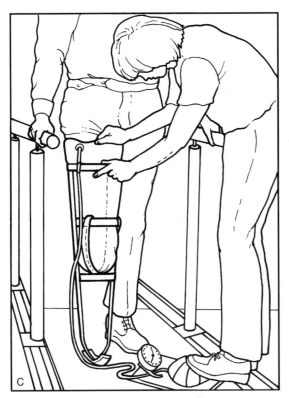

Figure 6.4 Method of application of the Ppam aid for the trans-femoral amputee: (A) with the large bag in place, the small one is pushed inside; (B) checking the length of the frame; (C) inflating the large bag while holding it as high as possible.

the bags, depending on the length of the residual limb.

7. The outer bag is then inflated to 40 mmHg pressure using the foot pump.

8. The shoulder strap gives added suspension, passing over the opposite shoulder to the amputated side.

Note: The position of the trans-femoral Ppam aid may need frequent adjustment during the treatment session.

Use of the Ppam aid

The following guidelines are offered for safe use of the Ppam aid.

1. The therapist must always inspect the residual limb and wound before, during and after using the Ppam aid.

2. For amputees whose wounds still contain sutures, show slow healing or for those with low Doppler readings, it is recommended that the Ppam aid is used only to aid standing briefly and possibly walking once the length of the parallel bars for the initial treatment sessions. For those whose wounds are healed but are still tender, it is recommended that for the first 2–3 days, the Ppam aid is not worn for more than 1 hour with frequent rest periods, during which time the bags are deflated and the residual limb is elevated.

For those whose residual limbs have healed satisfactorily with no signs of ischaemia, the treatment time can be increased up to 2 hours with less frequent rest periods. While the amputee is sitting down to rest between walking or standing periods, the large bag may be deflated to reduce constant pressure on the new wound and the Ppam aid should be elevated.

3. The condition of the wound must be checked daily under sterile conditions before and after treatment. Some oozing may have occurred or the dressing may have slipped and wound dressing will be required.

4. The elderly amputee should always remain in the parallel bars. The younger amputee with full strength in the upper limbs and good balance may progress from the parallel bars to walking with crutches. However, progression to stair climbing, steps and slopes is inadvisable as the Ppam aid is only a partial weightbearing device. The Ppam aid should never be used with walking sticks.

5. It is possible for bilateral amputees who have previously been successful unilateral amputees to use the Ppam aid, providing they are strong and can balance with their existing prosthesis. It may be necessary to reduce the length of the original prosthesis to lower the centre of gravity in order to assist balance and mobility.

Two Ppam aids should never be used on bilateral amputees because excessive pistoning occurs within the plastic bags and tissue breakdown can follow. Furthermore, the stability is insufficient for the amputee to use two Ppam aids.

Amputee mobility aid (AMA) (Fig. 6.5)

The AMA is a pneumatic temporary prosthesis similar to the Ppam aid. It is designed specifically for the trans-tibial amputee and allows the amputee to walk more naturally bending the knee during the gait cycle. It is manufactured in the UK by Vessa Limited.

The residual limb is supported by an inflatable plastic bag, which is sectioned to give selective inflation. It can be fitted 5–10 days postoperatively and, as with the Ppam aid, is a partial weightbearing device and should usually be used within the parallel bars. However, if an amputee has good balance, crutches can be used. Unlike the Ppam aid, there is a prosthetic foot, allowing the individual to wear their own shoe (see Fig. 6.6).

A disadvantage of the AMA is that high pressures are exerted on the residual limb, so care must be taken by dysvascular amputees, as with the Ppam aid.

The therapist must attend to the hygiene of the bags as for the Ppam aid.

Femurett (Fig. 6.7)

The Femurett is manufactured by LIC and provides greater stability than the Ppam aid for the trans-femoral amputee. The wound must be sufficiently healed to commence walking with a

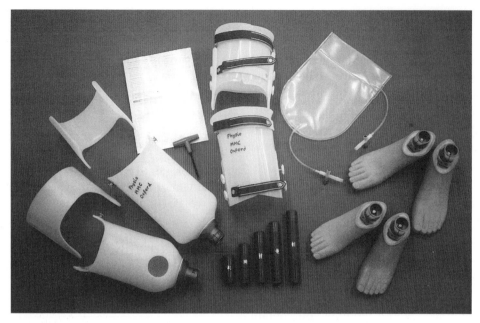

Figure 6.5 The components of the AMA showing the various sizes of component parts available. (Photograph by kind permission of the prosthetic physiotherapy service, Oxford.)

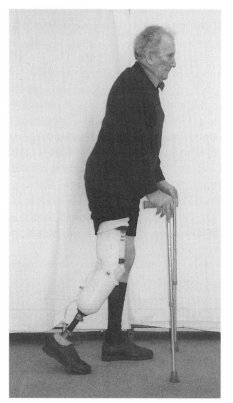

Figure 6.6 A trans-tibial amputee walking with the AMA. (Photography by kind permission of the prosthetic physiotherapy service, Oxford.)

rigid socket. There is an ischial seating area, firm lateral wall, basic knee mechanism and prosthetic foot. The socket comes in different sizes and can be easily adjusted to the individual. There is a basic alignment device, but care must be taken when making abduction/adduction adjustments that the nut does not become detached from the screw. The socket can be cleaned by wiping it with a cloth soaked in an appropriate cleaning solution.

Tulip Limb (Fig. 6.8)

The Tulip Limb is also manufactured by LIC and is a training device for trans-tibial amputees that can be used when the wound is sufficiently healed to tolerate a rigid interface. It consists of an inflatable sac and an outer rigid shell socket, with shank and prosthetic foot attached. As with the Ppam aid, the patient walks with a straight knee.

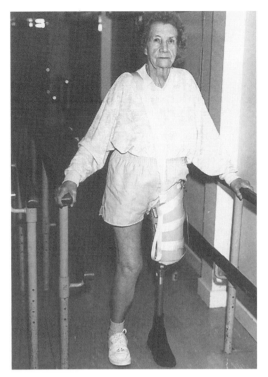

Figure 6.7 The Femurett. (Photograph by kind permission of Mrs M. Boultwood, LIC and Dr Morrison, Oxford DSC.)

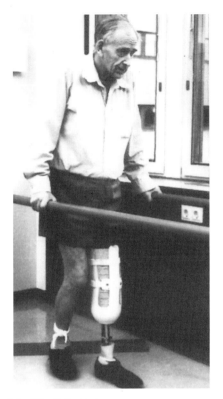

Figure 6.8 The Tulip Limb.

Above knee/below knee (AK/BK) temporary prosthesis

This temporary prosthesis for the trans-tibial amputee is custom made for an individual amputee by a prosthetist and is ischial weightbearing. A knee lock is present and the patient walks with a straight knee. Unlike the other early walking aids, which are for use in the therapy facility only, this prosthesis will be used by the amputee in their own home environment. It is only supplied for the following reasons:

- An unhealed residual limb, e.g. burns, skin grafts, open wounds, infection, dermatological conditions
- An unstable knee joint
- An excessively hypersensitive or painful residual limb
- Fractures of the femur or tibia of the affected side in the process of healing
- Knee flexion contracture more than 25°.

The advantage of this temporary prosthesis is that the amputee can be measured for it pre-operatively and therefore postoperative mobility is hastened. This prevents the complications resulting from a sedentary or bedfast existence and enables early discharge from hospital, even though healing is still in progress.

The disadvantages are that it is cosmetically very unacceptable and difficult to apply. The quadriceps muscle is inhibited and the knee joint immobilised.

Construction of the AK/BK temporary prosthesis (see Fig. 6.9)

Thigh corset. The thigh corset is a blocked leather, front-fastening thigh corset that partially supports the body weight; the principal weight transmission area is the ischial seating area on the posterior aspect of the corset.

Suspension. The two types of suspension used

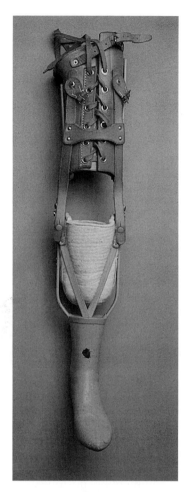

Figure 6.9   The above AK/BK temporary prosthesis.
(Photograph by kind permission of Richmond, Twickenham
and Roehampton Healthcare NHS Trust).

are either a rigid pelvic band with shoulder strap
or soft suspension.

Knee joint. The knee joint is a uniaxial joint
with a simple spring device that locks the prosthesis in extension. A manual release, either H-
strap or metal bar design, enables the amputee to
sit with a flexed knee.

Socket. The socket is made of soft felt with
a pad for distal tissue support. It is made sufficiently large to allow the residual limb to be
properly supported with either a bandage or
shrinker sock in order to prevent dependent
oedema. The felt socket protects the residual limb
as the amputee walks. No weight is transmitted

through this felt socket, which should merely
be regarded as a 'container'.

Base. The base can be either a uniaxial or
SACH foot (see Ch. 8)

Check of the AK/BK temporary prosthesis

The fit of the temporary prosthesis must be
checked by the therapist on the first attendance
for gait re-education and subsequently at regular
intervals. The amputee's skin must be checked
before and after each session.

Corset. With the amputee standing and suitably undressed, the therapist should check the
ischial seating and the adductor region in the
following ways:

The ischial seating is checked for correct weightbearing as described in Chapter 13. The leather
corset is checked for correct fastening.

If the ischium is not seated correctly the reason
may be that:

1. The corset is too large: this is determined
if the sides of the front opening are touching. To
remedy this, more stump socks can be added
to achieve a variety of thicknesses.
2. The corset is too small: this is determined if
the tongue of the leather is not covering the front
opening. To remedy this, the number of stump
socks and/or their thickness can be reduced.
It must be noted that the thigh corset must never
be tighter proximally than distally as this may
constrict circulation. If adjustments are needed,
the therapist should contact the prosthetist.

Adductor region. There should be no discomfort
in this area. Possible causes of discomfort may be
that:

1. The amputee is 'sinking' into the corset,
   which is probably a result of incorrect
   weightbearing on the ischium or incorrect
   fastening of the leather corset.
2. The stump sock is inadequately pulled up
   over the rim of the corset.
3. There is insufficient strength and function
   of the hip extensor muscles on the affected
   side, causing the amputee to flex at the hip
   and rub the skin area over the adductor

region. This can be a particularly common complaint by those wearing such a temporary prosthesis. If further adjustments are necessary the therapist should contact the prosthetist. The therapist should not be tempted to pad or cut down the adductor region of the socket, as this does not reduce the discomfort.

Length

Standing. The prosthesis may be about 2 cm shorter than the natural leg to allow hitch-through during swing phase. The method of checking the length is similar to that used for the trans-femoral prosthesis (see Ch. 13).
A common fault occurs when the amputee has fastened the residual limb either 'in' or 'out' of the corset, thus making the prosthesis either too long or too short.

Sitting. The amputee's knee should be free to flex to 90°. If the corset or the felt socket interferes with this action, the position of the residual limb within the socket should again be checked. The hinges of the prosthetic knee joint should lie about 1.5 cm above the knee joint line. (This is because the centre of rotation of the knee is situated near the centre of the medial femoral condyle). If the prosthesis is incorrectly positioned, the anterior aspect of the residual limb will knock against the felt socket when the patient is seated.

Felt socket. This should not constrict the residual limb: it is important to remember that the residual limb must be supported either by a bandage or a shrinker sock in this temporary prosthesis. There should be tissue support distally in the container. The restraining straps around the container prevent excessive flexion during walking.

If the patient complains of discomfort in this area the therapist should check that:

1. the socket is not too tight. Tightness may be a result of an oedematous residual limb or an excessive amount of dressing or bandage, which may be reduced.
2. the stump sock has not wrinkled within the socket and is causing constriction of the residual limb.

3. the prosthesis has been properly applied with the amputee's knee extended fully so that the residual limb becomes correctly positioned within the socket.

If adjustments are still needed then the therapist should contact the prosthetist.

Suspension. The method of checking the rigid pelvic band and shoulder strap is similar to that used for the trans-femoral prosthesis (see Ch. 13).

The soft suspension must be comfortable and the down straps from the belt to the socket must be firm when the patient is standing up. Very occasionally this temporary prosthesis is self-suspending, in which case the therapist should check that there is no excessive pistoning between the residual limb and the prosthesis during walking. This is best observed posteriorly with the amputee walking away from the therapist. If this occurs, the fastening on the corset should be checked to ensure that it is firm. On no account should the therapist or amputee tighten the corset so much that the residual limb becomes 'strangled', producing a tourniquet effect. This will damage the residual limb and prevent healing. If pistoning continues, auxiliary suspension is required and an appointment with the prosthetist must be made.

Knee lock. Before the amputee applies the prosthesis, the therapist should check the working of the knee lock mechanism to ensure that it locks and releases efficiently. The amputee should be observed operating the knee lock to ensure that the process is fully understood. With elderly people this may take several sessions to achieve.

Functional re-education with the AK/BK temporary prosthesis

Donning

1. The amputee should sit on a firm bed or chair, undressed apart from a vest.
2. The trans-tibial dressing/bandage/shrinker sock must be in place.
3. The sock must be pulled smoothly over the residual limb (see Fig. 6.10A). It may be difficult not to wrinkle the trans-tibial dressing.

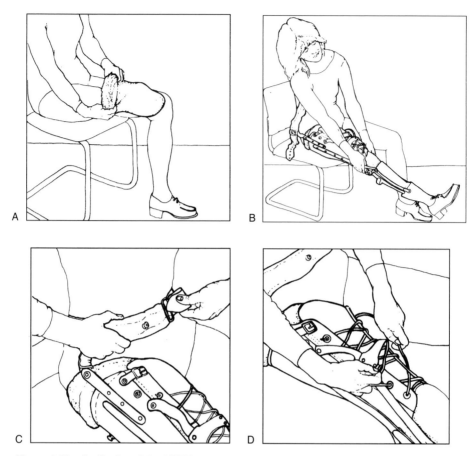

Figure 6.10 Application of the AK/BK temporary prosthesis.

4. With the prosthetic knee joint locked in full extension and the front fastening fully opened, the temporary prosthesis is eased up over the residual limb, which should fit into the felt socket and the prosthetic knee joint should be 1.5 cm above the knee joint line (see Fig. 6.10B).
5. If there is a rigid pelvic band this should now be fastened (see Fig. 6.10C).
6. The front of the leather socket should be fastened correctly (see Fig. 6.10D).
7. Any further auxiliary suspension should be fastened and adjusted when the amputee is standing.
8. The stump sock should be pulled up over the rim of the socket.

Doffing

1. The amputee should sit down on a firm surface.
2. The auxiliary suspension should be undone.
3. With the temporary prosthesis locked in extension, the front fastening of the leather socket should be undone completely and the residual limb eased out of the prosthesis. The natural knee joint must be maintained in full extension throughout this manoeuvre.
4. The stump sock should be pulled off.
5. The bandage or shrinker sock should be removed and the skin of the residual limb checked for any redness or rubbing; occasionally, the dressing over the wound

may need to be replaced after a period of gait re-education. The bandage or shrinker sock must be replaced.

6. The skin of the thigh should be checked for any areas of redness, rubbing or spots.

Dressing. The same method is used as for the trans-femoral prosthesis (see Ch. 13). The trouser leg width nearly always has to be widened, as the prosthetic knee and felt socket are very bulky.

Toilet. The same points apply for this prosthesis as for the trans-femoral prosthesis.

Gait re-education. As there is a long lever controlling the prosthesis, there is often a tendency to take too long a stride and to circumduct during the swing phase, instead of hip hitching. The same method of gait re-education is taught as for the trans-femoral prosthesis (see Ch. 13). The knee joint must be mobilised and the quadriceps and hamstring muscles strengthened with an exercise programme while this temporary locked knee prosthesis is being used, otherwise transition later on to a free knee prosthesis, e.g. a patellar tendon weightbearing prosthesis, will be very difficult.

BIBLIOGRAPHY FOR PREVIOUS EDITIONS

Abel E W, Frank T G 1991 The design of attendant propelled wheelchairs. Prosthetics and Orthotics International 15(1):38–45

Alexander A 1971 Immediate postsurgical prosthetic fitting: the role of the physical therapist. Physical Therapy 51(2):152–157

Bonner F J, Green R F 1982 Pneumatic airleg prosthesis: report of 200 cases. Archives of Physical Medicine and Rehabilitation 63:383–385

Booker H, Smith S 1988 The AK/BK revisited. Physiotherapy 74(8):366–368

Burgess E M, Zettl J H 1969 Immediate application of prostheses for amputations. In: Cooper P (ed) Surgery annual. Appleton-Century-Crofts Educational Division. Meredith Corporation, p 371–390

Dickstein R, Pillar T, Mannheim M 1982 The pneumatic post-amputation mobility aid in geriatric rehabilitation. Scandinavian Journal of Rehabilitation Medicine 14:149–150

Donn J 1991 Use of the TES Belt as an alternative means of suspension with the Ppam Aid. Physiotherapy 77(9):591–592

Liedberg E, Hommerberg H, Persson B M 1983 Tolerance of early walking with total contact among below-knee amputees – a randomized test. Prosthetics and Orthotics International 7:91–95

Little J M 1971 A pneumatic weight-bearing temporary prosthesis for below-knee amputees. Lancet 6 Feb:271–273

McLaurin C A, Brubaker C E 1991 Biomechanics and the wheelchair. Prosthetics and Orthotics International 15(1):24–37

Monga T N, Symington D C 1984 The airsplint as a pneumatic prosthesis in management of the elderly amputee. Physiotherapy Canada 36(2):61–65

Parry M, Morrison J D 1989 Use of the Femurett adjustable prosthesis in the assessment and walking training of new above-knee amputees. Prosthetics and Orthotics International 13:36–38

Ramsey E M 1988 A clinical evaluation of the LIC Femurett as an early training device for the primary above-knee amputee. Physiotherapy 74(12):598–601

Redhead R G, Davis B C, Robinson K P, Vitali M 1978 Post-amputation pneumatic walking aid. British Journal of Surgery 65(9):611–612

Van Ross E 1991 Pushchairs. Prosthetics and Orthotics International 15(1):46–50

BIBLIOGRAPHY FOR THE THIRD EDITION

Bumfrey E 1995 Out and about: solving problems of mobility. In: Community practice. Prentice Hall, London, ch 12

Burgess E M 1997 Guest editorial. Wound healing and tissue repair of the surgical amputation of limbs. Journal of Rehabiltation Research and Development 34(1):vii–ix

Flanagan M 1993 Pressure sore risk assessment scales: an introduction to the main risk assessment tools available to practitioners today. Journal of Wound Care 2(3):162–167

Norton D, McLaren R, Exton-Smith A N 1962 (reissue 1975) In: An investigation of geriatric nursing problems in hospital. Churchill Livingstone, Edinburgh

Ozyalcin H, Sesli E 1989 Temporary prosthetic fitting for below-knee amputation. Prosthetics and Orthotics International 13:86–89

Scott H, Condie E, Nicol S, Treweek S 1997 An evaluation of the Amputee Mobility Aid (AMA): an early walking aid for trans-tibial amputees. National Centre for Training and Education in Prosthetics and Orthotics, Strathclyde

Waterlow J 1985 A risk assessment card. Nursing Times 81:49–55

7

Assessment for lower limb prosthetic rehabilitation

PRIMARY AMPUTEE

There are different reasons why a primary amputee may be referred to the local prosthetic service:

1. For consultation as to the amputee's suitability and readiness for prosthetic rehabilitation. This is the most common reason for referral.

2. For the amputee to have an opportunity to see prostheses and, by meeting other amputees, to fully understand the implications of learning to use a prosthesis. This is most useful for amputees from hospitals where few amputations are performed.

3. For cast and measurement, fitting and subsequent delivery of the prosthesis.

Not every amputee referred to the prosthetic rehabilitation service will be fitted with a prosthesis. If the amputee is not accepted for prosthetic rehabilitation at the first visit, it must be remembered that this decision can be altered at a later date.

Early referral to the service is needed for amputees making an uneventful recovery from surgery. Referral can be made before removal of the sutures. Delay in referral causes an unnecessary postponement of the delivery of the prosthesis.

Later referral to the service is more advisable for the frail and for those with numerous medical complications or multiple physical problems and after a recommendation from the service outreach team who have assessed the individual in hospital. The amputee must be sufficiently fit to endure an ambulance journey to the centre, the somewhat exhausting day seeing unfamiliar faces and the journey home. Frail amputees must be able to cope with a full day's rehabilitation programme in hospital.

FACTORS INFLUENCING THE DECISION FOR REFERRAL

1. Does the amputee want to walk?

Does the amputee fully understand the procedures involved and the amount of personal effort required in prosthetic rehabilitation? If so, then referral must be made.

2. Will it be possible for the amputee to walk?

In assessing the amputee's potential for prosthetic mobility, the therapist has the following guidelines.
   The amputee must:

- Be independent transferring
- Be independent dressing
- Have sufficient manual dexterity to manage buckles and buttons
- Have adequate eyesight (blindness alone is not a contraindication)
- Be able to understand and remember instructions
- Have adequate oxygen perfusion for the increased energy consumption needed for walking with a prosthesis (see Ch. 9).

If amputees are unable to demonstrate these basic abilities it is unlikely that they will benefit from prosthetic rehabilitation.

3. Where will the amputee walk – who will help?

The amputee's accommodation and the help available must be considered. An early home visit may help to ensure that a realistic rehabilitation goal is set, whether this entails supply of a prosthesis, crutches or wheelchair; the visit will also establish whether relatives, carers, friends or neighbours are willing to give ongoing encouragement and support. Bilateral amputees must have sufficient room to walk with aids around furniture in their home.

It has been found that amputees who live in sheltered accommodation or continuing care facilities are most unlikely to use prostheses even if they are supplied, as mobility is safer and faster in a wheelchair.

Younger homeless people will find hostel accommodation easier if they are independent walking, even if the method used is unconventional.

4. Will prosthetic rehabilitation improve the amputee's quality of life?

Quality of life is an individual measure and varies with an individual at different stages of their development and life. Therefore the referring team must have had sufficient in-depth dialogue with the individual and their carers before making any judgement about this.

Visiting the prosthetic service will empower the individual to make their own judgement. The distance to travel to the service and the time needed to achieve prosthetic rehabilitation success must be weighed up with other things the individual wishes to do with their time and their remaining years.

For patients suffering from progressive disease, the stage of the disease must be identified and the prognosis considered in depth. Prosthetic rehabilitation can be a lengthy, tiring procedure and the overall benefits of the eventual outcome must be considered. For some, employment may rank above the need for prosthetic mobility. Bilateral amputees must consider this aspect very carefully (see Ch. 17).

PROCEDURE OF ASSESSMENT

Written referral is made to the prosthetic rehabilitation service, for whom the hospital notes must be available.

There are now local arrangements throughout the UK for prosthetic referral, which take different forms.

To a regional specialist prosthetic service

The amputee travels from the hospital to the centre and is examined by the primary referral team. This team can consist of the following:

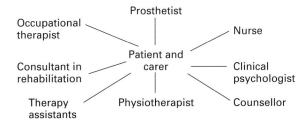

In addition, a medical geneticist should be available for the parents of children with congenital deficiency. Access to a specialist orthopaedic surgeon may also be necessary.

The carer can be either a relative, or a member of staff who has been caring for the amputee, or both. Written assessments from the hospital's nurse, therapists, and social worker must be taken along at the first visit.

A summary of the assessment and decision made is returned with the patient so that the hospital team remains fully informed.

To a satellite prosthetic clinic within the local district

A doctor and prosthetist can visit locally from the regional prosthetic centre, to see all amputees referred from the locality. There is a consulting room and workshop facility permanently available. The hospital team are therefore in closer contact and the service is integral to the total care in the district. This type of service improves the access for amputees and avoids lengthy tiring journeys, and greater continuity of care can be achieved.

Visiting team to the hospital

In some areas there are arrangements whereby a rehabilitation consultant can visit a patient in their hospital ward. This is particularly useful pre-operatively, when the patient may be very sick or infectious, and when an expert opinion on the level of amputation is needed.

Whatever local arrangement is in place, successful referral and rehabilitation will only occur if there is good communication between all involved. The hospital therapist should make

every effort to meet all the team members in order to facilitate subsequent telephone or written communication.

PROSTHETIC CONSIDERATIONS OF THE VARIOUS LEVELS OF AMPUTATION

Trans-tibial amputees

Almost all amputees with trans-tibial amputation can be successfully rehabilitated. Many of these amputees can manage without walking aids eventually, and should achieve a normal gait pattern. Age alone is not a contraindication (see Ch. 15).

Knee disarticulation and trans-femoral amputees

Lack of the natural knee joint requires complex prosthetic replacement that cannot totally replace the natural knee function. Therefore the gait can be slow, and there is a high energy consumption. Younger and fitter amputees should walk well without aids (see Chs 13 and 14).

Hindquarter and hip disarticulation

The majority of these amputees are young and have normal musculature and balance. Despite the presenting pathology, they are usually able to manage the large, complicated prosthesis, coping with prosthetic hip and knee joints. A few will require a walking aid (see Ch. 12).

Bilateral amputees

All these amputees must have their accommodation made suitable for wheelchair mobility before referral to the prosthetic centre.

All bilateral amputees must understand that prosthetic rehabilitation takes a long time and occurs in stages; great motivation and determination are essential. Most bilateral amputees will walk with two walking aids, and the hands are therefore not free to carry anything. This limits function.

Energy expenditure both for application of prostheses and walking is enormous (See Ch. 9) and above average upper limb strength must be present. Amputees must be able to lift their body weight using push-up blocks (see Fig. 5.2, p. 60) and much will depend upon their build and weight.

The presence of knee joints is a vital consideration, as illustrated in the following:

1. The majority of bilateral trans-tibial amputees will manage prostheses.

2. If there is only one knee joint present and the contralateral side shows no fixed hip flexion contracture, then prosthetic rehabilitation is possible.

3. Where no natural knee joints remain, prosthetic use is difficult, particularly if there are fixed hip flexion contractures, and if the amputee is obese. For this group of amputees, the wheelchair will be their main means of mobility.

Bilateral trans-femoral amputees who are not

suitable for prosthetic rehabilitation can be supplied with cosmetic prostheses, which are for wheelchair use only (see Fig. 7.1). These are of great psychological benefit to both the amputee and relatives as the complete body image is maintained. Some amputees and therapists, unaware of this option, may strive towards functional prostheses solely for the cosmetic benefit and not for mobility (Ch. 17).

Upper and lower limb combination

If there is one upper limb and one lower limb amputation present, the lower limb prosthesis is usually fitted first and the amputee taught to walk. Exercise to the upper residual limb and general postural correction take place while the lower limb prosthesis is being fitted and delivered. The upper limb prosthesis is supplied afterwards.

If there is one upper limb and bilateral lower

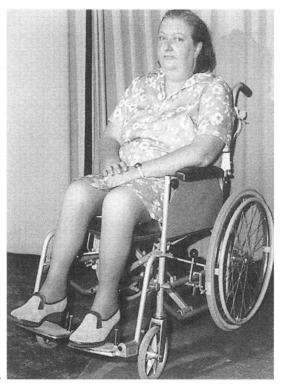
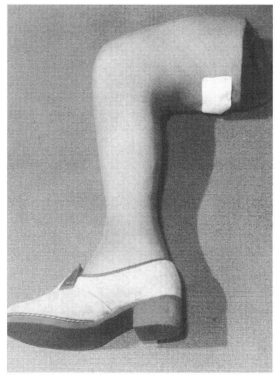

A

B

Figure 7.1 Cosmetic prostheses: (A) a bilateral trans-femoral amputee wearing cosmetic prostheses; (B) a cosmetic prosthesis with Velcro fastening for attachment to the wheelchair seat.

limb amputations, it is usual for the upper limb prosthesis to be fitted first. Functional activities from the wheelchair are then achieved. Lower limb exercises and balance training continue while this is taking place and the prostheses for the lower limbs are supplied subsequently.

All these individuals face a complicated prosthetic future and it is very important that they are referred to a prosthetic centre where there are full prosthetic and rehabilitation facilities (See Ch. 21).

PROSTHETIC CONSIDERATIONS WITH PRESENTING PATHOLOGY AND AGE OF THE AMPUTEE

(See Chs 1 & 2).

DECISION MAKING BETWEEN THE SPECIALIST TEAM AND THE PRIMARY AMPUTEE

After the assessment, the team will base the decision as to whether or not to supply a prosthesis on the balance of probable successful outcome when considering the parameters of pathologies present, level of amputation, length and condition of the residual limb, the amputee's home environment and individual wishes.

At this stage some amputees have to face the challenge of *not* becoming a limb wearer. This can be particularly traumatic if the amputee has been told, or has assumed throughout the process of their amputation that they will be given a prosthesis. While this situation is sometimes unavoidable, it is helpful to provide as much information as possible about their likely outcome from as early on as possible. This helps them to adjust gradually. This process is clearly facilitated where the surgeon has contact with the prosthetic rehabilitation team and can provide realistic outcome information. In a prosthetic centre, where new amputees may have watched others progress before them, it may be important to explain differences in situations that can affect outcome. New amputees will sometimes identify with established amputees (particularly with the same level of amputation, or of the same age or sex) and become disappointed when their own progress is not as rapid. Follow-up visits can be arranged for amputees where prosthetic rehabilitation is not at first considered viable.

If prosthetic rehabilitation *is* a viable option, the next consideration is the prescription of the first prosthesis. Amputees may experience considerable disappointment at this stage of their rehabilitation as the difference between reality and their expectations become clear. Having harboured hopes of 'bionic limbs', there may be transient distress or depression as they adjust to the feel of a new limb and its function. Component parts giving very similar function can vary widely in their price range; therefore in some places, a multidisciplinary approach to this has been to set a certain prosthetic prescription for amputees with a lower predicted mobility grade outcome. Care should also be taken to explain the attention to cosmesis, which occurs later in the process, in order to avoid unnecessary alarm.

FOLLOW-UP

Primary amputee

It is important that primary amputees are monitored at home following discharge from hospital. The community therapist, physical disability teams, district nurse and GP are in the best position to carry this out. Feedback from these professionals to the prosthetic centre doctor is essential and welcomed. Many small problems can occur in the first few weeks, such as alteration in residual limb volume, inability to operate joint mechanisms, uncertainty regarding social services or benefits, uncertainty as to how to increase and progress activity, and natural anxieties or depression that can occur after leaving a supportive environment. Very often these small issues, if not picked up quickly, can lead to lack of use of the prosthesis.

As the months go by, the need for retraining in domestic or leisure activities should be assessed, and the prosthetic prescription will need to be reviewed. When amputees have contacted self-help groups and/or sports or leisure organisations, they may have identified new areas of interest and need in their lives.

Fitting problems

Some individuals who are having difficulty adjusting to the psychological impact of their amputation may manifest this in presenting with fitting problems. Identification of this and redirecting the amputee toward the psychologist or counsellor can be more helpful for them and avoids wasted time with the prosthetist. However, some people who are psychologically disturbed may also have genuine fitting problems and these should not be overlooked.

Established amputee

Follow-up assessments may reveal that:

1. The amputee's needs may have altered due to an improvement in their physical abilities. Those who have become more active will need a reassessment of their prosthetic components as they now will gain the benefit from more sophisticated equipment. They may have found new avenues in their life, e.g. sporting activities, which require specialised prostheses (see Ch. 18).

The prosthetic manufacturers introduce new and improved components each year and the established amputee will need to keep abreast of items of benefit to their individual situation (see Ch. 22).

2. The amputee's needs may have altered due to a deterioration, e.g. change in body weight, loss of other leg or other physical deterioration such as concurrent pathology or a change in home environment. To actively manage a downward spiral of functional activity, reassessment of the prosthetic components may be required to ensure safety, stability and the ability to apply the prosthesis independently. A therapy reassessment will identify a need for a top-up therapeutic programme or the provision of additional aids and appliances.

3. The amputee may need to give up using

prostheses and therefore require help in achieving other forms of mobility for an independent and fulfilling lifestyle.

OTHER FORMS OF MOBILITY

Wheelchair (see Ch. 6)

It is likely that the amputee has already been supplied with a wheelchair, but if it was thought that the chair would only be used occasionally and that most of the time the amputee would walk, then reassessment must take place if prostheses are no longer the main method of achieving mobility.

Hopping

Hopping may have to be explored in combination with the wheelchair as some rooms may be inaccessible with the chair and structural alterations inadvisable or impossible (see Ch. 6).

Occasionally, hopping may be considered to be faster and easier than using a prosthesis, particularly for those with a painful residual limb or high level of amputation.

Walking directly on weightbearing residual limbs

The Symes and knee disarticulation amputees are ideal candidates for walking directly on weight-bearing residual limbs. Some form of residual limb cover should be supplied. Some trans-tibial amputees may walk around on their hands and knees, but care with the viability of the tissues of the residual limbs must be considered.

Other ideas

Occasionally the therapist must devise another system of mobility. It may be necessary to find a specialist disability service, where the therapists along with rehabilitation engineers and electronics experts can devises a solution to an individual mobility issue.

BIBLIOGRAPHY FOR PREVIOUS EDITIONS

Buttenshaw P J 1991 The multidisciplinary team approach for the assessment of primary amputees. Personal communication

Chilvers A S, Browse N L 1971 The social fate of the amputee. Lancet 27 Nov: 1192–1193, 1315–1316

Doherty S M, Nichols P J R 1974 Non-prosthetic problems of rehabilitation of the ischaemic lower limb amputee. Orthopaedics 7(2):77–85

Hamilton A 1981 Rehabilitation of the leg amputee in the community. Journal of Postgraduate Medicine 225:1487–1497

Hamilton A, Williams E, Nichols P J R 1974 The elderly lower limb amputee. Update 9:1641–1650

Hamilton E A, Nichols P J R 1972 Rehabilitation of the elderly lower-limb amputee. British Medical Journal 2:95–99

Hanspal R S, Fisher K 1991 Assessment of cognitive and psychomotor function and rehabilitation of elderly people with prostheses. British Medical Journal 302:940

Holden J M, Fernie G R 1987 Extent of artificial limb use following rehabilitation. Journal of Orthopaedic Research 5:562–568

Hubbard W A 1989 Rehabilitation outcomes for elderly lower limb amputees. Australian Journal of Physiotherapy 35(4): 219–224

Jain S K 1988 Rehabilitation of elderly amputees. Armed Forces Medical Journal India 44(1):15–20

Kay J 1991 Domiciliary rehabilitation of elderly amputees. Physiotherapy 77(1):60–61

Narang I C, Mathur B P, Singh P, Jape V S 1984 Functional capabilities of lower limb amputees. Prosthetics and Orthotics International 8:43–51

Parish J G, James D W 1982 A method for evaluating the level of independence during the rehabilitation of the disabled. Rheumatology and Rehabilitation 21: 107–114

Siriwardena G J A, Bertrand P V 1991 Factors influencing rehabilitation of arteriosclerotic lower limb amputees. Journal of Rehabilitation Research and Development 28(3):35–44

BIBLIOGRAPHY FOR THE THIRD EDITION

Anderson S P 1995 Dysvascular amputees: what can we expect? Journal of Prosthetics and Orthotics 7(2):43–50

Andrews K 1996 Rehabilitation in limb deficiency. 3. The geriatric amputee. Archives of Physical Medicine and Rehabilitation 77:S14–S17

Chakrabarty B K 1995 Lower limb amputation: striking the balance. Annals of the Royal College of Surgeons 77(2):157–158

Christensen B, Ellegaard B, Bretler U, Østrup E-L 1995 The effect of prosthetic rehabilitation in lower limb amputees. Prosthetics and Orthotics International 19:46–52

Cutson T M, Bongiorni D R 1996 Rehabilitation of the older lower limb amputee: a brief review. Journal of the American Geriatrics Society 44(11):1388–1393

Esquenazi A, Meier R H III 1996 Rehabilitation in limb deficiency. 4. Limb amputation. Archives of Physical Medicine and Rehabilitation 77:S18–S28

Gauthier-Gagnon C, Grise M-C, Potvin D 1995 The use of the prosthesis by the lower extremity amputee: a follow-up study of enabling factors. Proceedings of the 12th International Congress of the World Confederation for Physical Therapy, Washington

Greive A C, Lankhorst G J 1996 Functional outcome of lower-limb amputees: a prospective descriptive study in a general hospital. Prosthetics and Orthotics International 20:79–87

Ham R, de Trafford J, Van de Ven C 1994 Patterns of recovery for lower limb amputation. Clinical Rehabilitation 8:320–328

Jones L, Hall M, Schuld W 1993 Ability or disability? A study of the functional outcome of 65 consecutive lower limb amputees treated at the Royal South Sydney Hospital in 1988–1989. Disability and Rehabilitation 15(4):184–188

Leung E C-C, Rush P J, Devlin M 1996 Predicting prosthetic rehabilitation outcome in lower limb amputee patients with the functional independence measure. Archives of Physical Medicine and Rehabilitation 77:605–608

McCollum P T, Stonebridge P A, Holdsworth R J, Jain A 1995 Rehabilitation outcome 5 years after 100 lower limb amputations. British Journal of Surgery 82:567–568

Pederson P, Damholt V 1994 Rehabilitation after amputation following lower limb fracture. The Journal of Trauma 36(2):195–197

Pernot H F M, de Witte L P, Lindeman E, Cluitmans J 1997 Daily functioning of the lower extremity amputee: an overview of the literature. Clinical Rehabilitation 11:93–106

Pohjolarnen T, Alaranta H, Kärkkäinen M 1990 Prosthetic use and functional and social outcome following major lower limb amputation. Prosthetics and Orthotics International 14(2):75–79

Rommers G M, Vos L D W, Groothoff J W, Eisma W H 1996 Clinical rehabilitation of the amputee: a retrospective study. Prosthetics and Orthotics International 20:72–78

Sapp L, Little C E 1995 Functional outcomes in a lower limb amputee population. Prosthetics and Orthotics International 19:92–96

Subbarao K V, Bajoria S 1995 The effect of stump length on the rehabilitation outcome in unilateral below-knee amputees for vascular disease. Clinical Rehabilitation 9:327–330

8

Prosthetic services

The therapist working with amputees in either an acute, community or specialist service, needs to understand the inter-relationship between prosthetic provision, service funding, facilities and rehabilitation in their locality, and the need to provide a service that is good value for money.

While therapists are not expected to know every technical detail of prosthetic components, they need to understand biomechanics as applied to prosthetics; they are responsible for being aware of the technology available and for managing that technology. In order to achieve the optimal prosthetic care for their patients, they must work closely with the prosthetist at all stages in the amputee's rehabilitation. All manufacturers have written information about their components and other supplies, e.g. liners, sleeves and socks – therapists are advised to obtain these for reference concerning use. Components may be unavailable in a local facility, but available elsewhere in the market in that country. If the function of the amputee is limited by the available components, the therapist may investigate and enquire elsewhere and bring the information back to the multidisciplinary team for discussion as to whether supply is indicated and economically possible. Networking, within professional organisations, with centres of excellence and with individuals known to be expert in their field, is the recommended way of going about this. Alternatively, it is possible to approach the manufacturing companies directly (see Appendix 1 for addresses). Therapists must also realise that new developments in technology move faster than the ability of providers to supply them to the amputee, which often needs to be explained to the amputee.

The therapist (together with the prosthetist) will also need to act as the amputee's advocate to ensure their individual needs are met, ranging from a high level of sophisticated hardware to the simplest of prosthetic devices. Attitudes toward amputees in any country relate to the culture and social structure and there may be differences within different regions of a single country. In 1992, Poonekar listed prevailing factors that affect prosthetics and orthotics in India; these factors could also apply to much of the rest of the world:

- economic factors
- social factors
- cultural factors
- climatic factors
- locally available forms of technology
- time and distance constraints
- psychological factors
- materials and resources
- religious factors
- appropriate technology.

SERVICE FRAMEWORK

The United Kingdom

England, Wales and Northern Ireland

The local health authority has responsibility for purchasing all aspects of healthcare for their residents. They contract with 37 local health trusts (in 1998), across the regions that subcontract the prosthetic and technical elements of the service to a specialist company, with support from the NHS Supplies Authority. There are a variety of types of contract: some last for 3 years, others for longer; some include orthotic services with prosthetics, others do not. All contracts have quality measures against which they will be assessed. In recent years there has been more flexibility in the contracts, but each one is agreed individually. The contract covers services for the primary amputee, repairs and ongoing prosthetic supply and, in some cases, research and development. Healthcare providers may need to prioritise the

supply and availability of the variety of components in order to maximise the distribution within their budget.

Scotland

The local Health Boards purchase in a similar manner from five provider trusts (in 1998), supported by Scottish Healthcare Supplies. Commodity advisory panels, which include in their membership, representatives from all the provider trusts, provide guidance to Scottish Healthcare Supplies regarding the content and terms of these contracts.

Private supply

Some prosthetic companies have private service facilities either for private patients or for charities that are buying a particular prosthetic device for an individual amputee. It is advisable that the therapist seeks the best possible service and treatment for the individual amputee who chooses private supply, ensuring the correct balance between comfort, function and cosmesis; for this to occur, both the therapist and prosthetist must work together. In the UK, the majority of private supply orders are for overseas amputees; however there is a small but increasing demand from amputees requiring sophisticated or specialist activity prostheses that may not be available on the local contract. The amputee must be aware that, when using private facilities, ongoing maintenance will also have to be paid for privately.

Standards

The Medical Devices Directorate of the NHS Executive has the monitoring function for prosthetic manufacturing standards for the whole of the UK. All components placed on the market or assembled in the UK must be CE marked, a European Economic Community (EEC) standard, and comply with international standards, e.g. ISO 10328, an international structural testing standard for lower limb prostheses. Internationally, there is similar legislation to ensure patient safety.

Reciprocal arrangements

UK national amputees can attend any prosthetic service in the UK for emergency repairs if required.

Amputees from the EEC and some overseas countries can also attend these services as an emergency (as laid out in FDL(94)33); other overseas nationals must pay for help received.

Services to developing countries

Therapists and prosthetists trained in the developed countries may at some time in their career go to a developing country to help establish local prosthetic services. This work may be funded by organisations such as the United Nations High Commission for Refugees (UNHCR) or the International Committee of the Red Cross/Red Crescent (ICRC). In developing countries, enormous demand confronts a chronic lack of resources and trained personnel. In many cases, the intervention of a non-governmental organisation (NGO) provides the best possibility of initiating a prosthetic service but the development of national programmes and governmental support of NGO activities is essential to the achievement of long-term objectives.

The single most important issue facing the developing world is 'appropriate technology', previously a term sometimes used to describe primative or crude technology, when it should mean the application of the best that can be done with the resources of equipment, staff, materials and finance available. When applied to prosthetics, the technology must satisfy accepted biomechanical and functional principles, and this implies that the practitioners must be trained to a satisfactory level.

It is important that staff understand the parameters of the service offered, in the same way as in their own country. The present philosophy is to set up prosthetic facilities to be run and organised by the local population – a development model more than an emergency assistance model. This involves an extensive teaching commitment and an appreciation of the appropriate prosthetic techniques and cultural differences for the particular country, so adequate preparation before travelling abroad is necessary. The International Society for Prosthetics and Orthotics (ISPO) has developed workshops in some countries and a twinning system between a developed and a developing nation.

PROSTHETIC CONSTRUCTION

There are two distinct and comprehensive prosthetic systems: endoskeletal and exoskeletal.

Endoskeletal (modular prostheses)

Endoskeletal prostheses use the human skeleton as the model; a tube frame provides the weight-bearing function and a foam cover gives the prosthesis its near-natural appearance. The modular design incorporates a variety of joint components to suit the needs of the individual amputee, and changes may be generally achieved in a day's visit to the prosthetist (see Fig. 8.1).

Exoskeletal (conventional or crustacean prostheses)

The exoskeletal prostheses have a rigid outside shell as the supporting structure. They are generally less sophisticated and more difficult to adjust than the endoskeletal systems. In addition, many of the components available in endoskeletal limbs cannot be housed within their construction, and change of prescription cannot be achieved quickly. However, they are generally more durable (at the cost of function) and are useful for the developing countries as they are both simple and have a sturdy construction. Prior to the 1960s, these were the only type of prosthesis available and thus there may be some older, experienced amputees who are unable or unwilling to try other types of prostheses, so prosthetic services must be able to supply these if needed (see Fig. 8.2). Functional upper limb prostheses continue to be of this construction as are beach activity prostheses for lower limb amputees.

Most prostheses have common features as listed in Box 8.1

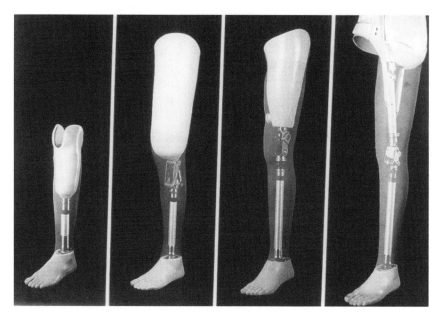

Figure 8.1 Endoskeletal prostheses. From left to right, for trans-tibial, knee disarticulation, trans-femoral and hip disarticulation levels of amputation. (Photograph by kind permission of Otto Bock UK Ltd.)

Box 8.1 Components of Prostheses
1. A prosthetic socket 2. Auxiliary suspension 3. Prosthetic joints 4. Inter-joint segments 5. For the lower limb, a base (foot) to contact the floor 6. For the upper limb, a hand or other terminal device 7. Cosmetic covering

Selecting the most appropriate components for prosthetic restoration is a challenging task due to the variety and complexity of prosthetic components and materials available, socket fabrication techniques and different suspension methods. Ideally this should be carried out by an expert multidisciplinary team working closely with the amputee.

Kristinsson observes 'there are conceptually different aspects to the quality of prosthetic fittings. First, there is the quality of the available components and materials, i.e. tools, database and the craftsmanship necessary to put them together as a functional unit. Second, there are the latest methods of fitting a socket and the involved prosthetist's skill'.

Note: Further detail of prosthetic construction can be found in the relevant chapters describing the levels of amputation (Chs 11–19).

Prosthetic socket

The socket is a critical element of a successful prosthesis. A good socket has the following characteristics:

- comfort for the amputee
- provision of an interface between the residual limb and the prosthesis, transferring load and energy
- maintenance of suspension for the prosthesis.

The contours of the socket should produce a comfortable and functional connection between the residual limb and the prosthesis. For details of specific sockets for each level of amputation, refer to Chapters 12–16 and Chapter 19.

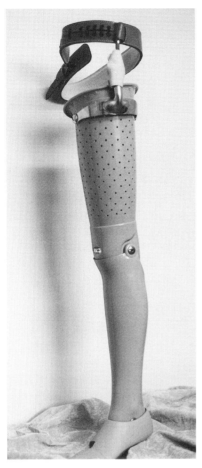

Figure 8.2   An exoskeletal prosthesis, for the trans-femoral amputee showing a double swivel rigid pelvic band auxiliary suspension. (Photograph by kind permission of Vessa Ltd.)

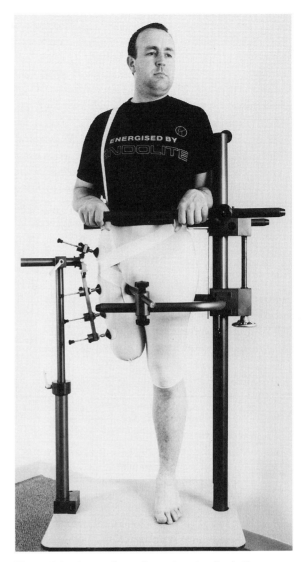

Figure 8.3   A trans-femoral amputee standing in the Endocast casting system. (Photograph by kind permission of CA Blatchford and Sons Ltd.)

Making the prosthetic socket

This is a skilled procedure carried out by the prosthetist. A negative plaster cast of the amputee's residual limb is usually taken, using either a wrap or pressure cast technique, or occasionally circumferential measurements are taken at regular intervals along the length of the residual limb. The more distal the amputation, the more choice of casting positions, e.g. lying, sitting or standing; however, for the higher levels, casting is generally done with the amputee standing (see Fig. 8.3). The negative cast is filled with liquid plaster to form a positive, which can then be modified (rectified) to suit the amputee's requirements. Reduction rectification increases the weightbearing on the pressure-tolerant areas and building up rectification decreases weightbearing on pressure-sensitive areas. Negative or positive casts can be digitised and modification (rectification) effected on a computer prior to socket manufacture (see CAD-CAM, page 109).

Shape

There is standard terminology referring to socket shape for all standard levels of amputation (as in Figs 1.1 and 1.2) but for each level there are several different shapes and variations. In all cases, the shapes are designed to relieve pressure-sensitive areas, increase contact for pressure-tolerant areas, to control rotation and to provide different levels of suspension. Some socket shapes offer total suspension, i.e. supracondylar (held on by the bony anatomical contours of the residual limb) and some shapes offer partial suspension and therefore require auxilliary suspension.

Suspension

Suspension is a key factor in prosthetic design; good suspension through the socket enhances efficient energy transfer, maximises control and minimises discomfort and abrasions. The total contact socket is one in which the area over which the force is applied is maximised. The advantages of this type of socket are:

- reduction in pressure on any localised part of the residual limb
- prevention of oedema by aiding venous return
- improved sensory feedback (some amputees have reported that the prosthesis 'feels lighter and more a part of them').

Not all residual limbs can take total suspension from the socket and will therefore need auxiliary suspension.

Materials used

Plastic. 80% of sockets are made of plastic and there are different types:

1. thermoplastic, normally draped to form sockets, a method using polypropylene plastic sheets of uniform thickness. Production time is quick. Some thermoplastics are flexible and transparent, e.g. Surlyn; the resulting sockets are flexible and change shape readily. They are needed where there is potential for excessive pressure. They are supported in a rigid frame connected to

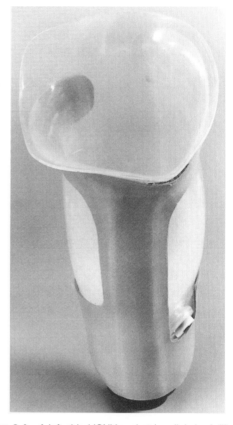

Figure 8.4 A left-sided ISNY socket (medial view). The carbon fibre reinforced medial strut carries the load, and the flexible inner liner is supported on two wings from the top of the strut. (Photograph by kind permission of C A Blatchford & Sons Ltd.)

the rest of the prosthesis, e.g. an ISNY frame for the trans-femoral amputee (see Fig. 8.4).

2. thermosetting, normally referred to as 'laminated' sockets, a method of using thermosetting resins in conjunction with reinforcing materials, e.g. glass fibre, carbon fibre, nylon, etc. These can be made to suit individual requirements.

Metal. Used mainly for exoskeletal prostheses in the UK.

Wood. Used mainly for exoskeletal prostheses worldwide.

Leather. Used for some sockets in conventional trans-tibial prostheses, or rarely in hip disarticulation, knee disarticulation or Symes levels of amputation.

Diagnostic (check) sockets

These are temporary sockets made of transparent material to give direct visualisation of the soft tissues and are for amputees who have particular difficulties with their residual limb, e.g. scarring, insensate or hypersensitive tissue, or alignment difficulties. It is a diagnostic aid that is used during controlled weightbearing while practising walking in the prosthetic or therapy facility under supervision.

Liners and socks

Liners are an integral part of some sockets, most commonly for the knee disarticulation levels of amputation and below. They are for comfort, and aid the prosthetist in making adjustments for amputees with volume and shape changes, or for those with marked bony prominences. They may also be part of the system of suspension, and can be made of silicone (e.g. the Iceross socket system see Fig. 8.5), or a combination of neoprene impregnated with gel (e.g. the Alpha liner), when mechanically attached to the socket.

Socks are used as an interface between the residual limb and the prosthetic socket to adjust both for the physiological changes that occur during the day and for comfort. They can be made of:

- wool, manufactured in a number of different thicknesses

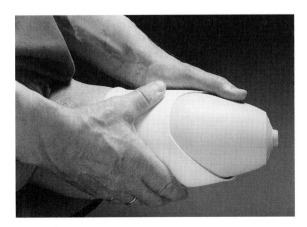

Figure 8.5 The Iceross socket system silicone sleeve being applied to a trans-femoral residual limb. (Photograph by kind permission of Ossür UK.)

- cotton, manufactured in one or two ply
- nylon, the thinnest type and used to remove friction between the skin and the socket interface or to facilitate application of the socket
- specialised socks impregnated with different types of gel, where particular skin protection is needed.

The addition of socks can be particularly useful when the volume of the residual limb is still decreasing, and conversely, use of thinner socks aids fitting when the volume of the residual limb increases.

Auxiliary suspension

The need for auxiliary suspension is determined by the shape of the residual limb, the socket design, and the assessment of the amputee particularly with regard to applying and removing the prosthesis and any concurrent pathology, e.g. stroke. There are varying designs depending on the amount of additional suspension required, from a simple cuff to a rigid pelvic band.

For upper limb amputees, means of auxiliary suspension are also known as 'appendages', and these often have dual functions of operating active movement and suspension. The design of the suspension is governed by the biomechanics of the individual situation and the manual dexterity and cognition of the amputee.

Materials used

Materials of construction can be either rigid or soft:

1. *Soft.* Neoprene is used in total elastic suspension (TES) belts for the trans-femoral level (see Fig. 13.3, p. 164), webbing is used in upper limb suspension and the Silesian belt for the trans-femoral level, soft leather is used for cuffs at the trans-tibial and trans-radial levels, a lanyard for securing an Iceross sleeve to the rigid socket at the trans-tibial level.

2. *Rigid.* Blocked leather is used for thigh corsets (see Fig. 15.8, p. 199), plastic is used for an articulating supracondylar suspension for the

trans-tibial level of amputation (see Fig. 15.6, p. 192), and metal is used in the rigid pelvic band for trans-femoral level of amputation (see Fig. 13.10, p. 172).

Prosthetic joints

Lower limb

There are more than 100 different prosthetic knee joints available for use with the levels of hip disarticulation, trans-femoral and knee disarti-culation, which form at least 50% or more of the amputee population requiring therapy. The therapist working in specialist prosthetic centres must develop a thorough understanding of their properties and function. The budget and local prescription practice of the prosthetic service may determine the range that can be offered locally, and therefore the type that the therapist will have most familiarity with, but an awareness of the total market in their own country is essential to ensure individual needs are catered for. The private patient has the ability to consider the widest possible range for their needs. There are a variety of hip joints, but they are less in number due to the lower prevalence of need for this level of amputation.

Knee joints may be locked (either manually or automatically) or free, and either single axis or polycentric, the latter more closely resembling the movement of the natural knee joint.

Free knees can be stabilised (either by their geometry or a weight-activated brake), have swing phase controls (which can be pneumatic, hydraulic, or micro-processor controlled, etc (see Fig. 8.15)) or have a combination of any of these features. There are a few separate ankle joints but they are often in combination with the foot component.

Upper limb

There are few shoulder joints available; they have passive movements and may be lockable. The elbow joint is usually free swinging and lockable by the remaining hand or with a trick movement of the shoulder. Electric power can be utilised to lock or move the elbow.

Humeral rotation is provided by a friction joint, which may be lockable and is part of the elbow unit.

There are few prosthetic wrists that provide flexion and extension. Most functional prostheses have pronation and supination in the wrist unit. It may have variable friction, or may be lockable in a variety of positions with a knob for quick release. Electric-powered wrist rotators can be used in conjunction with myoelectric control (See Ch. 19 for further details).

Interjoint segments

Materials used

1. carbon fibre
2. metal (e.g. titanium, aluminium).

Femoral component

1. For the hip disarticulation level, a degree of 'bounce' can be provided with a flexible com-ponent designed to bend on loading to absorb the ground reaction force and permit a more natural gait. The amputee, by varying the amount of pelvic thrust at toe off, can selectively release energy and control the forward speed of the knee. The result provides controlled foot rise and effective shortening of the prosthesis at mid-swing to allow variability in toe clearance.

2. A rotation aid device installed distally in the femoral component and activated manually permits 360° rotation for cross-legged sitting, squatting, etc. (See Figs 8.6 & 8.7).

Tibial component

1. Torque absorbers are useful to reduce the friction between the residual limb and the socket when the body is rotating over fixed feet, e.g. as in swinging a golf club.

2. Shock absorbers offer vertical shock ab-sorption and dissipation of torsional forces for improved comfort and gait. There are many different designs, some being combined tibia and foot components (See Fig. 8.8).

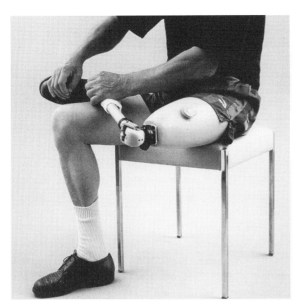

Figure 8.6   A trans-femoral amputee using the rotation adaptor for cross legged sitting. (Photograph by kind permission of Otto Bock UK Ltd.)

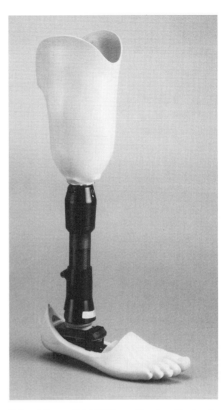

Figure 8.8   A trans-tibial PTB prosthesis with shock absorber in the tibial segment. (Photograph by kind permission of CA Blatchford and Sons Ltd.)

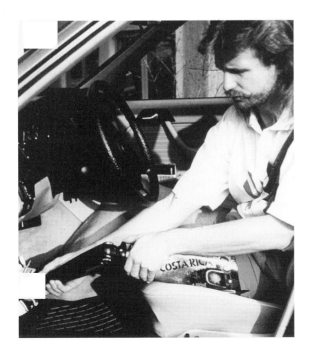

Figure 8.7   A trans-femoral amputee using the rotation adaptor to ease his prosthesis into a car. (Photograph by kind permission of Otto Bock UK Ltd.)

Upper limb

The interjoint segment for trans-humeral and higher levels of amputation may be endoskeletal for cosmetic prostheses. Forearm sections for functional prostheses are exoskeletal and are not custom made but chosen from an 'off-the-shelf' range.

Feet

Foot designs are being improved and upgraded constantly to reduce the energy required by the amputee to walk and to provide the athlete with greater performance. For the lower limb amputee there are a number of ankle/foot combinations, and some feet for use without an ankle component. An overview of the main types of foot design follows.

Jointed feet

Uniaxial ankle. The ankle movement is controlled by one or two rubber bumpers, one of which controls plantarflexion on heel strike and the other (if fitted) dorsiflexion during the last stages of stance phase. The foot can be made of wood covered with leather, but is more likely to be moulded urethane. The construction of a wooden forefoot permits flexion at toe off (see Fig. 8.9).

Multiaxial ankle. This enables a complete range of movements, i.e. plantarflexion, dorsiflexion, inversion and eversion, and rotation. These movements can be adjusted for each amputees' need, weight and activity level by increasing or decreasing the hardness of the rubber component and bumper in the ankle mechanism (see Fig. 8.10).

Jointless feet

These can be either the most basic of design or the most sophisticated.

Jaipur foot. This foot was designed for developing countries responding to the need for squatting, barefoot walking and cross-legged sitting. It is made up of three blocks simulating the anatomy of a normal foot. The forefoot and heel blocks are made of sponge rubber and the ankle block of light wood. The three components are bound together, enclosed in a rubber shell and vulcanised in a mould to give it the shape and cosmetic appearance of a real foot. It is cheap, durable, waterproof and supple, but heavier than some other prosthetic feet.

SACH (solid ankle cushion heel) foot. This is a simple foot with no ankle joint. The plastic foam of the foot has a wedge section in the heel that may be varied in density to suit the weight and activity of the amputee. This wedge absorbs the shock load at heel strike and simulates ankle movement. At toe off, the material used in the construction of the foot enables flexion to occur in the forefoot (see Fig. 8.11).

Dynamic elastic response feet. This is a term given to feet employing the concept of energy storing from heel strike to midstance and energy release during push off. There are many different designs available employing a one-piece keel (see Figs 8.12–8.13 and 15.2, p. 189) and the quantity of energy stored and released depends on the materials used in the construction, the weight and walking speed of the user and their footwear. Each will suit an individual need, such as fast walking, running and specific activities. (Examples are the Seattle Lightfoot, Quantum foot, Springlite, Dynamic Plus, Enhanced Dynamic Response Foot, Flex-Foot system). Much comparative research in gait analysis and energy

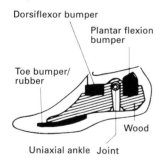

Figure 8.9 A cross-section of a uniaxial foot.

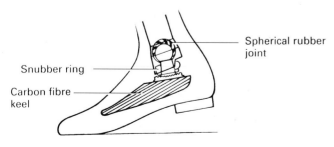

Figure 8.10 The multiaxial ankle.

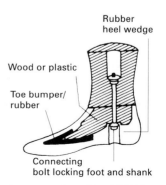

Figure 8.11 A cross-section of the SACH foot.

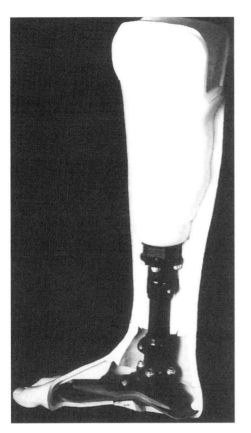

Figure 8.12   A trans-tibial prosthesis with a Quantum foot. (Photograph by kind permission of Vessa Ltd.)

expenditure is taking place; it is hoped that more precise indications for use will emerge, particularly for the athlete and the older user.

These are examples of some of the prosthetic feet that are available at present. There are many more with specific designs and variations. Some feet have the added adjustability in that the heel height can be altered by approximately 2 cm. This enables the amputee to wear shoes of different heel heights. (See Fig. 8.13) If the amputee has a fixed foot, they may require more than one prosthesis for use with different footwear. The foot prescription is also another option to improve socket comfort, as different designs and materials will affect the ground reaction force at heel strike and rotational forces when turning or twisting.

Terminal devices

For the upper limb amputee, there are cosmetic and functional terminal devices. Functional terminal devices may be activated either with body power (the most common being the split hook), or external power. If both function and cosmesis are required there will be a compromise between the two (for further details see Ch. 19).

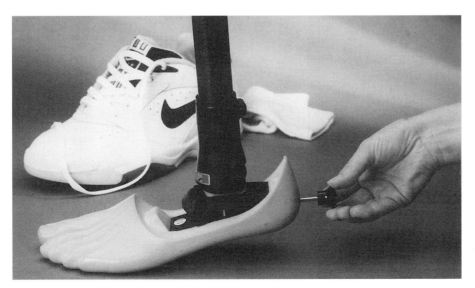

Figure 8.13   A dynamic response energy-storing foot showing the heel height adjustment. (Photograph by kind permission of CA Blatchford and Sons Ltd.)

Cosmesis

The individual amputee's attitude to the cosmetic appearance of their prosthesis varies; some demand a mirror image of the remaining limb (both shape and colour), while, at the other end of the spectrum, some are happy to have no cosmetic cover at all and indeed want to draw attention to the limb by employing a multicoloured socket.

Materials used in endoskeletal prostheses

Foam covers. These employ fire retardant materials and may be either one piece or two piece for the lower limb prostheses or the material used for a cosmetic hand. The cover may be completed with a stocking, skin-type spray or PVC to match the shade of the remaining limb. (Fig. 8.14). The one piece cosmesis may, when new, appear to hamper movement of a joint, particularly the knee. The therapist must note that when it is worn a few times, the joint will move more easily.

Silicone cosmetic cover. Bespoke covers are sculpted and colour matched to the contralateral side in detail, including nails, freckles, veins, hairs, etc.; they are available for those amputees who require a life-like finish. It is available for both lower and upper extremity prostheses including partial feet appliances and single phalanx replacement. As it is expensive, particularly for the time taken in the craftsmanship needed, it is not universally available from public health services.

A simple pull-on sheath-like silicone skin is available in several colours.

Thermoplastic, e.g. Plastazote. This material gives a good join at the ankle and is more durable than soft foam. It is usually covered with stockinette or may be spray finished with a silicone spray.

Coloured laminate socket. The amputee can choose from a wide range of colours and patterns (see Fig. 8.15) and the prosthetic components are exposed.

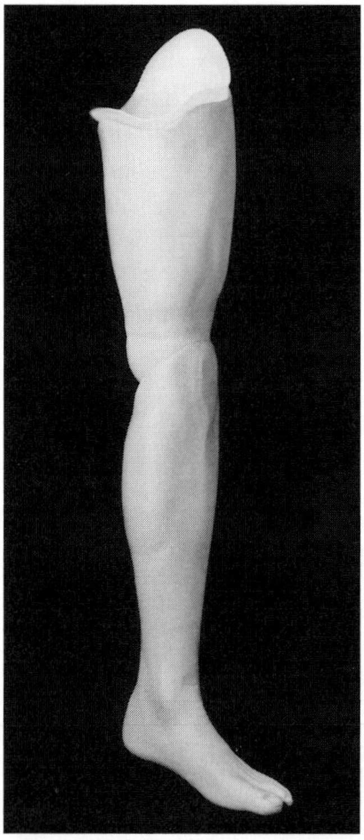

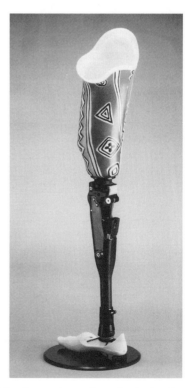

Figure 8.14 A trans-femoral prosthesis with discontinuous cosmesis (i.e. the knee is not enclosed). (Photograph by kind permission of CA Blatchford and Sons Ltd.)

Figure 8.15 A trans-femoral prosthesis showing a coloured laminate socket and microprocessor-controlled knee component. (Photograph by kind permission of CA Blatchford and Sons Ltd.)

Materials used in exoskeletal prostheses

The material of construction (plastic, wood or metal) may achieve a skin tone by either being painted, having a stocking or a laminated cover of a plastic material applied.

Materials used for prosthetic hands

PVC is the material of choice for hard use and active wearers as it is robust, but it does stain easily. Silicone is for the moderate user in both electric and passive hands. Because the hand is so visible, the shade of colour on both anterior and posterior aspects is important.

The therapist needs to learn the terminology of prosthetic components in order to communicate well with the prosthetists regarding the individual amputee's needs.

PROSTHETIC ASSEMBLY

Workshop assembly or central fabrication

The most important component of a prosthesis is the socket. This can either be made using a plaster-of-Paris cast (either with or without added pressure) or by taking circumferential and longitudinal measurements of the residual limb, as mentioned previously.

Most prosthetic centres will have workshop facilities to make the individual sockets on site and assemble the rest of the prescribed components for a modular prosthesis. However, some prostheses, particularly exoskeletal prostheses, may have to be made in a central fabrication unit off site. The balance between workshop assembly and central fabrication differs from country to country, which in turn has an effect on the skills and craftsmanship required by the prosthetist, the time allowed for individual amputee contact and the efficiency of the business.

Alignment

This is the term used in lower limb prosthetics to express the establishment of the position in space of the components of the prosthesis relative to each other and to the amputee (see Fig. 8.16A & B).

Static alignment is tested visually both with the prosthesis alone on the workshop bench (bench alignment), and when worn by the amputee standing still, or may be checked by the use of laser systems. Dynamic alignment is assessed by observation of the movement pattern during the gait cycle. Particular alignment difficulties can be resolved using the full technology and expertise present in a gait laboratory, or by a video/vector machine in the clinic (see Chs 9 & 10).

Malalignment can cause a significant increase in ground reaction force and stance phase time. This results in increased pressure on the residual limb and increased loading on the remaining limb, which in turn results in an uneven gait pattern and potential for damage to the weightbearing joints. In dysvascular amputees, the potential for damage to the remaining limb is high.

In upper limb prostheses, alignment is not adjustable. It is pre-determined and built into the prosthesis.

Computer-aided design/computer-aided manufacture (CAD-CAM)

Computerisation of the fabrication of casts for prosthetic sockets has met with some success. Either a negative plaster cast is made of the residual limb and a sensor scans the inner surface of the cast, or cast-free digitising is used (a sensor is directly applied to the residual limb) and this shape is then translated onto a software programme on which the prosthetist can make any alterations as necessary onto the image of the socket on the screen. When the correct shape is created, a signal is sent to a carving unit where a positive plaster mould is then carved to the required shape; the carving unit may be on site or some distance away in a central fabrication unit. Data is stored in the computer so this method makes it possible both to reproduce a prosthetic socket and be consistent in quality.

Prosthetic systems

These are the individual manufacturers' trade-names for their items in the same range. Blatchford's

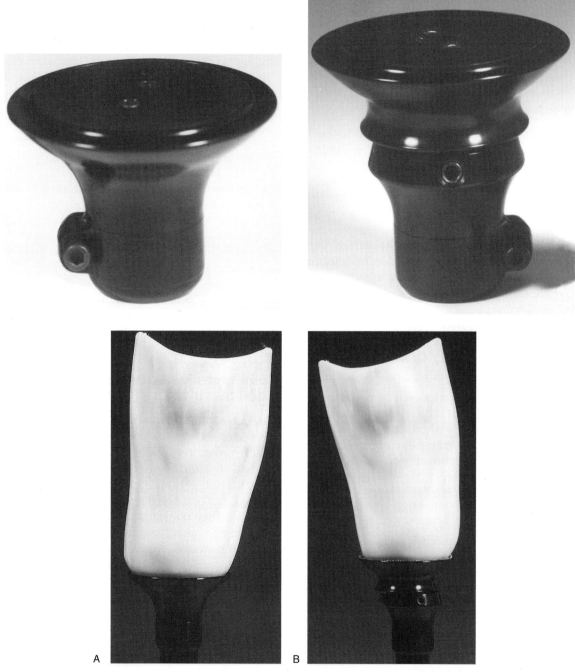

Figure 8.16 A PTB prosthesis showing two designs of alignment component: (A) shows the Ultimate Tilt that facilitates a 16° angulation; (B) shows the Ultimate Tilt and Slide, which combines the features of A with a total of 10 mm shift in anteroposterior and medial-lateral directions. (Photograph by kind permission of Ortho Europe.)

'Endolite', Otto Bock Modular System, Seattle Limb Systems, are a few examples. While a prosthetist can choose to assemble all components of a limb from the same system, it may be possible to interchange a range of components between systems, creating a hybrid prosthesis. However, not all components are interchangeable and the prosthetist is the expert in this matter. There are separate systems for adults and children with different testing standards to comply with.

RESEARCH AND DEVELOPMENT

Specialist therapists need to be involved in prosthetic research as they know the questions to be addressed with regard to function. However, many components become available on the market before guidelines are drawn up as to their recommended use, or research carried out on the outcome of their use by the amputee. Research and development (R&D) is a commercially sensitive area and professionals must often wait until the next national or international conference for details to emerge; therefore attending these events and reading current literature is an essential way to keep abreast of developments.

Prosthetic manufacturers and university departments of engineering and biomedical sciences tend to carry out the large-scale research programmes, looking at the strength of materials and components, and comparative studies of performance of components (often using energy consumption as the objective outcome), but individual prosthetists and inventors are also working on some innovations, the need for which is determined by close observation of clinical practice and amputee demand.

Application of high-level technology to lower limb prosthetics ensures greater control, ease of use and reduction of effort by amputees during walking activities. In upper limb prosthetics, it ensures greater function of grip/release and finer manual dexterity.

R&D for the developed world

Prescription

Prosthetic manufacturers have started to draw up prescription criteria for their components, based on the parameters of amputee body weight, level of amputation, stability and functional ability based on activity level. Therapists are also working to provide guidelines for prescription based on the therapy assessment prior to prosthetic rehabilitation (see Ch. 7). (Personal communications A. Lambert 1997, R McGregor 1997).

Components

1. Power-assisted gait and hand control devices are undergoing modification to improve prosthetic function and allow a more natural movement with varying speeds.

2. Specific individual requirements for function, e.g. for sports, are leading to the development of individual components and new systems.

3. Socket design to improve comfort and suspension is an area investigated widely.

4. Sensory feedback mechanisms in the foot and hand are being developed so that pressure is appreciated thus improving information to the amputee for balance and function.

5. Control systems are being developed for upper limb prostheses, utilising the link between the prosthesis and the remaining neural network in the residual limb.

6. Improvements in battery life, size and weight for upper limb will improve external power.

7. Mechanical grasp patterns of prosthetic hands are also being developed.

8. The technique of osseointegration (see Ch. 21) could obviate the need for a prosthetic socket, so modular components that screw directly into the bone of the residual limb will be developed.

Materials

Silicone, either in sheet form or as a gel, has transformed comfort, suspension and cosmesis in recent years and further uses are being investigated for this material.

Design

Knee joint design including microprocessors, different geometry and pneumatic and hydraulic developments are advancing rapidly.

Gait analysis

The kinetics of gait are being examined with various types of functional components and prosthetic feet to determine their performance and thus inform prescription more accurately.

R&D for the developing world

Some examples of R&D for the developing world are:

- Low-cost, direct-fitting socket techniques

- Internationally affordable, durable prosthetic systems and mobility aids using thermoformable plastics such as polypropylene.

The need is to develop very low-cost technologies without sacrificing quality. Using computer models and other analytical tools, systems that are appropriate and effective in different economic and physical environments are being examined.

BIBLIOGRAPHY FOR PREVIOUS EDITIONS

Buttenshaw P 1991 Amputees benefit from teamwork. Therapy Weekly 17(41):2

Canby T Y 1989 Reshaping our lives. National Geographic 176(6):746–760

English A W G, Gregory Dean A A 1980 The artificial limb service. Health Trends 12:77

Fernie G R, Halsall A P, Ruder K 1984 Shape sensing as an educational aid for student prosthetists. Prosthetics and Orthotics International 8:87–90

Fillauer C E, Pritham C H, Fillauer K D 1989 Evolution and development of the silicone suction socket (3S) for below-knee prostheses. Journal of Prosthetics and Orthotics 1(2):92–103

Foort J 1979 Modular prosthetics – a philosophical view. Prosthetics and Orthotics International 3:140–143

Hirons R R 1991 The prosthetic treatment of lower limb deficiency. Prosthetics and Orthotics International 15:112–116

Hughes J 1978 Education in prosthetics and orthotics. Prosthetics and Orthotics International 2:51–53

Kabra S G, Narayanan R 1991 Ankle-foot prosthesis with articulated human bone endoskeleton: force-deflection and fatigue study. Journal of Rehabilitation Research and Development 28(3):13–22

Limb M, Calnan M 1990 Artificial limbs: a real need. Health Service Journal 100(15 Nov) 5227:1696–1697

Menard M R, McBride M E, Sanderson D J, Murray D D 1992 Comparative biomechanical analysis of energy-storing prosthetic feet. Archives of Physical Medicine and Rehabilitation 73(5):451–458

Mensch G 1986 Aids and equipment. Prosthetic update. Physiotherapy Canada 38(6):369–371

Michael J W 1992 Prosthetic feet: options for the older client. Topics in Geriatric Rehabilitation 8(1):30–38

Murphy E F 1984 Sockets, linings and interfaces. Clinical Prosthetics and Orthotics S(3):4–10

Nielsen C C 1991 A survey of amputees: functional level and life satisfaction, information needs and the prosthetist's role. Journal of Prosthetics and Orthotics 3(3):125–129

Redhead R G et al 1991 Prescribing lower limb prostheses.

Royal College of Physicians 1986 Physical disability and beyond. Reprinted from Journal of The Royal College of Physicians of London 20(3) (complete report)

Southwell M 1983 The history and design development of artificial limbs. Thesis, Department of Industrial Design, Manchester Polytechnic

Taylor J S 1979 Modular assembly above-knee prostheses. Prosthetics and Orthotics International 3:144–146

Topper A K, Fernie G R 1990 An evaluation of computer aided design of below-knee prosthetic sockets. Prosthetics and Orthotics International 14(3):136–142

Torburn L et al 1990 Below-knee gait with dynamic elastic response prosthetic feet: a pilot study. Journal of Rehabilitation Research and Development 27(4):369–384

Van Jaarsveld H W L et al 1990 Stiffness and hysteresis properties of some prosthetic feet. Prosthetics and Orthotics International 14(3):117–124

BIBLIOGRAPHY FOR THE THIRD EDITION

Allard P, Trudeau F, Prince F, Dansereau J, Labelle H, Duhaime M 1995 Modelling and gait evaluation of asymetrical-keel foot prosthesis. Medical and Biological Engineering and Computing 33:2–7

Boonstra A M, Schrama J, Fidler V, Eisma W H 1995 Energy cost during ambulation in trans-femoral amputees: a knee joint with a mechanical swing phase control versus a knee joint with a pneumatic swing phase control. Scandinavian Journal of Rehabilitation Medicine 27:77–81

Buckley J G, Spence W D, Solomonidis S E 1997 Energy cost of walking: comparison of intelligent prosthesis with conventional mechanism. Archives of Physical Medicine and Rehabilitation 78(3):330–333

Casillas J-M, Dulieu V, Cohen M, Marcer I, Didier J-P 1995 Bioenergetic comparison of a new energy-storing foot and SACH foot in traumatic below-knee vascular amputations. Archives of Physical Medicine and Rehabilitation 76:39–44

Dewar M 1997 CAD/CAM systems in pedorthics, prosthetics and orthotics. International Society for Prosthetics and Orthotics UK Newsletter Summer:13–14

Datta D, Vaidya S K, Howitt J, Gopalan L 1996 Outcome of fitting an ICEROSS prosthesis: views of trans-tibial amputees. Prosthetics and Orthotics International 20:111–115

Esquenazi A, Meier III R H 1996 Rehabilitation in limb deficiency. 4.Limb amputation. Archives of Physical Medicine and Rehabilitation 77:S18–S28

Gailey R S, Lawrence D, Burditt C, Spyropoulos P, Newell C, Nash M S 1993 The CAT-CAM socket and quadrilateral socket: a comparison of energy cost during ambulation. Prosthetics and Orthotics International 17:95–100

He P, Xue K, Murka P 1997 3-D imaging of residual limbs using ultrasound. Journal of Rehabilitation Research and Development 34(3):269–278

Köhler P, Lindh L, Netz P 1989 Comparison of CAD-CAM and hand made sockets for PTB prostheses. Prosthetics and Orthotics International 13:19–24

Korver A J H 1993 Amputees in a hospital of the International Committee of the Red Cross. Injury 24(9):607–609

Kristinsson O 1993 The ICEROSS concept: a discussion of a philosophy. Prosthetics and Orthotics International 17(1):49–55

Lake C, Supan T J 1997 The incidence of dermatological problems in the silicone suspension sleeve user. The Journal of Prosthetics and Orthotics 9(3):97–106

Lilja M, Öberg T 1995 Volumetric determinations with CAD/CAM in prosthetics and orthotics: errors of measurement. Journal of Rehabilitation Research and Development 32(2):141–148

McCurdie I, Hanspal R, Nieveen R 1997 ICEROSS – a consensus view: a questionnaire survey of the use of ICEROSS in the United Kingdom. Prosthetics and Orthotics International 21(2):124–128

Meanley S 1995 Different approaches and cultural considerations in third world prosthetics. Prosthetics and Orthotics International 19(3):176–180

Miller L A, Childress D S 1997 Analysis of a vertical compliance prosthetic foot. Journal of Rehabilitation Research and Development 34(1):52–57

Mullick S 1997 Efficacy of silicone-gel impregnated prosthetic sock in optimisation of interface problems of ambulatory trans-tibial amputees wearing patellar tendon bearing prostheses. Proceedings ISPO UK NMS Annual Scientific Meetings, England, 36–37

Narita H, Yokogushi K, Shii S, Kakizawa M, Nosaka T 1997 Suspension effect and dynamic evaluation of the total surface bearing (TSB) trans-tibial prosthesis: a comparison

with the patellar tendon bearing (PTB) trans-tibial prosthesis. Prosthetics and Orthotics International 21(3):175–178

Pinzur M S, Cox W, Kaiser J, Morris T, Patwardhan A, Vrbos L 1995 The effect of prosthetic alignment on relative limb loading in persons with trans-tibial amputation: a preliminary report. Journal of Rehabilitation Research and Development 32(4):373–378

Postema K, Hermens H J, De Vries J, Koopman H F J M, Eisma W H 1997 Energy storage and release of prosthetic feet. Part 1: biomechanical analysis related to user benefits. Prosthetics and Orthotics International 21:17–27

Reynolds J P 1995 Prosthetics under management care. Magazine of Physical Therapy November 3(11):58–62

Sabolich J A, Ortega G M 1994 Sense of feel of lower-limb amputees: a phase-one study. Journal of Prosthetics and Orthotics 6(2):36–41

Sanders J E, Lam D, Dralle A J, Okumura R 1997 Interface pressures and shear stresses at thirteen socket sites on two persons with trans-tibial amputation. Journal of Rehabilitation Research and Development 34(1):19–43

Sharp M 1994 The Jaipur limb and foot. Medicine and war 10:207–211

Silver-Thorn M B, Steege J W, Childress D S 1996 A review of prosthetic interface stress investigations. Journal of Rehabilitation Research and Development 33(3):253–266

Simpson D, Convery P 1997 Aspects of prosthetic socket design. British Association of Chartered Physiotherapists in Amputee Rehabilitation, Newsletter 6:8–9

Snyder R D, Powers C M, Fontaine C, Perry J 1995 The effect of five prosthetic feet on the gait and loading of the sound limb in dysvascular below-knee amputees. Journal of Rehabilitation Research and Development 32(4):309–315

Taylor M B, Clark E, Offord E A, Baxter C 1996 A comparison of energy expenditure by a high level trans-femoral amputee using the intelligent prosthesis and conventionally damped prosthetic limbs. Prosthetics and Orthotics International 20:116–121

Torburn L, Powers C M, Guiterrez R, Perry J 1995 Energy expenditure during ambulation in dysvascular and traumatic below-knee amputees: a comparison of five prosthetic feet. Journal of Rehabilitation Research and Development 32(2):111–119

Zahedi S 1996 Advances in external prosthetics. Current Opinion in Orthopaedics 7(vi):93–98

9

Normal locomotion and prosthetic replacement

Revised by Nicky Thompson

Normal human locomotion is the product of many complex interactions between the forces generated within the body and external forces acting upon it. It has been described as a series of rhythmical, alternating movements of the extremities and trunk that result in the forward movement of the centre of mass. In this chapter, it is not the intention to describe locomotion in anything like its actual complexity, but to present fundamental facts in order to gain an understanding of the gait of the amputee and some aspects of prosthetic design. Gait re-education requires the ability to analyse each phase of the gait cycle with its integrated motions of the various segments of the body. Success relies on the accurate knowledge of the functional characteristics of the normal locomotor system. Considering the complexity of movement in normal locomotion, prosthetic technology has resulted in surprisingly good gait patterns in the lower limb. However the amputee does have to adapt their gait to the individual design, components and alignment of the prosthesis supplied.

GAIT TERMINOLOGY

In analysing pathological gait, normal function is the model against which it is judged. In order to apply the terminology of the normal gait cycle to patients with a wide variety of pathologies, generic terminology has developed to describe the phases of the gait cycle. Thus, 'heel strike' is more widely applicable as 'initial contact' and 'push off' as 'terminal stance'. While wishing to adopt this generic terminology, the term 'heel strike' has been deliberately retained throughout this book, since it is an important action that significantly influences the stability of prosthetic gait.

Gait cycle

A single gait cycle or stride begins when one foot strikes the ground and ends when it strikes the ground again (Fig. 9.1). Events in the gait cycle are defined sequentially as occurring at specific percentages of the gait cycle. Heel strike occurs at 0% and 100% of the cycle. During normal walking, toe off occurs at approximately 60% of the gait cycle. Therefore stance accounts for approximately 60% of the gait cycle and swing 40%. Opposite toe off and opposite heel strike occur at 10% and 50% of the cycle, respectively. Double support periods occur twice during the gait cycle and each phase of double support lasts about 10% of the cycle. The length of the double support period is directly related to walking speed: as speed increases the period of double support decreases. The absence of double support indicates that a person is running rather than walking.

Stance phase

This begins at heel strike on one leg and ends at toe off on the same leg.

Initial contact (heel strike): instantaneous event when the heel touches the ground. (Time and location of contact is less well defined in those patients with foot clearance problems).

Loading response (0–10%): body weight is transferred onto the forward limb. The foot is lowered to the ground and the knee is flexed for shock absorption.

Mid-stance (10–30%): the limb and trunk advance over the stationary foot.

Terminal stance (push off) (30–50%): the heel of the supporting extremity leaves the ground and the body is propelled forwards by the powerful action of the plantarflexors.

Pre swing (toe off) (50–60%): body weight is unloaded and transferred to the contralateral limb and the toe begins to lift off the ground.

Swing phase

Swing phase begins where stance phase ends and is the period between toe off on one leg and heel strike on the same leg:

Initial swing (60–73%): The instant the toe leaves the ground the limb must be accelerated to advance the body in preparation for the next heel strike.

Mid-swing (73–87%): This continues the task of limb advancement and foot clearance.

Terminal swing (87–100%): This occurs as the forward motion of the limb is decelerated to control its position for heel strike.

Velocity

The average horizontal speed of the body along the plane of progression measured over one or more strides.

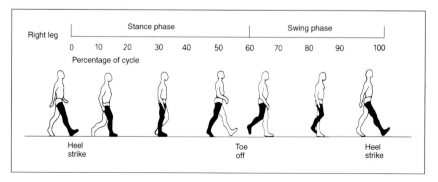

Figure 9.1 The gait cycle.

Cadence

The number of steps per unit time usually represented as steps per minute.

Planes of motion

Coronal plane: when the subject is viewed from the front – the vertical plane divides the body into anterior and posterior parts.

Sagittal plane: when the subject is viewed from the side – the vertical plane divides the body into right and left parts.

Transverse plane: when the subject is viewed from above – the horizontal plane divides the body at right angles to the coronal and sagittal plane.

CLINICALLY OBSERVABLE CHARACTERISTICS OF GAIT

The centre of mass (COM) of the body is a point at which all the weight of the body may be assumed to be concentrated at a certain instant. Its location is not fixed but changes with movement. In the normal body standing erect, its location is slightly anterior to the second sacral vertebra.

Walking may be viewed as the displacement of the body COM from one point to another. To walk with a minimum expenditure of energy, it is necessary to minimise variation of the instantaneous velocity and vertical and lateral displacement of the body COM. The principal motions and the velocity of the COM in normal walking are determined by a number of observable gait characteristics.

Vertical displacement of the body COM (Fig. 9.2)

In the normal walking pattern, the body's COM undergoes a rhythmic upward and downward motion as it moves forward. The body's COM is at its lowest and therefore its most stable during double support, while the body's COM rises to its highest position during mid-stance when the walker is least stable.

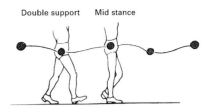

Double support   Mid stance

Figure 9.2   Vertical movement of the COM while walking.

The normal vertical displacement of the body's COM is approximately 5 cm and the most significant clinically observable factor limiting this excursion is the coordinated function of the knee and ankle. During loading response, when the knee begins to flex and the ankle begins to plantarflex, the net result is a reduction in the extent to which the COM displaces upwards as the pelvis moves over the supporting leg. The transfemoral amputee walking with a locked knee will therefore display a greater vertical displacement of the body COM, significantly raising the energy cost of walking.

Lateral displacement of the body COM (Fig. 9.3)

As weight is transferred from one leg to the other there is a shift of the pelvis and trunk to the weightbearing side. The body COM as it moves forward, not only undergoes the vertical motion already described, but also moves from side to side.

The normal lateral COM displacement, walking on level ground, is approximately 5 cm, and the following clinically observable factors limit this excursion.

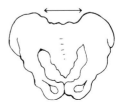

Figure 9.3   Lateral displacement of the COM is approximately 5 cm with each stride.

Width of the walking base (Fig. 9.4)

In normal walking, one foot is placed ahead of the other in the line of progression. If a line is drawn through successive mid-points of heel strike of each foot, the distance between these parallel lines represents the width of the walking base. In normal subjects, this varies between 5 and 10 cm. The lateral displacement of the body COM is such that it remains over the supporting leg. If an amputee walks with an abducted gait the lateral displacement increases and therefore the energy cost increases.

Pelvic obliquity (Fig. 9.5)

This is the angular motion of the pelvis in the coronal plane. The pelvis tilts at mid-stance by

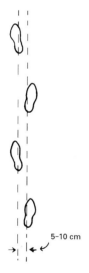

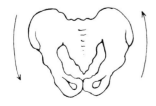

Figure 9.4 The width of the walking base controls the lateral displacement of the pelvis.

Figure 9.5 Pelvic obliquity on the unsupported side is controlled by the hip abductors on the opposite side. This controls lateral displacement of the body COM.

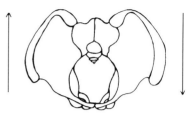

Figure 9.6 Transverse rotation of the pelvis permits one leg to move forwards while the other is fixed with minimal lateral displacement of the body COM.

about 5°, listing downwards from the weight-bearing limb.

Pelvic rotation (Fig. 9.6)

The pelvis appears to rotate about a vertical axis, which assists the advancement of one limb while the other is fixed to the ground. This minimises the width of the walking base. The rotation occurs at each hip joint, which passes from relative external rotation to relative internal rotation during stance phase. The femur rotates approximately 10° with respect to the pelvis. Torque transmitted through the femur generates a relative rotation between the femur and the tibia.

Velocity of body COM

This refers to the instantaneous speed and direction of the COM. This is constantly changing during the gait cycle as weight is applied and removed from each leg.

A normal subject tends to walk at a fairly well-defined average velocity of 1.2 m/s (velocity = step length × no. of steps/s). It is assumed that this speed is optimal such that the energy consumption is minimal. One of the most important factors is the weight distribution of the segments of the limb, which in swing phase act as a pendulum.

If restraints are imposed or abnormal function occurs, changes in the instantaneous velocity of the COM will be necessary to maintain any particular average velocity. The distribution of weight in the leg segments will affect this velocity. For example, the weight distribution will be different for a trans-femoral amputee wearing a prosthesis with a very sophisticated knee mechanism and SACH foot compared to one wearing a lightweight, simple knee mechanism and light DER foot (see Ch. 8).

Arm swing

The trunk and shoulders rotate during walking and these rotations are approximately 180° out of phase with the pelvic rotation and appear to provide a balancing effect that smoothes the forward progression of the body as a whole. This rotation is affected either by upper limb amputation or brachial plexus lesion.

ANALYSIS OF MOTIONS AND FORCES

Internal and external forces cause and control movement – known as 'kinetics'. In walking, the internal forces are generated from muscle activity and stabilising ligaments while the external forces are due to gravity and the reaction of the ground on the foot. The ground reaction force (GRF) can be measured using a force platform and is equal in magnitude and opposite in direction to the force exerted by the weightbearing limb.

If a force is applied at a distance from the centre of an axis of rotation or a joint centre, this creates a moment that must be balanced by an equal and opposite moment at that joint. The result is a 'couple' (two parallel forces acting in opposite directions, which combine to produce a moment) which will cause angular acceleration of the limb segment unless resisted by an opposing moment at the joint. In walking, the *external* moments about a joint in the weightbearing limb can be estimated from the product of the GRF and the perpendicular distance to a joint centre (Fig. 9.7). This allows the relative magnitudes of the moments about joints to be readily appreciated but has limitations in that it does not account for gravitational or inertial forces of the limb segments. In order to account for all components of force, a procedure known as 'inverse dynamics' is required (Winter 1991) which is the method used in modern 3-dimensional gait

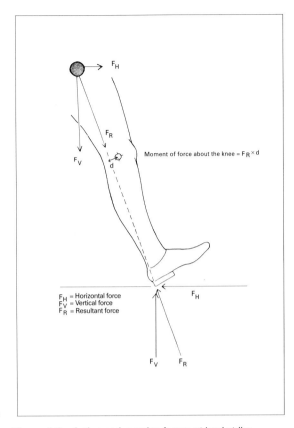

Figure 9.7 Action and reaction forces at heel strike.

analysis systems that calculate the net *internal* joint moments.

Figures 9.8–9.15 illustrate the ground reaction vector (a line indicating the magnitude and direction of force) superimposed on the weight-bearing limb thus allowing visualisation of external joint moments throughout the gait cycle. In normal gait, the GRF acts close to the hip, knee and ankle joint centres thus minimising moments about these joints and the corresponding energy expenditure.

Analysis in the sagittal plane

Initial contact (heel strike) (Fig. 9.8)

Heel strike is a momentary event as the foot strikes the ground and it initiates the period of stance. The leg is optimally positioned to initiate progression and knee stability. The ankle is

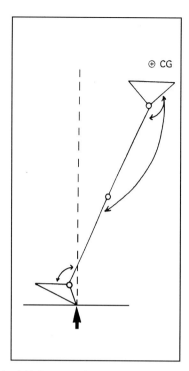

Figure 9.8 Initial contact. (Reproduced from Hughes J, Jacobs N 1979 Normal human locomotion. Prosthetics and Orthotics International 3:4–12, by kind permission of the authors and publishers.)

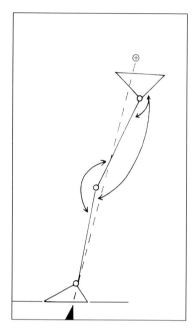

Figure 9.9 Loading response. (Reproduced from Hughes J, Jacobs N 1979 Normal human locomotion. Prosthetics and Orthotics International 3:4–12, by kind permission of the authors and publishers.)

in neutral dorsiflexion, the knee extended and the hip flexed approximately 30°. The impact of striking the floor creates a momentary, abrupt vertical ground reaction force that is posterior to the ankle joint causing a plantarflexor moment, anterior to the knee causing an extensor moment, and anterior to the hip causing a flexor moment. The foot is held in the neutral position by the ankle dorsiflexors. Knee extension is passive as a result of the anterior GRF, and the hip extensors (hamstrings and gluteus maximus) decelerate the thigh at this point.

Loading response (Fig. 9.9)

Loading response is the initial period of double support, during which weight is transferred onto the stance limb. This drives the forefoot towards the floor resulting in ankle plantarflexion and knee flexion. The knee flexion provides valuable

shock absorption to lessen the effect of this rapid weight transfer and the external knee flexor moment is controlled by eccentric contraction of the quadriceps while maintaining knee stability. The external plantarflexor moment at the ankle is controlled by eccentric contraction of the ankle dorsiflexors lowering the foot to the ground. During loading response hip extension is initiated by concentric contraction of the hip extensors.

Mid-stance (Fig. 9.10)

Mid-stance progression is dependent on the pivotal action of the ankle rocker to advance the limb over the supporting foot. Eccentric contraction of the ankle plantarflexors advances the tibia over the foot achieving approximately 5° dorsiflexion by the end of mid-stance. Progression is assisted by momentum of the contralateral swinging limb. The ground reaction vector is moved anterior to the ankle and knee joint so assisting progressive knee extension by what is known as the 'plantarflexion/knee extension

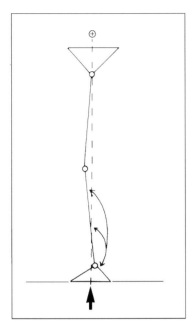

Fig. 9.10 Mid-stance. (Reproduced from Hughes J, Jacobs N 1979 Normal human locomotion. Prosthetics and Orthotics International 3:4–12, by kind permission of the authors and publishers.)

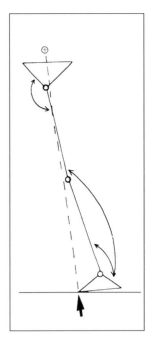

Figure 9.11 Terminal stance. (Reproduced from Hughes J, Jacobs N 1979 Normal human locomotion. Prosthetics and Orthotics International 3:4–12, by kind permission of the authors and publishers.)

couple'. By the end of mid-stance, the ground reaction vector is posterior to the hip joint necessitating minimal muscle activity to extend the hip from 30° to 10° of hip flexion. As the opposite foot leaves the ground, the hip abductors contract to maintain a stable pelvis.

Terminal stance (push off) (Fig. 9.11)

During terminal stance, the body is advanced ahead of the stationary foot achieving maximum dorsiflexion and the heel rises. Passive hip and knee extension allows forward progression of the trunk and the ground reaction vector moves toward the metatarsal heads generating a large dorsiflexor moment at the ankle. This moment is counteracted by powerful contraction of the plantarflexors, which assist in accelerating the body forwards. Gastrocnemius also acts as a knee flexor and initiates the second wave of knee flexion, which begins at the end of terminal stance.

Pre-swing (toe off) (Fig. 9.12)

Pre-swing is the final phase of stance ocurring at 50–60% of the gait cycle. During this period, the ground reaction force loses its significance as body weight is unloaded and transferred to the contralateral limb. The critical action during this period is the rapid initiation of knee flexion contributing to limb advancement in swing. Peak plantarflexion of approximately 20° is reached at the end of this phase but ankle plantarflexor activity is rapidly decreasing as the limb is being unloaded.

Initial swing (Fig. 9.13)

The moment of toe off signifies the onset of swing phase and the actions occurring during initial swing are designed to facilitate limb advancement. Momentum generated in pre-swing continues in initial swing and is facilitated by hip and knee flexor activity. In order to assure foot

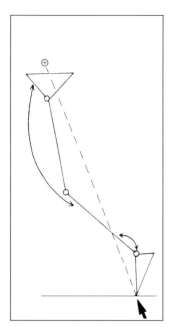

Fig. 9.12 Pre-swing. (Reproduced from Hughes J, Jacobs N 1979 Normal human locomotion. Prosthetics and Orthotics International 3:4–12, by kind permission of the authors and publishers.)

clearance, the knee reaches peak swing phase knee flexion of approximately 60° and the ankle rapidly begins to dorsiflex.

Mid-swing (Fig. 9.14)

Mid-swing continues the task of limb advancement and foot clearance. Hip flexion and knee extension are essentially passive. The hip continues to flex, and the knee begins to extend assisted by gravity once the knee flexors relax. The ankle continues to actively dorsiflex to neutral.

Terminal swing (Fig. 9.15)

This is the transition phase between swing and stance and muscle activity is intense. Limb advancement is completed by active knee extension to neutral. Eccentric contraction of gluteus maximus and the hamstrings decelerate the hip and knee in readiness for heel strike and neutral ankle dorsiflexion is maintained.

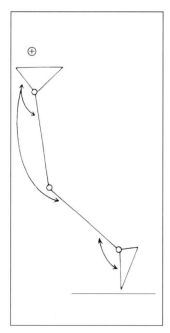

Figure 9.13 Initial swing. (Reproduced from Hughes J, Jacobs N 1979 Normal human locomotion. Prosthetics and Orthotics International 3:4–12, by kind permission of the authors and publishers.)

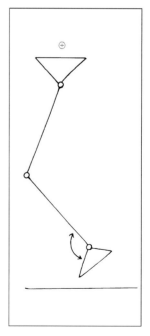

Fig. 9.14 Mid swing. (Reproduced from Hughes J, Jacobs N 1979 Normal human locomotion. Prosthetics and Orthotics International 3:4–12, by kind permission of the authors and publishers.)

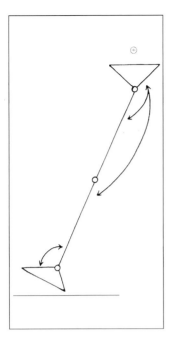

Fig. 9.15 Terminal swing. (Reproduced from Hughes J, Jacobs N 1979 Normal human locomotion. Prosthetics and Orthotics International 3:4–12, by kind permission of the authors and publishers.)

Prosthetic considerations

It is not possible to replace all movements with prosthetic components. Also, the individual amputee is not always capable of managing sophisticated components. The prosthetist will try and match the amputee's abilities with the components available and the therapist must retrain the gait, bearing in mind the amputee's physical ability and the design of the prosthesis supplied. The diagrams in Tables 9.1 and 9.2 attempt to show the prosthetic components currently available that act during the gait cycle in the sagittal plane.

Gait analysis techniques have allowed the quantification of compensatory mechanisms in amputee gait, which have implications for rehabilitation programmes. For example, in a study on trans-femoral amputee subjects, Seroussi et al reported significantly increased concentric hip extensor work in early stance, and increased ankle push off power on the intact limb, compensating for decreased ankle push off on the prosthetic limb. They also suggested that these

muscle groups may benefit from a strengthening programme.

Analysis in the coronal plane (Fig. 9.16)

Moments in the coronal plane are products of the ground reaction force that passes from a point under the supporting foot through the COM. All external moments will be in the direction of adduction at hip and knee and principally inversion at the ankle.

At the hip, the maximal adduction moments occur just before foot flat, when maximal vertical load is being applied and maximal lateral displacement of the pelvis occurs. The patient must therefore have strong abductor muscles to overcome this adductor moment, otherwise a Trendelenburg gait is produced. At the knee the adductor moment is controlled by the integrity of the ligaments, rather than muscular control. At the ankle, the movements of inversion and eversion, which take place mainly at the subtalar joint, control foot position in this plane.

Prosthetic considerations. At the hip, the transfemoral socket design and suspension will assist the control of the adductor moment.

At the foot, the multiaxial ankle and DER feet (see Ch. 8) will help to absorb inversion and eversion, as will the type of shoe worn.

Analysis in the transverse plane

A set of complex, transverse rotations take place in the pelvis, hip joint, femur and tibia. The swinging limb pivots about its long axis in an outward direction and is suddenly pivoted in the opposite direction at full weightbearing or at the moment of foot flat.

Swing phase is characterised by the external rotation of all segments. The leg segments rotate in the same direction as, and in phase with, pelvic rotation.

Stance phase from heel strike to foot flat is characterised by internal rotation of the segments of the leg.

Prosthetic considerations. The rotation factor is of great importance to the amputee, as in all but the hip disarticulation levels of amputation

Table 9.1 Prosthetic components available during the stance phase.

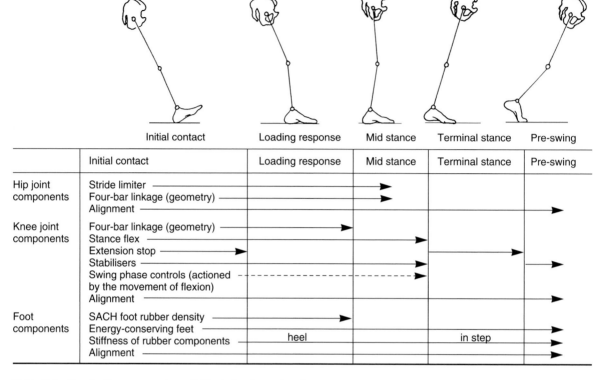

	Initial contact	Loading response	Mid stance	Terminal stance	Pre-swing
Hip joint components	Stride limiter ⟶ Four-bar linkage (geometry) ⟶ Alignment ————————————————⟶				
Knee joint components	Four-bar linkage (geometry) ⟶ Stance flex ——————————————⟶ Extension stop ⟶ Stabilisers ——————————————⟶ Swing phase controls (actioned - - - - - - - - ⟶ by the movement of flexion) Alignment ————————————————⟶				
Foot components	SACH foot rubber density ⟶ Energy-conserving feet ————————⟶ Stiffness of rubber components ——— heel ——————— in step ——⟶ Alignment ———————————————————————⟶				

Table 9.2 Prosthetic components available during the swing phase.

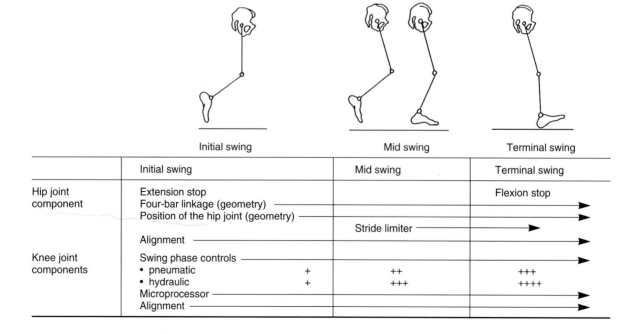

	Initial swing	Mid swing	Terminal swing
Hip joint component	Extension stop Four-bar linkage (geometry) ⟶ Position of the hip joint (geometry) ⟶ Alignment ———————————————⟶	Stride limiter ⟶	Flexion stop
Knee joint components	Swing phase controls ———————⟶ • pneumatic + • hydraulic + Microprocessor ———————————⟶ Alignment ——————————————⟶	++ +++	+++ ++++

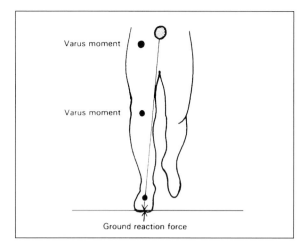

Figure 9.16 Frontal analysis.

the kinetic factors of hip motion are still present. When the amputee walks in a prosthesis, these rotation forces are transmitted down through the prosthesis to the ground, tending to rotate it in the transverse plane. These forces are absorbed at the residual limb/socket interface where friction can result, and this may be a major source of discomfort and skin breakdown. The amputee may then display various gait abnormalities to try and reduce this socket discomfort. This is why socket design is of the utmost importance (see Ch. 8).

Prosthetic components available to absorb some of the rotation forces are silicone sockets, torque absorbers, multiaxial foot and DER feet.

ENERGY COST OF AMBULATION

Much research has been carried out on the amount of energy required by physically fit people when they are walking; this has been compared with the amount of energy required by amputees walking similar distances. The amount of energy required by amputees is greater than that required in normal gait and it varies depending upon the level of amputation, the length of the residual limb, the reason for the amputation, the prosthetic design, the age of the patient and the speed of walking. Average adult human walking speed is 1.2 m/s. Any disabled person

with gait problems will require more energy to walk the same distance at a similar speed, and amputees as well as other disabled people, tend to walk more slowly than their natural walking speed in order to keep their energy expenditure to a minimum. As the amputation level ascends, the average walking speed progressively decreases resulting in an overall increased energy expenditure (Waters et al). Not surprisingly, bilateral amputees expend more energy than unilateral amputees. Interestingly, unilateral amputees using a prosthesis, without crutches, have a lower rate of energy expenditure than non-amputees using crutches.

Examples of the energy consumption required at different levels of amputation will be found in many research papers, although the findings will vary depending upon the factors measured. However, in general, the following applies:

- Unilateral trans-tibial amputees require up to 9% more mean oxygen consumption than normal.
- Unilateral trans-femoral amputees require up to 49% more mean oxygen consumption than normal.
- Bilateral trans-femoral amputees require up to 280% more mean oxygen consumption than normal (Huang et al 1979).

PREREQUISITES OF NORMAL GAIT

The prerequisites of normal gait are (Gage 1991):

Stability in stance

The stance foot needs to be stable on the floor. The major lower extremity joints need to function in a normal fashion to allow advancement of the limb in swing, to allow balance and to provide propulsion. The COM must remain within the base of support while standing, and move forward from one base of support to the next while walking. Stability in stance requires trunk stability and adequate central balance.

Clearance in swing

This requires stability of the stance foot, appropriate positioning and power of the ankle, hip and knee on the stance side and adequate ankle dorsiflexion, knee flexion and hip flexion on the swing side.

Pre-position of the foot in terminal swing

On the stance side, this requires adequate stability, power and positioning of the limb. On the swing side, adequate ankle dorsiflexion and appropriate knee and foot positioning is necessary.

An adequate step length

This requires a stable and appropriately positioned stance limb, while the swing limb needs adequate hip flexion, relatively complete knee extension and neutral dorsiflexion.

Energy conservation

To conserve energy, the body uses several biomechanical mechanisms including joint stability provided by the GRF in conjunction with ligaments wherever possible. As discussed earlier, the COM excursion is minimised in all three planes to minimise energy expenditure.

TECHNIQUES OF GAIT ANALYSIS

'Clinical gait analysis' is a term that can be applied to numerous methods of evaluating a subject's walking pattern. Traditionally busy clinicians perform gait analysis by visual observation, however the complex nature of gait dysfunctions often defy simple observation and provide no quantitative basis for treatment. Recent advances in technology allow a more precise measurement of gait variables and methods include video-taping, kinematics, kinetics, electro-myography and energetics (Table 9.3). Modern gait analysis is based on the integration of these component methods of measurement and the data is used to help determine the surgical, orthotic, prosthetic and therapeutic treatment of a patient with ambulatory problems or to document the outcome of treatment.

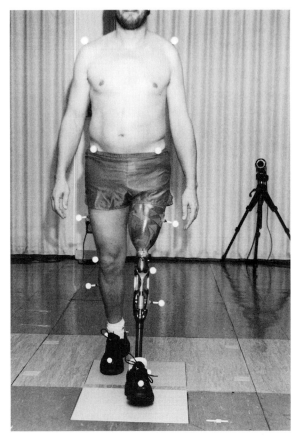

Figure 9.17 A trans-tibial amputee on the walkway of a gait laboratory. Note the markers attached to bony anatomical landmarks tracked with multi-camera system to give 3-dimensional analysis. (Photograph by kind permission of the Oxford Gait Laboratory).

Gait analysis has been found to be of great value in many pathologies, but at the present time is perhaps most highly developed clinically in neurological conditions, such as cerebral palsy and adult-onset hemiplegia, where complex gait deviations occur simultaneously in three planes of motion and primary deviations are often confounded with compensatory postures. A more scientific evaluation provided by gait analysis techniques has led to the development of new treatment protocols in this area. Gait assessment has also been widely used for evaluating the effectiveness of prosthetic limbs, including their alignment and performance, leading to improvements in prosthetic design.

Table 9.3 Techniques of gait analysis

Analysis	Technique	Comments
Visual	Observation	Subjective. Dependent on skilled clinician. Rapid, complex or subtle events missed. No permanent record
	Video	Descriptive, 2-dimensional in sagittal and coronal planes – complex rotations distorted. Slow motion analysis possible. Standardised technique will improve repeatability
Temporal and distance parameters	Stopwatch	Velocity = measured distance over time taken. Cadence = No. of steps per unit of time Interpret in relation to subject's age and sex
	Foot placement	Patient steps in ink/talcum powder then across floor. Measures taken of step and stride length, width of walking base and foot contact pattern
	Foot switches	Attach to soles of feet or shoes and record using computer. Measure cadence, stance and swing phase times, single and double support times. Awkward to position, especially if patient has abnormal foot contact pattern and switches can influence gait pattern
Foot pressure distribution	Static	Low technology systems such as Harris-Beath mat give semi-quantitative recordings of pressure distribution
	Dynamic	A number of quantitative force sensor systems available. Possible to measure pressure inside shoes, but technically more difficult than barefoot. Measurement of foot pressure can be particularly valuable in conditions where pressure likely to be excessive, e.g. diabetic neuropathy or rheumatoid arthritis
Kinematics	Electrogoniometry	Device strapped to the limb to make continuous measures of joint angles in one or more planes. Subject to alignment errors
	Passive and active marker systems (see Fig. 9.17)	Modern systems utilise 2-dimensional and 3-dimensional analysis using lightweight external markers attached to bony anatomical landmarks tracked with multi-camera systems
Electromyography (EMG)		Dynamic EMGs record muscle action potential during gait cycle. Provides information on phasic activity of muscle but not on strength. Particularly useful in neurological disorders where muscle transfers are considered
	Surface EMG	Surface electrodes attached to skin suitable for recording large superficial muscles. 'Cross-talk' with adjacent muscles can be a problem
	Fine-wire EMG	Fine wire inserted via needle suitable for recording small or deep muscles. Electrode placement confirmed with stimulation
Kinetics (measurement of force)	Force platforms	Measures resultant ground reaction forces on load-bearing limb. Force information combined with kinematics allows for internal moments to be calculated
	Video-vector generator	Allows for visual appreciation of external joint moments when real-time ground reaction vector superimposed on video by processing force-plate and video signals – useful for tuning orthoses and prostheses
Energy expenditure	Heart rate	Gives an indirect indication of the energy being expended in walking with limited reliability
	Oxygen uptake/ CO_2 output	Gives an almost direct measurement of the energy being expended in walking

BIBLIOGRAPHY FOR PREVIOUS EDITIONS

Bard G, Ralston H J 1959 Measurement of energy expenditure during ambulation with special reference to the evaluation of assistive devices. Archives of Physical Medicine and Rehabilitation 40:415–420

Fisher S V 1978 Energy cost of ambulation in health and disability. A literature review. Archives of Physical Medicine and Rehabilitation 59:124–133

Gailey R, Kirk N 1991 Energy expenditure of below-knee amputees during unrestrained ambulation. WCPT 11th International Congress Proceedings Book II:650–652

Ganguli S, Datta S R, Chatterjee B B, Roy B N 1974 Metabolic cost of walking at different speeds with patellar tendon-bearing prosthesis. Journal of Applied Physiology 36(4):440–443

Huang C T, Jackson J R, Moore N B et al 1979 Amputation: energy cost of ambulation. Archives of Physical Medicine and Rehabilitation 60:18–24

Hughes J, Jacobs N 1979 Normal human locomotion. Prosthetics and Orthotics International 3:4–12

Little H 1981 Gait analysis for physiotherapy departments: a review of current methods. Physiotherapy 67(11):334–337

Netz, Weisen, Wetterberg 1981 Videotape recording – a complementary aid for the walking training of lower limb amputees. Prosthetics and Orthotics International 5:147–150

Nowroozi F, Salvenelli M 1983 Energy expenditure in hip disarticulation and hemipelvectomy amputees. Archives of Physical Medicine and Rehabilitation 64(7):300–303

Patla A E, Proctor J, Morson B 1987 Observations on aspects of visual gait assessment: a questionnaire study. Physiotherapy Canada 39(5):311–316

Robinson J L, Smidt G L 1981 Quantitative gait evaluation in the clinic. Physical Therapy 61(3):351–353

Rose G K 1983 Clinical gait assessment: a personal view. Journal of Medical Engineering and Technology 7(6):273–279

Saunders J B de C N, Inman V T, Eberhart H D 1953 The major determinant in normal and pathological gait. Journal of Bone and Joint Surgery 35-A:543–548

Sethi P K 1977 The foot and footwear. Prosthetics and Orthotics International 1(3):173–182

Smith D M, Lord M, Kinnear E M L 1983 A video aid to assessment and retraining of standing balance. In: Perkins W J (ed) High technology aids for the disabled. Butterworths, London

Winter D A 1980 Overall principle of lower limb support during stance phase of gait. Journal of Biomechanics 13:923–927

BIBLIOGRAPHY FOR THE THIRD EDITION

Bohannon R W, Andrews A W, Thomas M W 1996 Walking speed: reference values and correlates for older adults. Journal of Orthopaedic and Sports Physical Therapy 24(2):86–90

Czerniecki J M 1996 Rehabilitation in limb deficiency. 1. Gait and motion analysis. Archives of Physical Medicine and Rehabilitation 77(3):S3–S8

Czerniecki J M, Gitter A, Weaver K 1994 Effect of alterations in prosthetic shank mass on the metabolic costs of ambulation in above-knee amputees. American Journal of Physical Medicine and Rehabilitation 73(5):348–352

Engsberg J R, Lee A G, Tedford K G, Harder J A 1993 Normative ground reaction force data for able-bodied and trans-tibial amputee children during running. Prosthetics and Orthotics International 17:83–89

Gage J R 1991 Gait analysis in cerebral palsy. MacKeith Press, London

Gailey R S 1997 Prosthetic and orthotic assessments: lower extremity prosthetics. In: Van Deusen J, Brunt D Assessment in occupational therapy and physical therapy. WB Saunders Company, Philadelphia

Gitter A, Czerniecki J, Meinders M 1997 Effect of prosthetic mass on swing phase work during above-knee amputee ambulation. American Journal of Physical Medicine and Rehabilitation 76(2):114–121

Gitter A, Czerniecki J, Weaver K 1995 A reassessment of center-of-mass dynamics as a determinate of the metabolic inefficiency of above-knee amputee ambulation. American Journal of Physical Medicine and Rehabilitation 74(5):332–338

Hurley G R B, McKenny R, Robinson M, Zadravec M, Pierrynowski M R 1990 The role of the contralateral limb in below-knee amputee gait. Prosthetics and Orthotics International 14(1):33–42

Seroussi E, Gitter A, Czerniecki J M, Weaver K 1996 Mechanical work adaptations of above knee amputee ambulation. Archives of Physical Medicine and Rehabilitation 77: 1209–1214

Waters S R L, Perry J, Antonelli D, Hislop H, Downey P 1976 Energy cost of amputees: the influence of level of amputation. Journal of Bone and Joint Surgery 58A:42–46

Winter D A 1991 The biomechanics and motor control of human gait, 2nd edn. University of Waterloo Press, Waterloo, Ontario

10

Gait re-education and prosthetic functional activity

Ideally, prosthetic rehabilitation should take place as part of inpatient care, as a more successful functional outcome is achieved and the amputee is discharged with a 'complete' body image. However, many hospitals have constraints on their beds and prosthetic rehabilitation takes place on an outpatient basis.

As the amputee will have been mobile using an early walking aid, e.g. Ppam aid, and will have had gait re-education within the limits of the device, it is important there is continuity from this stage to the prosthetic stage. If there is a delay in organising an appointment the amputee may attempt to use the prosthesis, and as a result will usually produce a poor walking pattern that is difficult to alter later on, even with expert tuition. Some older amputees will sit and await instruction; delay will result in their physical condition deteriorating and the prostheses will no longer fit them. Therefore, the hospital therapist must keep in contact with amputees, whether they are still in hospital or at home and be aware of all prosthetic appointments and delivery dates.

Planning of transport arrangements to the therapy facility must be made. Not all therapy facilities are able to arrange gait re-education (this is usually because of transport difficulties) so that referral to another location must be made. These arrangements are time-consuming and difficult but must be pursued with vigour. If none of these arrangements are possible then referral to the community therapist can be made. Indeed, the home environment can be the most relevant place for retraining functional activity.

Treatment should be given on a daily basis, but it may be necessary to fit the therapy around visits from community services and clinic appointments. Amputees should attend for a whole morning or afternoon, or both, so that sufficient time is given to exercise, walking, rest periods and socialising with other amputees, gaining advice from either them, the therapist or counsellor regarding other rehabilitation matters. Treatment does not have to be on a one-to-one basis; a rehabilitation environment is preferable, e.g. in a gymnasium where several amputees can be treated simultaneously.

The advantages of daily treatment are:

1. Continuity of treatment improves prosthetic re-education and acceptance of the prosthesis by the amputee.
2. The amputee adjusts more quickly to the new body image.
3. The skin toughens more quickly to tolerate new weightbearing areas.
4. Functional activities other than walking are practised, e.g. donning and doffing the prosthesis, attending meals and sitting in different chairs, using the lavatory, carrying out functional tasks and walking outside the actual treatment area. All activities must be relevant to the amputee's individual needs.
5. Independence using the prosthesis is achieved more quickly. For example, a unilateral trans-tibial amputee may only need 1 week of gait re-education; the unilateral trans-femoral amputee may only need 2 weeks of gait re-education, but the bilateral amputee, particularly without natural knee joints, is more likely to take over 1 month to walk with reasonable independence. (see Ch. 7)

GOAL PLANNING

The pattern of walking exhibited by an individual represents their solution to the problem of how to get from one place to another with minimum effort, adequate stability and acceptable appearance. The relative importance attached to each of these aspects differs from one individual to another.

As stated in Chapter 9, the appearance of normal gait is the sum total of the various characteristic determinants of human locomotion. The gait of an amputee will depend upon the condition of the determinants remaining, e.g. joints, skeletal links, muscles, body shape and weight, the extent to which the prosthetic replacements mimic the original body parts and the interface between body and prosthesis.

Before starting gait re-education it is important that the therapist has realistic goals in mind and discusses these with the amputee. The following points should be considered while assessing the amputee at the first treatment session (see Chs 2 and 7):

— Diagnosis
— Concurrent medical problems
— Life expectancy
— Age
— Physical state and functional capabilities
— State of psychological adjustment
— Social and housing situation
— The amputee's expectations with the prosthesis supplied.

Initial stages

The therapist must follow an organised sequence of re-examination of the amputee and detailed inspection of the prosthesis even before applying the prosthesis.

Examination of the amputee

All the features of the original examination database (see Ch. 2) are re-checked or, if the amputee is new to the therapist, carried out in full. Particular emphasis is now paid to the mobility of the trunk, which plays such a large part in the maintenance of a symmetrical gait pattern.

Inspection of the residual limb

In addition to the general examination of range of movement and muscle power, the residual limb should be inspected for shape, muscle cover, distal bone bevelling, areas of skin redness or breakdown and a close inspection is made of any scars. If the amputation scar is unhealed, or adherent to the underlying soft tissue or bone, it will suffer trauma when in the close fitting socket of the prosthesis and therefore the length of time that the prosthesis is worn must be limited. This is particularly important with the trans-tibial level of amputation in a patellar tendon bearing prosthesis (see Ch. 15).

Check of the prosthesis

The prothesis is checked on its own, *before* the amputee dons it. Unless all the features of the prosthesis are understood by the therapist, correct gait training will be impossible. A careful inspection must be made of the:

- *suspension, joints and socket* (see Chapters 12–16 for specific details concerning the level of amputation)
- *static alignment and shoe.* A prosthesis should stand in a vertical position on a flat surface without any support. If the shoe heel height is not the one for which the limb was made, the prosthesis will appear to incline either forwards or backwards, as the keel of the prosthetic foot will not be correctly balanced by the heel height of the shoe.

The stump sock

There are many different types of sock (see Ch. 8) and the first prosthesis for a primary amputee should ideally fit with one sock, but as residual limb volume varies considerably in the early stages, a variety of socks should have been supplied. The therapist can then experiment with them in order to achieve the correct fit of the socket (see Chapters 12–16 for specific details).

Check fit of the prosthesis

The weightbearing areas, suspension, length, alignment and comfort must all be checked prior to gait re-education (see Chapters 12–16 for specific details).

In the parallel bars

All gait re-education should start in the parallel bars. However, if these are not available, e.g. in an amputee's home, a suitably safe support should be devised, such as holding a fixed work surface or chair back.

With the feet at a normal base width (i.e. 5–10 cm) and with both hands holding the bars, weight transference is attempted over the prosthesis. The aim is for the supporting limb to be in the mid-line of the body. This can be assisted by the therapist directing the movement of the pelvis and shoulder manually and progressing to a resisted movement. This side-to-side weight transference is then practised with the contralateral hand only holding the bar and progressed to the ipsilateral hand only, which is more difficult. Rhythmic stabilisations in standing with a normal base width, and then stride standing are practised to encourage balance.

After these preliminary exercises, and frequent rests if required, walking is then started holding both bars, and stepping off with the sound limb. The aim is for a symmetrical gait pattern; this is achieved when the pelvis moves forward over the supporting limb, equal stride length is made, correct reciprocal trunk movements occur and the hands are advanced in the correct rhythm. The therapist must be inside the parallel bars either in front or behind the amputee. The therapist will be able to work comfortably here and avoid back strain, by sitting on an adjustable stool on wheels, easily scooting along to accommodate the velocity of the amputee's gait, giving guidance to the pelvis, shoulder or prosthesis and either assisting the movement or resisting it.

Many amputees find achievement of a symmetrical gait pattern difficult, and unless sufficient time and manual guidance are given at this early stage, gait faults appear. Walking must continue in the bars in a forward, sideways and backwards direction, paying particular attention to reciprocal trunk rotation.

Progression out of the parallel bars

Progression from here is dependent on the general capabilities of the individual amputee. Most primary amputees of all levels should aim to walk with two sticks, progressing to one or none when the skin of weightbearing areas has more tolerance and strength, and balance and confidence have improved. If crutches are used, little of the progression described above occurs and progression in amputee gait training is inhibited; however, crutches may be needed for painful residual limbs. The walking frame is the walking aid of last resort for the amputee, as it forces the hips into flexion, causing incorrect weight-bearing areas on the socket; the pelvis does not move vertically over the supporting limb, the trunk cannot rotate and a symmetrical pattern is impossible.

The gait pattern that is adopted in the early stages of rehabilitation becomes fixed in the amputee's mind; therefore it is worth all the time and resource implications in these early sessions to aim for a good gait pattern with walking sticks. Retraining the amputee with sticks after they have used crutches or a frame is extremely difficult and often unsuccessful.

Prosthetic functional activity

When the amputee is walking out of the parallel bars, standing activities and functional walking can be started. Work in the kitchen is applicable to most amputees and practise of a familiar or necessary activity will build confidence (see Fig. 10.1). Initially, all equipment can be on the work surface so no reaching or bending is required; as confidence grows, the task can be made more complex.

As the amputee thinks about the task rather than their walking, their gait may become more spontaneous and natural, or the pattern may deteriorate. It is important to encourage the best possible gait pattern and to stand with weight evenly distributed between both feet. If an amputee uses walking aids, the use of a trolley at home may be necessary for moving items around the kitchen or to other rooms and they should be taught the correct way to use it.

Activities can be graded so there is more walking required, reaching, bending, lifting, walking in confined spaces, through doorways and on different floor surfaces; all these activities prepare the amputee for use of their prosthesis in their daily lives.

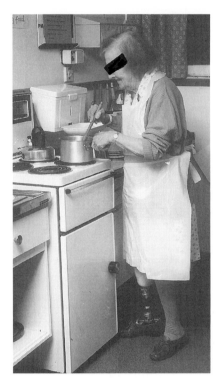

Figure 10.1 A trans-tibial amputee engaged in functional domestic activity. (Photograph by kind permission of Richmond, Twickenham and Roehampton Healthcare NHS Trust).

More active amputees benefit from more vigorous activities such as woodwork or gardening, involving transferring weight evenly, reaching up and down, sitting on the floor, kneeling and getting up, and lifting objects. Walking outside in public environments, e.g. walking on pavements, crossing roads, entering shops and buildings, using public transport, using stairs and escalators, should be practised with a therapist first, so that possible hazards are identified and overcome before the amputee attempts them alone (see Ch. 18).

Young fit unilateral amputee

The aim of re-education for this amputee is always to attain a normal gait pattern. Full strength of all muscle groups and full mobility of trunk and all joints are essential to achieve this.

The exercise programme should be concurrent with prosthetic education.

Observation of the amputee can only be carried out if the amputee is suitably undressed in order that arms, trunk, spine, hips and knees are clearly visible. Observation of the whole body should be made, from head to foot, from the front, the sides and from behind.

The amputee then progresses to using two sticks; these aids are necessary to prevent any gait deviation as a result of skin soreness from the weightbearing areas. Sticks should not be discarded too quickly as deterioration of the gait pattern can occur.

Visual feedback of performance can be aided by the use of mirrors or video equipment to reinforce the therapist's instructions.

The rehabilitation programme must be fitted around other important aspects of the amputee's life, e.g. school, college or employment. The importance of follow-up visits is discussed so that checks on the gait pattern are maintained; the young amputee can easily adopt an incorrect gait pattern during the early stages of prosthetic use. Also, progression of mobility into leisure activities and sports can be advised at the right time (see Ch. 18).

There is, however, a group of amputees whose gait pattern deteriorates after discharge from therapy. This is thought to be because of a psychological need to present to others a visible disability. These individuals are often quite capable of walking normally but choose not to do so. The therapist must be aware of this so that at follow-up visits the emphasis is on psychological support with a clinical psychologist or counsellor's help, rather than criticism of the observed gait. This may gradually improve as the amputee adjusts to the new situation.

Older unilateral amputee

The aim for this amputee is to attain the best possible gait pattern, bearing in mind that certain physical problems (e.g. flexion contracture, claudication, cardiorespiratory limitation) may limit normal pattern. A daily exercise programme will minimise their effects.

First, a check is made to see if the amputee can don and doff the prosthesis, and advice is given if there are clothing difficulties. After initial instruction from the therapist, amputees can be left to practise gait on their own for short periods when it is safe to do so; rest periods should be allowed as much as required. Further instruction and correction are given as necessary. The use of mirrors at this stage helps some, giving visual feedback of the gait pattern.

For these amputees, progress is slow but steady. It has been found that daily attendance for gait re-education hastens mobility and the use of just one, or two, sticks can be achieved. Social activities and activities of daily living should then be encouraged. Consideration of home environment and confidence levels are as important as physical ability.

Following discharge, review and treatment are necessary when the prescription of the prosthesis changes, or if the medical condition alters. Consideration can be given to suitable sports or social activities as the amputee becomes more confident (see Ch. 18).

Frail elderly amputee and those with multiple medical problems

The rehabilitation aims for these amputees are safety and function. The actual gait pattern achieved is irrelevant and formal gait training unnecessary. The most important task is to identify the individual's needs by visiting the home environment.

In the therapy department, the amputee first learns how to don and doff the prosthesis. This process may take some time to achieve and adaptations to the suspension of the prosthesis may be helpful. There is little point in continuing with the prosthesis if the amputee cannot don it independently when no help is available at home.

The amputee must not only learn to walk, but must be able to stand up from and sit down on a chair without overbalancing. Transfers must be performed safely; these amputees cannot afford to fall as the result may prove to be catastrophic.

Short treatment sessions spaced throughout

the day, with simple but repetitive activity, have been found to achieve the best result. This group needs to be treated symptomatically; if they are unwell for the occasional session they should be allowed to rest. However, a little activity should be tried each day.

The therapist must be aware that this group of amputees may not succeed in using a prosthesis. If there is no indication that independence will be achieved, even after a fair trial, then a positive decision must be made with the individual and carer to stop gait re-education. Wheelchair re-education continues and each functional activity necessary to the individual along with leisure activities are explored.

For those who are progressing, the walking aid chosen must be the safest in the home surroundings: for many this will be a walking frame.

Once a comfortable fit of the prosthesis has been achieved, and the amputee is safe while walking, the community therapist should re-educate for functional activities within the home: other members of the primary healthcare team can give support. Treatment in the therapy facility then ceases but may be restarted, for a short intensive period, if referral back from the community is made. An example of this is if the amputee stops using the prosthesis because of a short illness, e.g. chest infection, abdominal operation or immobility following a fall, etc.

Those with progressive disease and the frail elderly may find that prostheses are of no functional use and in no way enhance the quality of their life. Careful assessment and exploration of their thoughts and feelings should be sensitively made before returning the prosthesis to the prosthetic centre. Some feel that their prosthesis, which they have had for some time, is a real part of them and suffer a reaction if it is removed against their wishes.

Bilateral amputee

The aim of gait re-education is governed by:

- the presence of natural knee joints
- the ability to don the prostheses
- associated diseases
- adequate cardiorespiratory status

- home environment and carer support
- the individual's motivation

The bilateral trans-tibial amputee will achieve a normal gait pattern but other levels will almost always appear laboured. The gait pattern achieved and successful prosthetic outcome will depend on the levels of amputation.

In the therapy facility, the amputee is taught how to don and doff the prostheses. This requires time, patience, perseverance and much practice. The amputee then dresses and commences walking in the parallel bars. Standing up and sitting down can be difficult and requires considerable practice and experimentation using different chair designs. The bilateral amputee remains in the parallel bars for many treatment sessions, as balance takes some time to achieve and skin tolerance takes time to build up.

Bilateral amputees find standing difficult due to continuous weight bearing on their residual limbs. It is necessary to practice standing for short periods initially with support, doing simple unilateral activities and progressing to more complex bilateral tasks.

The energy required to use two prostheses is very high and time should be allowed for amputees to gradually increase their stamina: the higher the levels of amputation, the greater the energy cost when walking.

Once some balance has been achieved, the bilateral amputee progresses to using walking aids: the choice is between quadrapods and walking sticks. It is not safe for a bilateral amputee to use a frame as the base is not always wide enough for their stance; there is a tendency for the bilateral amputee to fall backwards whilst lifting the frame and the considerable side-to-side trunk sway required to initiate swing phase may make the frame tip sideways. The advantages of quadrapods are that they are stable, free standing and can be correctly positioned before the amputee stands up. The disadvantage is that the combined width of the bilateral amputee and quadrapods is considerable; this is a point to consider if they live in a small home. Also, some find their appearance unacceptable.

If, after a fair trial of gait re-education throughout several sessions, the bilateral amputee is unable to walk outside the parallel bars using aids, then it is obvious that prosthetic use will not enhance their lifestyle. A positive decision must be made with the individual to stop using prostheses, to continue rehabilitation in a suitable wheelchair and explore leisure activities.

For those amputees who are able to walk with aids, functional tasks should be practised, walking in confined spaces and on different floor surfaces and the therapist must visit their homes to see if they can manage. It may be apparent that even though the amputee can walk well in the therapy facility, prosthetic use at home may be a hindrance.

For those who manage well, follow-up treatment sessions will be necessary when the prosthetic prescription changes or there are changes in health status and new social activities wish to be tried.

Bilateral amputees require a great deal of time (2–3 hours) for each treatment session. The therapist must take this into account when organising the place and time of treatment. The exercise programme should continue concurrently with prosthetic education.

OBSERVATIONAL GAIT ANALYSIS

The gait should first be analysed visually in the parallel bars. An overall view of the whole patient is taken from the front, at the side and from behind. It is often helpful if the therapist sits on a low stool to observe movement of the pelvis and legs. The analysis then proceeds to observing the gait pattern during both stance and swing phases. This analysis is carried out at every treatment session. Slow motion video recordings in the frontal and sagittal planes may be helpful in the analysis of gait deviation. A table of detailed gait analysis techniques is given in Chapter 9. Common gait faults are given in Tables 10.1 and 10.2, pp 136–140.

Any observed deviation should be noted. It is important that these deviations are expressed in standard terminology used by a prosthetist, so that discussion between the therapist and the prosthetist is readily understandable.

Causes of gait abnormalities

These may be:

1. The general condition of the amputee
2. The shape, length and size of the residual limb and any discomfort present
3. Prosthetic malfunction
4. Inadequate or incorrect re-education
5. Psychological, social or economic reasons.

The purpose of identifying gait deviation and its cause is to improve the gait pattern towards the normal. This may be achieved by medical or surgical treatment, therapeutic measures, psychological help, prosthetic alteration, or by gait re-education. These treatments are to the amputee's advantage because the nearer to normal the gait pattern becomes, the less energy is consumed. Therefore, the exercise tolerance is extended, and as a result the individual feels less disabled. However, the therapist often treats the amputee during the early stages in which the residual limb is still maturing and it will be found that many gait deviations will be caused simply by residual limb discomfort and volumetric changes.

Compensatory patterns

Each amputee's gait is individual and has its own compensatory pattern. This may have been present before the amputation, but it may have been caused by walking in an uncomfortable prosthesis at an earlier stage without adequate rehabilitation. The former pattern cannot usually be evaluated but the latter should have been avoided. Exceptionally, some amputees have never been referred for gait re-education and will have taught themselves and managed the best they can.

ACKNOWLEDGEMENTS

The authors acknowledge teaching material from the University of Strathclyde, Glasgow, New York University and Northwestern University, Chicago, USA.

Table 10.1 Gait abnormalities of the trans-tibial type level using a patellar tendon bearing (PTB) prosthesis

Deviation	Amputee cause	Prosthetic cause
1. *Excessive knee flexion* during stance phase	1. Fixed flexion of knee and hip joint 2. Compensatory pattern 3. Pain	1. Excessive dorsiflexion of prosthetic foot 2. Socket incorrectly aligned: either insufficient flexion set in the socket, or set too far forward on the foot 3. Socket ill-fitting 4. Cuff suspension faulty 5. Excessively stiff plantar flexion of prosthetic foot
2. *Insufficient knee flexion or hyperextension* during the stance phase N.B. PTB sockets are aligned with 5° flexion	1. Quadriceps too weak to support flexed knee 2. Knee joint instability 3. Residual limb discomfort 4. Particularly common if amputee is used to a thigh corset prosthesis as the patient has difficulty establishing this new knee pattern	1. Excessive plantar flexion of foot 2. Too hard a plantar flexion resistance 3. Socket incorrectly aligned: either too flexed or socket set too far back on the foot
3. *Rotation of foot*	1. Weak muscles around the hip 2. Knee joint instability combined with knee muscle weakness 3. Pain	1. Too hard a plantar flexion resistance 2. Ill-fitting socket 3. Poor suspension
4. *Lateral shift of the prosthesis* during stance phase	1. Residual limb pain 2. Knee joint instability	1. Incorrect alignment of prosthesis: socket too abducted or the foot is set too far medially
5. *Lateral bending of the trunk* during stance phase (patient leans towards the prosthesis)	1. Painful stump or pain in the remaining leg 2. Lack of balance 3. Lack of confidence 4. Muscle imbalance, weakness at the hip joint 5. Compensatory pattern	1. Prosthesis too short 2. Incorrect alignment: socket too adducted or the foot is set too far laterally
6. *Drop off* Knee flexion occurs too early in stance phase	1. No identifiable cause	1. Excessive dorsiflexion of foot 2. Incorrect alignment: socket set too far forward
7. *Delayed knee flexion* during the swing phase	1. Problems with pelvic and hip movements 2. Knee joint stiffness 3. Compensatory pattern, after having used a thigh corset prosthesis	1. Inadequate suspension 2. Excessive plantar flexion of prosthetic foot
8. *General deviations*	1. Uneven arm swing 2. Uneven timing 3. Uneven steps 4. Amputee too tired to maintain a good gait pattern	

Table 10.2 Gait abnormalities of the trans-femoral and knee disarticulation levels of amputation. Each individual can only be expected to walk within their capabilities. Some gait deviations may occur because the prosthesis is too complicated for the individual. After a fair trial of gait re-education, the therapist should contact the prosthetist if there are problems, and suggest either modifications or a change of prescription

Deviation	Stiff knee gait		Free knee gait	
	Amputee causes	Prosthetic causes	Amputee causes	Prosthetic causes
1. *Abducted pattern* Amputee walking with wide base with prosthesis held away from the mid-line	1. Abduction contracture of residual limb 2. Adductor roll	1. Prosthesis too long 2. Medial brim of socket too high therefore causing discomfort on the pubic ramus 3. Lateral wall of socket giving insufficient support to femur 4. Rigid pelvic band alignment incorrect 5. Prosthesis incorrectly aligned: socket too adducted	Same reasons	Same reasons
2. *Lateral or side bending of the trunk* during stance phase	*Towards prosthetic side* 1. Abduction contracture of residual limb 2. Very short residual limb 3. Painful or sensitive residual limb 4. Weak hip abductors in residual limb *Away from prosthetic side*	*Towards prosthetic side* 1. Lateral wall of the socket may give insufficient support to the femur 2. Prosthesis too short 3. Prosthesis incorrectly aligned: socket too adducted 4. Medial brim of the socket giving discomfort causing pattern to lean away from it *Away from prosthetic side* 1. Prosthesis too long 2. Prosthesis incorrectly aligned: socket too abducted	Same reasons	Same reasons
3. *Rotation of foot at heel strike* usually outwards	1. Poor muscle control of the residual limb, extensors and medial rotators	1. Plantar flexion resistance too hard in prosthetic foot 2. Socket may be too loose 3. Prosthesis incorrectly aligned (too much toe out)	Same reasons	Same reasons
4. *Circumduction* Prosthesis is swung in a wide arc during swing phase	1. Abduction contracture of residual limb 2. Muscle imbalance: weak adductors of the residual limb and inability to hip hitch	1. Prosthesis too long 2. Inadequate suspension	1. Same reasons 2. Muscle weakness 3. Lack of confidence in flexing the knee	1. Same reasons 2. Too much stability, or too much friction in the knee mechanism

Table 10.2   (cont'd)

Deviation	Stiff knee gait — Amputee causes	Stiff knee gait — Prosthetic causes	Free knee gait — Amputee causes	Free knee gait — Prosthetic causes
5. *Vaulting* The amputee rises up on the toe of the remaining leg to swing the prosthesis through from toe off to heel strike	1. Fear of catching the toe of the prosthesis 2. Very short residual limb 3. Poor muscle control (hip hitching)	1. Prosthesis too long 2. Inadequate suspension	1. Same reasons 2. Poor muscle control of hip flexion	1. Same reasons 2. Too much stability or friction in the knee mechanism
6. *Uneven step length*	*Prosthetic step too long* (most common) 1. Inability to extend hip over prosthesis during stance phase, due to hip flexion contracture and weakness of hip and back extensors 2. Lack of confidence 3. Compensation, especially if initial gait rehabilitation was using a frame for aid *Short prosthetic step* 1. Lack of confidence 2. Pain	*Prosthetic step too long* (most common) 1. Flexion contracture not accommodated prosthetically 2. Prosthesis too long *Short prosthetic step* 1. Ill-fitting socket causing discomfort 2. Alignment incorrect: socket too flexed	*Prosthetic step too long* 1. Same reasons 2. Habit, to ensure prosthesis is flung into extension *Short prosthetic step* (most common) 1. Amputee feels insecure with the knee mechanism	*Prosthetic step too long* 1. Same reasons *Short prosthetic step* (most common) 1. Prosthetic knee may buckle because of incorrect alignment or adjustment: socket too flexed
7. *Uneven timing* Steps of unequal length usually characterised by a very short stance phase on the prosthesis	1. Lack of balance 2. Lack of confidence 3. Weak residual limb, trunk and remaining leg muscles 4. Compensatory pattern 5. Pain on the ischial tuberosity	1. Ill-fitting socket causing discomfort	Same reasons in free knee gait as 6	Same reasons in free knee gait as 6
8. *Uneven arm swing* The arm on the prosthetic side is usually held stiff to that side of the body. There is no natural swing	1. Lack of balance 2. Lack of confidence	1. Ill-fitting socket causing discomfort	Same reasons in free knee gait as 6 & 7	Same reasons in free knee gait as 6 & 7

N. B. Uneven step length, uneven timing and uneven arm swing are often seen in combination and are often a result of the same cause

Table 10.2 (cont'd)

Deviation	Stiff knee gait Amputee causes	Prosthetic causes	Free knee gait Amputee causes	Prosthetic causes
9. *Lumbar lordosis* During stance phase there is excessive curvature of the lumbar spine	1. Hip flexion contracture 2. Weak hip extensors 3. Weak abdominal muscles 4. Attempt to move centre of gravity forwards to improve stability	1. Insufficient flexion in socket alignment 2. Discomfort on ischial weightbearing area 3. Heel of shoe on prosthesis too high	Same reasons	1. Same reasons 2. Insufficient stability in knee mechanism
10. *Forward trunk flexion*	1. Weak hip extensors 2. Hip flexion contracture 3. Poor general posture 4. Kyphosed spine 5. Compensation, looking at feet, from walking with a frame, or because of poor eyesight	1. Insufficient flexion built into socket 2. Socket discomfort	Same reasons	1. Same reasons 2. Insufficient stability in knee mechanism
11. *Drop off* There is a downwards movement of the body as weight is transferred forwards over the prosthetic foot	1. Wearing the incorrect heel height of shoe	1. Too soft a dorsiflexion resistance in prosthetic foot 2. Socket too anterior to the foot	Same reasons	Same reasons
12. *Foot slap* Prosthetic forefoot audibly slaps down onto floor at heel strike	1. Driving prosthetic heel into ground excessively because of fear of instability of the knee 2. Wearing incorrect shoe for the set of prosthetic foot	1. Plantar flexion resistance too soft. It does not offer sufficient resistance as weight is transferred onto the prosthesis	Same reasons	Same reasons
13. *Uneven heel rise* Heel of prosthesis rises upwards excessively when knee flexes at beginning of swing phase	N/A	N/A	1. Too much hip flexor muscle power used to flex the prosthetic knee	1. Prosthetic knee flexes too easily 2. Swing phase controls adjusted incorrectly

Table 10.2 (cont'd)

Deviation	Stiff knee gait		Free knee gait	
	Amputee causes	Prosthetic causes	Amputee causes	Prosthetic causes
14. a. *Medial whip* Heel travels medially on initial flexion at beginning of swing phase	N/A	N/A	*Medial* Walking habits caused by residual limb discomfort or a problem in the remaining leg	*Medial* Excessive external rotation of prosthetic knee *Lateral* Excessive internal rotation of prosthetic knee *Generally* 1. The socket may be too tight a fit 2. The socket may be too loose 3. Incorrect alignment at toe off 4. Excessive valgus or varus set into the prosthesis at the knee level
b. *Lateral whip* Heel travels laterally on initial flexion at beginning of swing phase	N/A	N/A	*Lateral* Same as above	
15. *Terminal swing impact* Knee reaches extension too quickly prior to heel strike	N/A	N/A	1. Residual limb forcibly flexes to produce full extension of the knee to ensure safety 2. Compensatory pattern 3. Lack of confidence This is often seen in combination with too long a prosthetic step	1. Incorrect adjustment of swing phase controls

BIBLIOGRAPHY FOR PREVIOUS EDITIONS

Breakey J 1976 Gait of unilateral below-knee amputees. Orthotics and Prosthetics 30(3):17–24

Buttenshaw P Dolman J 1992 The Roehampton approach to rehabilitation: a retrospective survey of prosthetic use in patients with primary unilateral lower limb amputation. Topics in Geriatric Medicine 8(1):72–78

Culham E G, Peat M, Newell E 1984 Analysis of gait following below-knee amputation: a comparison of the SACH and single-axis foot. Physiotherapy Canada 36(5):237–242

Day H J B 1981 The assessment and description of amputee activity. Prosthetics and Orthotics International 5:23–28

Foort J 1979 Alignment of the above-knee prosthesis. Prosthetics and Orthotics International 3:137–139

Friberg O 1984 Biomechanical significance of the correct length of lower limb prostheses: a clinical and radiological study. Prosthetics and Orthotics International 8:124–129

Ishai G, Bar A, Susak Z 1983 Effects of alignment variables on thigh axial torque during swing phase in AK amputee gait. Prosthetics and Orthotics International 7:41–47

Kay J 1991 Domiciliary rehabilitation of elderly amputees. Physiotherapy 77(1):60–61

Klenerman L, Dobbs R J, Weller C et al 1988 Bringing gait analysis out of the laboratory and into the clinic. Age and Ageing 17:397–450

Lord M, Smith D M 1984 Foot loading in amputee stance. Prosthetics and Orthotics International 8:159–164

May D R W, Davis B 1974 Gait and the lower-limb amputee. Physiotherapy 60(6):166–171

Murray M P et al 1983 Gait patterns in above-knee amputee patients: hydraulic swing control vs constant-friction knee components. Archives of Physical Medicine and Rehabilitation 64:339–345

Patrick J H 1991 Movement analysis improves diagnostic ability. Medical Audit News 1(6):91–92

Saleh M, Murdoch G 1985 In defence of gait analysis: observation and measurement in gait analysis. Journal of Bone and Joint Surgery 67B(2):237–241

Stillman B 1991 Computer-based video analysis of movement. Australian Journal of Physiotherapy 37:219–227

Wall J C, Charteris J, Turnbull G I 1987 Two steps equals one stride equals what?: the applicability of normal gait nomenclature to abnormal walking patterns. Clinical Biomechanics 2:119–125

BIBLIOGRAPHY FOR THE THIRD EDITION

Cobb J W 1992 Models for delivery of prosthetic services to geriatric patients. Topics in Geriatric Rehabilitation 8(1):59–63

Collin C, Collin J 1995 Mobility after lower-limb amputation. British Journal of Surgery 82:1010–1011

Dingwell J B, Davis B L, Frazier D M 1996 Use of an instrumented treadmill for real-time gait symmetry evaluation and feedback in normal and trans-tibial amputee subjects. Prosthetics and Orthotics International 20:101–110

English R D, Hubbard W A, McElroy G K 1995 Establishment of consistent gait after fitting of new components. Journal of Rehabilitation Research and Development 32(1):32–35

Hunter D, Smith Cole E, Murray J M, Murray T D 1995 Energy expenditure of below-knee amputees during harness-supported treadmill ambulation. Journal of Orthopaedics and Sports Physical Therapy 21(5):268–276

Jaegers S M H J, Arendzen J H, de Jongh H J 1995 Prosthetic gait of unilateral trans-femoral amputees: a kinematic study. Archives of Physical Medicine and Rehabilitation 76:736–743

Lemaire E D, Fisher F R, Robertson D G E 1993 Gait patterns of elderly men with trans-tibial amputations. Prosthetics and Orthotics International 17:27–37

Lemaire E D, Fisher F R 1994 Osteoarthritis and elderly amputee gait. Archives of Physical Medicine and Rehabilitation 75:1094–1099

Powers C M, Boyd L A, Fontaine C A, Perry J 1996 The influence of lower-extremity muscle force on gait characteristics in individuals with below-knee amputations secondary to vascular disease. Physical Therapy 76(4):369–377

Rossi S A, Doyle W, Skinner H B 1995 Gait initiation of persons with below-knee amputation: the characterization and comparison of force profiles. Journal of Rehabilitation Research and Development 32(2):120–127

Sener G, Yigiter K, Erbahceci F, Uygur F 1995 The effect of the prosthetic training based on proprioceptive feedback on weight bearing and gait biomechanics of above knee amputees. Proceedings of the 12th International Congress of the World Confederation of Physical Therapy, Washington

Shephard R J, Kavanagh T, Campbell R, Lorenz B 1994 Net oxygen costs of ambulation in normal subjects and subjects with lower limb amputations. Canadian Journal of Rehabilitation 8(2):97–107

Ward K H, Meyers M C 1995 Exercise performance of lower-extremity amputees. Sports Medicine 20(4):207–214

11

Practical advice for the amputee

The following advice is given to new amputees before discharge from therapy and is applicable throughout their whole life.

CARE OF THE RESIDUAL LIMB

Hygiene

The amputee should be made aware that there may be increased perspiration over the whole area of the residual limb that is encased in the prosthesis. Skin problems may occur if meticulous hygiene is not carried out.

The residual limb should be washed daily with mild soap and water and dried thoroughly with a clean towel, paying particular attention to skin folds; preferably this should be done in the evening, as a damp residual limb inserted into a socket at the start of the day can cause skin damage. In hot weather, the residual limb will need to be washed several times a day.

The skin of the residual limb must be examined daily for signs of chafing, using a mirror where necessary. If there is any skin break, blistering or other problems, it should be reported to the therapist or prosthetist at once; the prosthesis should not be worn until advice has been given.

No sticking plaster, spirit, cream, oil or medication should be put onto the residual limb unless advised to by a doctor.

To avoid skin problems, consider the following:

Stump sock: This must be clean and correctly pulled up so that there are no wrinkles inside the socket. Some amputees may have a skin sensitivity to certain materials, such as wool.

Prosthesis: A correct fit is essential.

Skin: If there is a skin problem, the amputee must seek medical advice; simple remedies are often successful but occasionally advice must be sought from a dermatologist. This is needed, in particular, for allergic and fungal skin conditions which residual limbs are prone to when encased in a prosthetic socket.

Residual limb complications

Examples are as follows:

- open wound
- wound sinus
- bone infection
- exostosis
- dermatitis
- oedema with suspected underlying pathology
- soft tissue lesion
- necrosis
- neuroma.

Often complications occur as a result of an ill-fitting prosthesis. The therapist can carry out simple measures to correct them (e.g. by altering the number of socks), but it may be necessary for the doctor and prosthetist in the prosthetic centre to carry out major adjustments or order a new prosthesis. Both the therapist and the amputee must be aware that seemingly minor residual limb problems can escalate drastically if they are not dealt with promptly. Occasionally it may be necessary to refer amputees back to their hospital surgeon.

When a prosthesis is not worn

The residual limb should be supported with a shrinker sock and elevated on a stump board.

CARE OF THE REMAINING LIMB

All lower limb amputees need to be aware that their ability to walk depends on the condition of the remaining limb. This is particularly vital for those suffering from peripheral vascular disease (PVD) and diabetes. It should also be noted that smoking tobacco is damaging to the remaining limb as well as the lungs.

Hygiene

The foot and leg should be washed daily with warm water and mild soap. After rinsing thoroughly, careful drying must be carried out and a soft towel used to blot in between the toes. The skin should not be rubbed vigorously. The community nurse or carer should be asked to carry out this procedure if the amputee is unable to do so.

Toenails should be cut with great care. After bathing, the nail is softer and easier to manage. The edge should be cut following the shape of the toe; the corners of the nails should never be cut back into the nail grooves. The nails should not be cut too short. If there is any difficulty, a qualified chiropodist must be consulted particularly for diabetic patients.

When the amputee is sitting down at home it is advisable to elevate the leg on a stool to prevent oedema. The legs must not be crossed. The heel should be protected to avoid heel ulceration from concentrated pressure. To keep warm, a rug should be used; avoid sitting with the remaining limb close to a fire.

Upper limb amputees who have a prosthesis with a set of appendages should take particular care of the hygiene of the axilla of the sound limb where the axilla loop is situated. Also, cutting fingernails is difficult and care should be taken using nail clippers on a board pressed down with the residual limb.

Peripheral neuropathy

One of the main problems for the diabetic patient is peripheral neuropathy. No opportunity should be lost by therapists, nurses or chiropodists to emphasise the danger of this lack of sensation to the patient.

The following advice must be given:

- Visually check the remaining foot daily. If the amputee has visual impairment the check should be made by a relative or community nurse.

- Use a thermometer to test the temperature of bath water, which must not exceed 40°C.
- Avoid hot water bottles; wrap a warm rug around the leg in bed. Similarly, do not sit close to a fire; use a rug instead.
- Avoid sunburn to the lower leg.
- Check the inside of shoes daily for foreign bodies or protruding tacks, nails, etc.
- Never wear new shoes for longer than 2 hours to begin with, even if they have been made to measure.
- Do not try instant foot 'cures' advertised in newspapers as they rarely work.
- If the foot gets wet, it must be dried thoroughly and put into dry hose and shoes.
- Corn pads, plasters and other dressings should not be applied without the advice of a chiropodist.

Chiropody/podiatry

The chiropodist will diagnose foot disorders, implement treatment programmes, relieve foot pain and provide advice on footwear and footcare.

The amputee must only seek the advice of a state-registered chiropodist (SRCh), who may work within the NHS or be in private practice. Those suffering from diabetes, PVD and rheumatoid arthritis must be seen regularly by a chiropodist. Elderly persons who cannot attend to their own foot care must also have their feet checked regularly, either by the chiropodist or community nurse.

Many large hospitals have a chiropodist who will treat patients considered to be at risk and who have been referred by a consultant; these patients include diabetics and those with PVD, etc. In the community, chiropody treatment is usually carried out in health centres and there is a domiciliary service for the housebound. The amputee's GP can generally supply details about local facilities. Conditions commonly dealt with by the chiropodist include:

- corns
- bunions

- callosities
- ingrowing toenails
- thick horny toenails
- skin problems on the foot
- toe and foot deformities.

The chiropodist must contact the amputee's GP or hospital doctor if there are any untoward signs in the remaining foot.

Footwear

Socks or stockings should allow movement of the toes and not be pulled tightly over them, nor should they have a restrictive elasticated top or be supported by a garter or elastic band. They must be washed daily. Natural fibres are preferable to nylon.

Shoes must be well fitting, in a good state of repair and with soles that bend easily. A natural material such as leather or canvas is advisable as it permits the foot to 'breathe'. Low heels are advisable and a lace-up design is useful for accommodating any oedema. Sandals should be avoided as the straps may cause lesions when the foot swells, particularly in the summer. There are many shoes available, either from shops or orthotic departments, which have a wide range of widths, depths and weight to suit individual needs. It may take a great deal of effort from the amputee, therapist, orthotist or chiropodist to find suitably comfortable and cosmetically acceptable footwear. This must be pursued with great vigour to achieve good results.

If the amputee or therapist observes any untoward signs or symptoms in the remaining foot or leg, a doctor must be consulted immediately.

Backcare

Footwear and heel height can alter the alignment of the prosthesis, which in turn may affect the lumbar spine, particularly in the trans-femoral levels and above. Shoes must be kept in a good state of repair; badly worn soles and heels cause a change in the alignment. The height of the heel of the shoe should not be changed from that for which the prosthesis was designed, unless the prosthesis has an adjustable foot (see Ch. 8), as this also alters the alignment. If an amputee presents with back pain, both musculoskeletal and prosthetic causes should be investigated.

Upper limb amputees should be encouraged to maintain a symmetrical posture and as much mobility of their back and shoulder girdle as possible.

Strength and mobility

The amputee must be taught a regime of maintenance exercises for the hip, knee and foot of the remaining limb. The elderly should perform these exercises daily. Other amputees need to re-start this exercise programme if they are forced to rest for a period of time because of illness or fitting problems with the prosthesis. The community therapist may need to visit these amputees at home, or the amputee may need to re-attend the therapy facility (see Ch. 5). Some upper limb amputees suffer from overuse of their remaining arm. It is extremely difficult for them to rest, but this may be the only way to resolve soft tissue discomfort. Prosthetic use does not appear to predetermine if overuse syndrome of the remaining arm is going to affect the individual.

CARE OF THE PROSTHESIS

The prosthesis will require maintenance periodically, particularly if it is used extensively.

Whenever the amputee has any queries concerning the fit, length, suspension, mechanical function or general state of repair of the prosthesis, the prosthetist must be contacted. Alterations, repairs or lubrication should not be carried out by the amputee. The amputee is never discharged from the care of the prosthetic service.

If either the foot or knee mechanism becomes wet or clogged with dust or foreign material, the limb must be checked. The amputee should not walk in water without a special protective covering, shower or water activity prosthesis (see Ch. 18).

If the amputee has a fall, particularly one that involves the prosthesis, this should be checked immediately by the prosthetist for safety, even if there appears to be no damage.

The prosthetic foot must be regularly checked for wear with the shoe and sock removed, particularly in the case of heavy and active users. The prosthesis should be kept away from any fire or naked flames.

Cleaning

Any metal or plastic socket should be wiped clean with a damp cloth at night and then dried thoroughly. Soap should not be used.

Leather sockets cannot be cleaned; they may need to be renewed frequently. The thigh corset, in particular, needs to be renewed if the amputee is incontinent or sweats excessively.

The liners of patellar tendon bearing (PTB) and prosthèse tibiale supracondylienne socket (PTS) prostheses can be wiped with a damp cloth but they may need frequent renewal. Liners made of Pelite can be washed with soap flakes, rinsed out and hung up to dry away from direct heat. Silicone sleeves and TEC liners must be washed daily in warm soapy water, rinsed and dried well.

The valve of self-suspending sockets (see Ch. 13) must be kept free from dust with a small soft brush, as powder and dust can collect in it. Cross-threading must be avoided.

The cosmetic cover (stocking or PVC) should be cleaned with a damp, slightly soapy cloth. If a dirty mark proves troublesome, or the cover is damaged, contact the prosthetic centre.

Upper limb amputees who do not wear stump socks must be particularly careful with socket hygiene. 'Wet wipes' or baby wipes can be used and occasionally an old toothbrush needs to be used to remove dead skin.

Body weight

Any change in the amputee's body weight will cause an alteration in the fit of the socket. This can be a particular problem when weight increase produces a tight socket.

The obese amputee finds it more difficult to use a prosthesis skillfully and effectively, e.g. bulging fatty tissue in the adductor region causes discomfort and chafing.

Those who lose weight will find that the socket becomes far too loose and requires adjustment. The method of suspension may need to be altered. All bony prominences should be checked for rubbing and increasing the number of socks should be considered.

CARE OF THE STUMP SOCK

A clean, dry stump sock should be worn daily. During hot weather, stump socks may need to be changed more than once a day. Some very active limb users may need to do this in cooler weather as well.

Socks come with washing instructions which the therapist should check to ensure that the amputee can follow them. Biological detergents should not be used in case of an allergic skin reaction.

The socks should be dried flat on a towel, away from direct heat to prevent shrinkage. Spin dryers and tumble dryers also shrink the socks and mat the fibres.

The amputee must be aware of the several types of stump sock available; sometimes different combinations of materials need to be tried out to achieve a comfortable fit (see Ch. 8).

GENERAL HEALTH

Keeping healthy is particularly important for amputees, especially if the amputation was due to a dysvascular or diabetic condition. Tobacco smoking should be avoided as should eating fatty foods. Eating a balanced diet (high in fibre, low in fat) is generally recommended for main-taining an optimum weight and the advice of a dietician should be obtained if the individual has problems with this.

Getting as much exercise as is possible also helps control weight. Specific prescribed exercises should be continued and reviewed by the therapist as necessary.

DRIVING

If the amputee hopes to return to driving, the specific legal requirements for the countries in which they intend to drive must be obtained from the national authorities. In the UK:

- the GP should be consulted
- the Driver and Vehicle Licensing Centre (DVLC) should be informed in writing of the level of amputation
- advice from the local prosthetic service can be obtained on car adaptations suitable for the amputee
- the amputee's insurance company must be informed of the amputation and any adaptations made to the car (see ch. 18).

LAND, SEA AND AIR TRANSPORT

For information concerning other forms of travel, and leisure and sport activities, see Chapter 18.

FURTHER INFORMATION

Local prosthetic centres supply a wide range of information leaflets and can provide advice on all aspects of aftercare for the amputee.

BIBLIOGRAPHY FOR PREVIOUS EDITIONS

Barnett A, Odugbesan O 1987 Foot care for diabetics. Nursing Times 83(22):24–26
Brooks A P 1981 The diabetic foot. Hospital Update May: 509–514
Disabled Living Foundation 1991 Footwear: a quality issue. Disabled Living Foundation, London
Finlay O E 1986 Footwear management in the elderly care programme. Physiotherapy 72(4):172–178
Hoile R 1981 Managing the ischaemic limb in the community. Community View 10:10–12
Levy S W 1980 Skin problems of the leg amputee. Prosthetics and Orthotics International 4(1):37–44
Stokes I A F 1977 The effect of shoe inserts on the load distribution under the foot. Chiropodist January:5–12

BIBLIOGRAPHY FOR THE THIRD EDITION

Ahmed A, Baylol M G, Ha S B 1994 Adventitious bursae in below knee amputees. Case reports and a review of the literature. American Journal of Physical Medicine and Rehabilitation 73(2):124–129

Ibbotson S H, Simpson N B, Fyfe N C M, Lawrence C M 1994 Follicular keratoses at amputation sites. British Journal of Dermatology 130:770–772

Levy S W 1995 Amputees: skin problems and prostheses. Cutis 55:297–301

Ravidran N D, Sreenivasan A, Marks L J 1997 Skin lesions in residual limbs following amputations. Proceedings of the Annual Scientific Meeting of ISPO UK NMS, England

12

Hindquarter and hip disarticulation levels of amputation

The majority of hindquarter and hip disarticulation levels of amputation are performed for malignant bone tumours in the lower limb. Occasionally, severe vascular disease, osteomyelitis and very rarely severe trauma may also result in the selection of this level of amputation. In exceptional cases it has been known for bilateral hip disarticulation to be caused by trauma.

These are extensive amputations involving the large muscle groups around the pelvis. There is no residual limb to act as a lever for prosthetic control and mobility is slow, functionally difficult to achieve and energy consumption is high. In some cases such extensive surgery may result in slow wound healing and the need for secondary skin grafting. Those who are undergoing chemotherapy and radiotherapy may also have wound healing problems and these patients often feel tired and unwell.

These are very mutilating procedures and many amputees find psychological adjustment difficult. All those suffering from malignancy require an enormous amount of psychological help at all stages of their care. Relatives and carers may require even more help and support (see Ch. 3).

Hindquarter

Generally, half the pelvis is removed, as well as the total lower limb. It is important to have X-ray confirmation of the extent of bony removal.

Hip disarticulation

This is a true disarticulation of the femur from the acetabulum; the total lower limb is removed, leaving the whole pelvis intact. Some surgeons leave the head of the femur in situ; this can cause great difficulty with socket fitting. This is not a true hip disarticulation but prosthetically is treated as one.

PROSTHESES

As soon as the amputee's wound is healed, assessment for casting can be made by the prosthetic rehabilitation team. Provided the amputee is sufficiently fit, the prosthetist will take a plaster-of-Paris cast embracing the site of amputation. It is essential that the amputee is able to stand for the period of time necessary for this procedure, at least half an hour. Figures 12.1 and

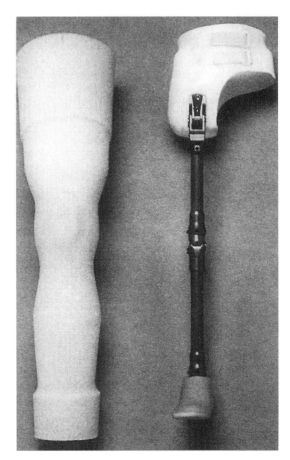

Figure 12.2   Modular hip disarticulation prosthesis for children. (Photograph by kind permission of Otto Bock Orthopaedic (UK) Ltd.)

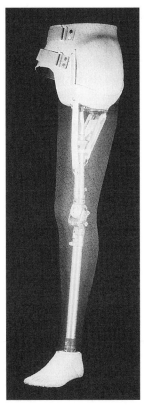

Figure 12.1   A modular hip disarticulation prosthesis. (Photograph by kind permission of Otto Bock UK Ltd.)

12.2 illustrate lightweight prostheses supplied for this level of amputation.

Socket

The shape of the socket depends always upon the plaster cast of the amputee's pelvis. It is usually a totally embracing socket, enclosing the iliac crests for hip disarticulation (and one iliac crest and the remaining pelvis for hindquarter), made of various materials including plastic laminates, thermoplastic drape and leather. For the hindquarter amputee, this contains and supports the abdominal and pelvic contents.

The weightbearing areas of the socket are different for each level of amputation:

Hindquarter: the amputee's weight has to be transferred over to the ischial tuberosity and buttock of the remaining leg.

Hip disarticulation: the amputee's weight is taken through the ischium and buttock of the amputated side.

Suspension

The suspension of these sockets is achieved through the total tissue contact, locking over the iliac crests; occasionally, extra suspension may be supplied by adding a shoulder strap.

Hip components

Hip limiter

The mechanism is placed anteriorly on the socket. It allows movement at the hip during the swing phase. Movement is controlled by a limiter, which can be adjusted as the amputee becomes more active by the prosthetist to increase or decrease the stride length. This component can be supplied either with or without a locking

mechanism: this is dependant on the functional ability of the amputee.

Four-bar linkage

The geometric design of this joint gives the advantage of the instantaneous centre of rotation occurring at the natural hip joint level. It therefore gives a smooth and easy gait pattern as it shortens the length of prosthesis during the swing phase, thus ensuring safe foot clearance of the floor. The component is on the anterior aspect of the socket and fits right out of the way when sitting, making it the most comfortable design (see Fig. 12.3).

Interjoint segment

One hip disarticulation system is available in an energy storing configuration. Energy in the form of flexion is introduced into the composite hip strut during weightbearing. The amputee, by varying the amount of pelvic thrust at toe off, can selectively release energy and control the forward speed of the knee. The result provides

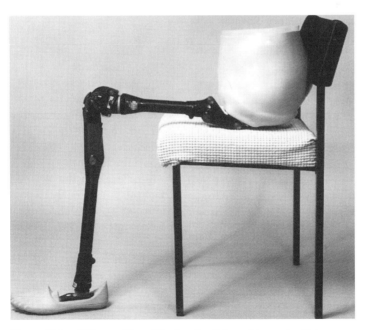

Figure 12.3   Sitting position of the four-bar linkage hip mechanism. (Photograph by kind permission of C. A. Blatchford & Sons Ltd.)

controlled foot rise and effective shortening of the prosthesis at mid-swing to allow variability in toe clearance.

With a strut system, a prosthesis can be made nearer to the length of the contralateral side and the need for vaulting should be completely eliminated.

Knee components

For a fuller explanation of these mechanisms see Chapter 13.

Stability in stance phase is very important to amputees at these levels and the polycentric designs have the added benefit of effectively shortening in swing phase therefore increasing ground clearance. Prostheses supplied for the hindquarter and hip disarticulation levels of amputation may have a combination of the hip and knee components. It is important that the therapist understands the various components and looks at them in detail, in order that the amputee can be instructed correctly.

CHECK OF THE PROSTHESIS

The fit of the prosthesis must be checked by the therapist on the first attendance for gait re-education and subsequently at regular intervals.

The amputee's skin must be checked before and after each session; this is particularly important if the amputee is having chemotherapy or radiotherapy. There may be a variance of body weight, which for such an extensive amputation will have a direct bearing on the fit of the socket.

The component parts of the prosthesis are then examined before applying it to the amputee so that their method of operation is understood by the therapist; the shoe is also checked to ensure it is the one for which the prosthesis was made.

Socket

With the amputee standing wearing the prosthesis and suitably undressed, the therapist should check the fit of the socket for the following:

- The iliac crests are accommodated within the socket

- The ischial weightbearing area is correctly postioned, i.e. for the hindquarter, on the ischium and buttock of the remaining limb; for the hip disarticulation, on the ischium of the amputated side
- The socket contains the pelvis with no excess flesh over the brim of the socket and no obvious gaps between the socket walls and the amputee
- The amputee is wearing suitable underclothes (see p. 154) and a pair of shoes.

Once the check of the fit of the socket is complete with the amputee standing, it should be checked with the amputee sitting:

- The upper brim of the socket should not bite into the flesh
- The upper brim of the socket should have adequate clearance of the lower ribs
- There should be clearance and comfort for the contralateral thigh
- The gluteal and perineal areas should be comfortable
- The foam cosmetic covering of the prosthesis should not restrict flexion of the knee joint.

Problems that may be encountered with the socket

Socket too large. There may be excessive movement between the socket and the amputee's tissues. This may be tested by asking the amputee to take weight through the remaining leg and lift the prosthesis. If the prosthesis drops excessively then the socket is too large. (This is important because the socket provides suspension for the prosthesis in addition to containing the tissues.) Gaps between the socket and the amputee's tissues, and excessively rubbed areas on the amputee's skin, are also indications that the socket is too large.

The therapist should check:

- that the prosthesis has been correctly applied
- that the fastenings are as tight as necessary for a snug fit
- whether the amputee has lost weight
- what type of underwear is worn.

If the socket is too large the therapist must contact the prosthetist for an urgent appointment and must not add pads or sponges to alter the socket.

Socket too small. There will be rolls of flesh over the brim of the socket, which will be excessively uncomfortable, especially when the amputee sits. In addition, the amputee's pelvis may not be contained within the socket; this will be particularly noticeable on the lateral aspect of the amputated side. The fastenings will be at their full length.

If the socket appears too small, the therapist should check:

- that the prosthesis has been correctly applied
- that the fastenings cannot be released further
- whether the amputee has put on weight
- what type of underwear is worn.

If the socket is too small the therapist must contact the prosthetist for an urgent appointment.

It should be noted that if the fit of the socket is grossly incorrect, the alignment of the prosthesis will also be affected.

Suspension

As the suspension is maintained by the socket, correct fit of the socket is essential. Auxiliary suspension in the form of a shoulder strap may be required by some amputees. This is placed over the opposite shoulder to the amputated side and should be adjusted to a firm suspension when the patient is standing.

Length

The prosthesis is made slightly shorter than the natural leg length. Adjustment can be made at the fitting stage to ensure a safe and smooth swing through, depending on the ability of the amputee and the environmental needs, e.g. rough ground, uneven pavements.

Prosthesis too long

The therapist should check:

- the fit of the socket

- that the shoes are a pair
- the posture of the amputee (some acquire a postural abnormality and pelvic drop with these high levels of amputation)
- that suspension of the prosthesis is maintained.

As a temporary measure a raise can be added to the shoe of the remaining foot. The length should be checked by the prosthetist as soon as possible.

Prosthesis too short

The therapist should check:

- the fit of the socket
- that the shoes are a pair
- the posture of the amputee.

As a temporary measure a raise can be added to the shoe on the prosthetic foot. The prosthesis must be checked by the prosthetist as soon as possible.

Alignment

The prosthesis will have been aligned by the prosthetist to give stability during the stance phase so that the amputee can control the hip, knee and foot mechanisms and a good sitting posture. When viewed from the lateral side the knee of the prosthesis appears hyperextended (Fig. 12.4).

If the alignment of the prosthesis appears incorrect, i.e. the amputee feels unstable during the stance phase or there is an uneven swing phase of the prosthesis, the therapist should check:

- the fit of the socket
- that firm suspension is maintained
- that the amputee has not changed the shoes (i.e. altered the height of the heel)
- that the length of the prosthesis is correct.

When the amputee is sitting, the position of the knee centre and the lower shin alignment should be observed. The therapist should contact the prosthetist if it is felt that the alignment is incorrect.

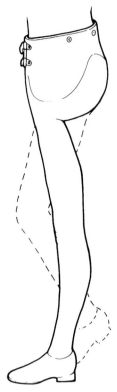

Figure 12.4 Correct alignment of the hip disarticulation prosthesis. This permits the ground reaction force to pass anterior to the knee causing an extension moment and thus stability during the stance phase.

FUNCTIONAL RE-EDUCATION WITH THE PROSTHESIS

Most amputees with hindquarter or hip disarticulation amputation regain their balance easily. Much of their rehabilitation depends on the confidence and experience of the therapist, as psychological adjustment and acceptance of the large cumbersome prosthesis, slow gait and certain lack of speed of function (e.g. turning round, sitting, climbing stairs or inclines) forms the larger part of their prosthetic rehabilitation.

Amputees with these levels of amputation may not wear stump socks. The sockets of their prostheses give a large amount of tissue support and the skin often becomes hot and sweaty. Therefore during treatment the prosthesis should be removed several times to check the skin condition. It is important that smooth cotton underwear with no seams or creases is used to prevent this. A long vest, smooth cotton pants or a body stocking are all suitable. However, it is often difficult to persuade some younger amputees not to wear nylon briefs and to wear long cotton vests.

The amputee should be given short, clear instructions at all stages of functional re-education. Competence in the use of the prosthesis is more quickly achieved if each stage is taken in turn.

Donning (see Fig. 12.5)

The amputee must learn to put on the prosthesis independently, carrying out the following tasks:

1. Stand, back against a wall, with bars, frame or furniture at either side.
2. Wear suitable underwear correctly.
3. Grasp the socket of the prosthesis and thrust the pelvis laterally into the socket. The prosthesis should be rotated slightly laterally at this stage. The pelvis must be in total contact with the socket.
4. Fasten the straps of the socket; this will rotate the prosthesis slightly medially
6. Secure the shoulder strap, if used, adjusting it whilst still standing.

Doffing

The amputee must be able to remove the prosthesis as follows:

1. Stand and unfasten the straps.
2. Remove the prosthesis by grasping the socket and easing the pelvis away from it.
3. Examine the skin for any redness, rubbing or spots. A mirror may be needed.

Dressing

1. Dress the prosthesis first (if trousers are being worn).
2. Place remaining leg through trousers.
3. Apply prosthesis.
4. Check the shoes are a pair and have the same heel height for which the prosthetic foot was measured.
5. Dress the top half of the body.

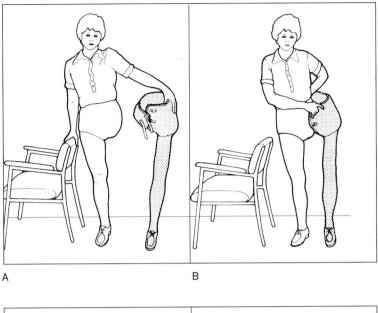

A   B

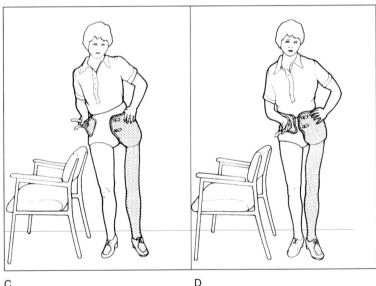

C   D

Figure 12.5   Donning the hip disarticulation prosthesis. (A) preparing to don prosthesis; (B) applying prosthesis; (C) adjusting prosthesis; (D) fastening prosthesis.

It must be remembered that the socket will increase the size of the amputee's pelvis. This must be taken into account when buying clothes, choosing a suitable armchair and measuring for a wheelchair.

Using the toilet

Men manage to stand and urinate with few problems wearing their prostheses.

It is often uncomfortable to sit on a lavatory

seat and inconvenient to remove underwear, so most people have to remove their prosthesis before using the lavatory.

Standing from a chair

1. Push up using both hands and the remaining leg.
2. Stand erect, thrusting pelvis forward, checking that the knee has stabilised before stepping forward.

Sitting down

This is more difficult than standing and walking. It may be necessary to practise without clothes on, so that the amputee can visualise the release mechanism (if present).

Sitting down with hip limiter (Fig. 12.6)

1. The amputee should stand erect with hip neutral in order to release the limiter mechanism. The button or lever must be maintained in the release position, otherwise it will latch again in extension. The buttocks should be thrust backwards and the trunk bent forwards with both knees flexed in order to sit. The thigh section may need to be pushed forward with the hand (see Fig. 12.6).
2. If no lock is present the amputee should lean backwards slightly to release the hip limiter, then push the thigh section forward with the hand in order to sit.

Sitting down with joints without limiters

The amputee should tilt the pelvis backwards, extend the lumbar spine, then flex the hip in order to sit. This flowing S-shaped movement takes practice and the amputee needs to sit with a purposeful action.

Standing exercises

The amputee stands with feet approximately 15 cm apart. The therapist should teach the following:

1. Hip hitching (this may not be possible with the hindquarter level of amputation)
2. Pelvic tilt or flick
3. A combination of hip hitching and pelvic tilt
4. Stepping forwards with remaining leg

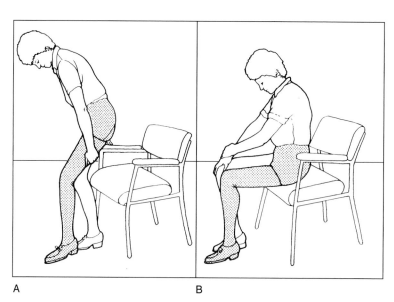

A   B

Figure 12.6   A: Preparing to sit; and B: sitting down with a hip disarticulation prosthesis.

5. Hitching, pelvic tilt and initiation of the swing of prosthesis from toe off to heel strike.

The amputee should not take too long a step initially in order to achieve stability when first learning to use the prosthesis. The length of the stride can be altered by the prosthetist by adjusting the hip limiter, if fitted. Some experienced amputees may be taught to do this themselves.

Walking

The therapist should:

1. Encourage small and equal steps and emphasise weightbearing through the prosthesis by encouraging the amputee to step forwards with the remaining leg first. It is sometimes difficult to transfer weight through the prosthesis at first as the amputee is so used to hopping on the remaining leg.

2. During the stance phase, encourage use of the back extensor muscles and the hip extensors of the remaining leg in order to maintain an erect trunk posture. This is to prevent excessive movement of the upper trunk and shoulders during the gait cycle.

3. Discourage vaulting on the remaining leg. However, some hindquarter amputees are unable to prevent this, and some amputees of these levels will vault to some extent in order to gain higher walking speed and for ground clearance.

Walking aids

Once the amputee has mastered a safe gait pattern in the parallel bars and can sit down and stand up, progression to walking aids is made.

In spite of the large prosthesis, the amputee learns to control the joint components easily, usually progressing to walking sticks. This can be commenced using one stick and one bar and then progressing to two sticks within the bars. Many may use one stick within approximately 1 week, if attending daily for treatment.

One of the problems discovered in using the prosthesis is that the walking speed is slow. This is especially true of the young amputee who is speedy and mobile when hopping using elbow crutches. This has to be recognised by the therapist and discussed. It is important that amputees realise that although they are faster on crutches, there is less independence using two hands for propulsion, and standing on one leg for a length of time is tiring and may cause early degenerative changes to the weightbearing joints, or soft tissue discomfort. It may be more desirable for the amputee's comfort and posture to stand on two legs.

Activities of daily living

Functional activity is the most relevant form of gait re-education for high-level amputees, both within the home and outside in the local environment.

Walking on different surfaces

This must be practised both inside and outside the hospital under the supervision of a therapist; linoleum, shiny wood floors, different thicknesses of carpet, pavement, grass, gravel and rough ground must all be attempted. The amputee must be confident on these surfaces both alone and when outside in crowded situations, e.g. busy streets, shops, etc.

Different surfaces will transmit different sensations up through the socket. The amputee must learn to recognise these new feelings and adapt accordingly. The amount of hitching and pelvic tilt required during the swing phase of the prosthesis will be different for each surface, and balance reactions will be varied.

Stairs

The same method for climbing stairs is used here as for the trans-femoral amputees (Ch. 13, p. 173). The remaining leg goes up first and the prosthesis down first.

Step/kerb

Again, when the amputee is negotiating steps the remaining leg goes up first and the prosthesis down first (Ch. 13, p. 173).

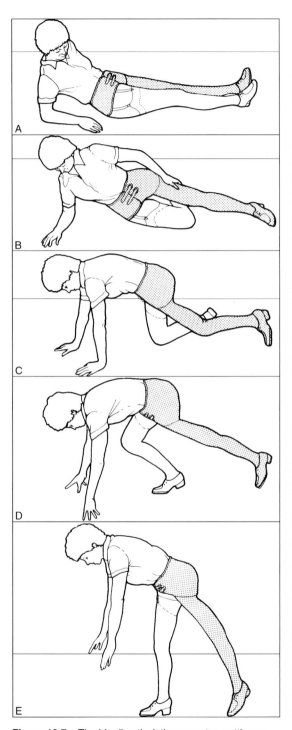

Figure 12.7 The hip disarticulation amputee getting up from the floor (Method 1).

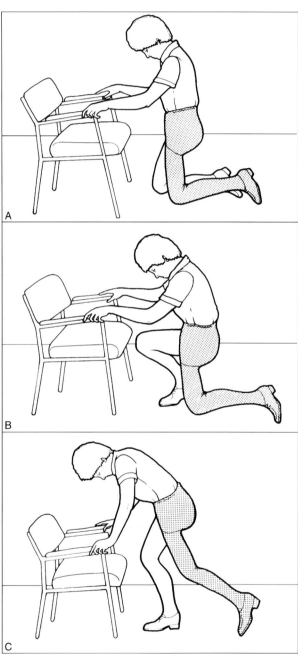

Figure 12.8 The hip disarticulation amputee getting up from the floor (Method 2).

Ramps/hills

The remaining leg leads when going uphill and the prosthesis is hitched up level with the remaining foot. When descending, the sticks are placed forwards first, followed by the prosthesis, and then the remaining foot is brought level with the prosthetic foot (see Ch. 13, p. 173).

When the gradient is steep amputees must learn to control the movement of the hip and maintain it in extension during the stance phase on descending. If there are problems with descending ramps it may be that the prosthetic foot does not have a soft enough action. Flat shoes are a distinct advantage. Walking sideways up and down a slope may offer a safer alternative.

Whilst the amputee should obviously be taught the skills to cope with gradients, ramps are not necessarily helpful for them. Stair climbing with an adjacent handrail is often much easier.

Getting up from the floor

It is rare that amputees with these levels of amputation fall, as their cadence is slow and they are careful and controlled when walking. However, they may choose to sit on the floor and should therefore practise getting up from it.

Method 1 (see Fig. 12.7)

1. Lie supine and gather the walking sticks (if used).
2. Release hip limiter, if present.
3. Roll over, leading with prosthesis, onto natural knee.
4. Push up on both hands, or use sticks and remaining leg to steady.
5. Stand upright.

Method 2 (see Fig. 12.8)

This is the same as Method 1 except a chair can be used to push up from.

PROSTHETIC INFORMATION

Detailed information regarding prostheses available in the UK can be obtained from the manufacturers. The addresses are listed in Appendix 1.

BIBLIOGRAPHY FOR PREVIOUS EDITIONS

Shurr D G, Cok T M, Buckwalter J A, Cooper R R 1983 Hip disarticulation: A prosthetic follow-up. Orthotics and Prosthetics 37(3):50–57
van der Waarde T 1984 Ottawa experience with hip disarticulation prostheses. Orthotics and Prosthetics 38(1):29–35
Walden J D, Davis B C 1979 Prosthetic fitting and points of rehabilitation for hindquarter and hip disarticulation patients. Physiotherapy 65(1):4–6

BIBLIOGRAPHY FOR THE THIRD EDITION

Lawless M W, Laughlin R T, Wright D G, Lemmon G W, Rigano W C 1997 Massive pelvis injuries treated with amputations: case reports and literature review. The Journal of Trauma: Injury, Infection and Critical Care 42(6):1169–1175

13

Trans-femoral level of amputation

The trans-femoral level is a common level of amputation; its great advantage is that for the dysvascular patient, complete healing occurs in a short space of time. This means that the amputee can be discharged home quickly with few surgical complications. There is a higher mortality rate at this level than for more distal levels and the amputee will have to cope with an artificial knee joint, which consumes more energy: on average 49% more mean oxygen consumption than normal. It is not a suitable level of amputation for children as the lower epiphyseal plate is removed and the residual limb does not grow with the child.

It is possible to fit a prosthesis to a very short residual limb, but the muscle control and leverage is greater with a longer residual limb and the prosthetist will have a greater choice of components. In the adult, a gap of at least 13 cm is needed between the distal end of the residual limb and the natural knee joint line to allow consideration of all the various knee components to be fitted and to avoid knee protrusion when sitting; anything less that 13 cm will restrict the prescription of knee components.

It is also possible to accommodate within the prosthesis a moderate amount of fixed flexion at the hip, but this will not permit a natural gait pattern; the cosmesis tends to be poor and at times unacceptable. For these amputees there will be an individual acceptable degree of fixed hip flexion, dependent upon body proportions, flexibility of the lumbar spine and importance of function and cosmesis. For these reasons it is difficult to state specific angles; however, approximately 25° hip flexion can be accommodated within the prosthesis. It is still possible to make a prosthesis with between 25° and 50° hip flexion, but the thigh section will obviously protrude making dressing difficult.

PROSTHETIC SOCKETS

Self-suspending sockets

Self-suspending sockets are given to amputees with stable mature residual limbs, good muscle control, full hip joint mobility, no oedema and no gross scarring. The advantages of these sockets are that:

- through the intimate contact with the amputee's skin, sensory feedback is enhanced.
- muscle contraction provides an instant prosthetic movement, with no time lapse or pistoning.

Another method of improving suspension is to use a silicone socket, such as Iceross.

Total surface bearing (TSB) sockets

TSB sockets are made of various plastic materials with or without flexible properties.

The amputee's weight is taken through the whole socket as well as the ischial weightbearing area. The residual limb tissues are in contact with all aspects of the socket; the fit is extremely accurate and a stump sock is not worn. The valve permits only a one-way flow of air outwards from the socket. This exclusion of air, as well as the active contraction of the residual limb muscles, maintains the suspension of the prosthesis. There is no negative pressure; therefore the distal tissues are supported. Occasionally, auxiliary suspension, such as a Silesian belt, may be required.

The suction socket

The amputee's weight is taken mainly through the ischial seating area and tissue support is given by the walls of the socket. The valve permits a two-way air flow, and the method of application of this socket creates sufficient vacuum to maintain suspension with the aid of active muscle contraction in the residual limb. The valve is either a screw-in or push fit design. Occasionally, auxiliary suspension is required.

Contour adducted trochanteric/controlled alignment method (CAT–CAM) socket

This is an intimately fitting socket containing the ischial ramus within the socket and fitting to within 1.5 cm of the anus. It has been evolving since the late 1970s after its development by John Sabolich in Oklahoma, USA. The casting procedure requires specific skills of the prosthetist and may take longer than that for other sockets.

The socket itself is contoured around the skeleton and muscle groups, relying on a total contact fit for its weightbearing (see Fig. 13.1). There is a high lateral wall extending above the greater trochanter of the femur. Because of the high medial wall, the ischial tuberosity is locked in the socket. The femur is held in marked adduction preventing lateral femoral shift. Weight is taken on the shaped subtrochanteric area as well as throughout the socket.

Sockets requiring auxiliary suspension

Quadrilateral and Health (H-type) sockets

Although these sockets vary slightly, they have a similar design that allows transmission of most of the body weight through the ischial seating. Their shape prevents the residual limb from slipping downwards giving the 'plug fit'. In both sockets the anterior and lateral walls are sufficiently high to maintain the tissues over the posterior weightbearing area. However, during stance phase, the hip abductors pull the distal femur against the lateral wall of the socket, causing the ischial tuberosity to move medially along the socket seat.

In the quadrilateral socket (see Fig. 13.2) weight is taken on the posterior brim of the socket. In the H-type socket, weight is taken on the postero-medial brim of the socket.

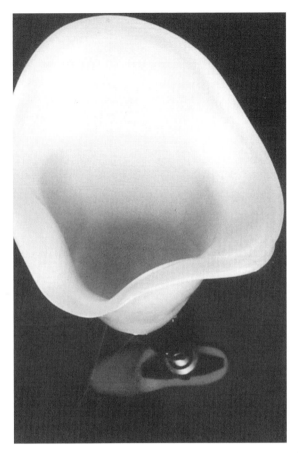

Figure 13.1 The CAT-CAM socket. (Reproduced with permission from Redhead et al 1991.)

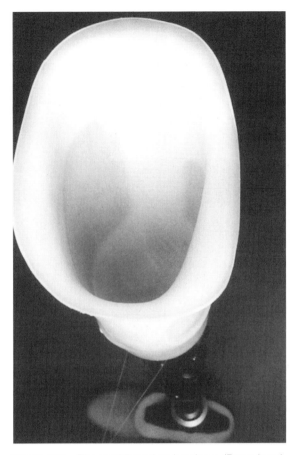

Figure 13.2 The quadrilateral socket shape. (Reproduced with permission from Redhead et al 1991.)

Conventional socket

This socket has an ill-defined shape but allows weightbearing both through an ischial seating area and through the brim and walls of the socket. This is often termed the 'plug fit'. This variety of socket suits both the obese amputee who has a shapeless residual limb and the amputee with a short, flexed residual limb. It is generally supplied only as a replacement socket for an established wearer.

AUXILIARY SUSPENSION

Soft suspension

All soft suspensions need to be adjusted when standing. Therefore good balance, hand grip and hand-eye coordination are necessary.

There are many variations of soft suspension made by different manufacturers for individual needs.

Total elastic suspension (TES) (see Fig. 13.3)

This is made of Neoprene or a similar material and can be hot to wear. It does not fully control rotation of the prosthesis or lateral drift of the socket, but does provide comfort. Amputees rarely have an allergic reaction to Neoprene.

Silesian belt

This is a simple wraparound strap connected to the anterior and lateral sides of the socket. It is usually used as an auxiliary suspension for a suction or self-suspending socket.

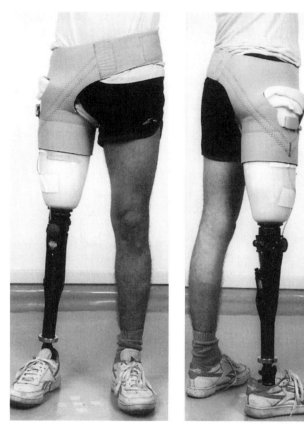

Figure 13.3   The total elastic suspension (TES). (Photograph courtesy of Richmond, Twickenham and Roehampton Health Authority Medical Photography Department.)

Roehampton soft suspension (RSS)
(see Fig. 13.4)

This is a leather waist belt with two diagonal down straps to the anterior and lateral sides of the socket. A well-defined waist is needed.

Rigid suspension

Rigid pelvic band (RPB) (see Fig. 13.10, p. 172)

This fits snugly around the contours of the pelvis. There is a uniaxial joint between the RPB and its attachment to the lateral brim of the socket that allows for only flexion and extension of the hip joint. In the majority of cases, a shoulder strap over the contralateral shoulder gives additional support.

KNEE COMPONENTS

The function of the knee joint is vital to the overall performance of the trans-femoral amputee. During stance phase, knee stability is the most important aspect; at heel strike and subsequent loading, the knee joint must not buckle. During swing phase, the forward motion of the shin section of the prosthesis must be controlled in order to produce a smooth natural-looking gait.

The design features chosen for an individual will depend on the amputee's weight, functional ability, terrain/environment over which they will walk and their leisure/sports requirements. It must be remembered that the more components that are added, the heavier the prosthesis becomes. Knee joints have evolved from the

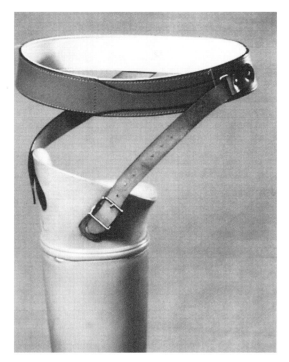

Figure 13.4   Roehampton soft suspension. (Photograph by kind permission of C. A. Blatchford & Sons Ltd.)

simplest single-axis free swing to the most sophisticated swing and stance phase control by microprocessor, and are constantly undergoing further development. Therapists must keep abreast of these developments.

Stance phase controls

Locked

Semi-automatic knee lock (SAKL). This spring-loaded mechanism automatically locks in extension. There is a manual control to release it so that the knee is flexed when sitting. This is the simplest knee mechanism available. It is also the safest knee mechanism and therefore most suitable for the unsteady or frail patient.

Manual knee lock. These mechanisms can be added to some knee designs.

Stabilised

There are a variety of stabilised knee designs, all of which are weight activated to 'lock' at

between approximately 0–25° flexion (depending on the individual amputee's needs and the component) thus cushioning heel strike and giving a feeling of security with a near normal gait.

A variety of swing phase controls can be added to this design, e.g. pneumatic swing phase, internal calf spring.

Polycentric knees. There are a variety of designs using from 4–6 axes of movement. They provide stability in extension through their geometry. They also can have swing phase controls added. They are suitable for the long trans-femoral level and those associated with knee disarticulation, as the moving instantaneous centre of rotation lies proximal and posterior to the anatomical knee centre, maintaining it posterior to the weightbearing axis of the lower limb. This provides an extension moment at the knee, decreasing the risk of the prosthetic knee buckling (see Fig. 14.1, p. 181).

Swing phase controls

These components will control the rate of swing of the lower leg during swing phase, depending on the muscle action of the residual limb and the forward momentum of the amputee.

Pneumatic control (i.e. air control) will adjust to variations of gait cadence in a limited range.

Hydraulic control (i.e. fluid control) has a broad range of variation to gait cadence. Examples are the Mauch and Otto Bock units. There are separate adjustment valves for flexion control and extension control (see Fig. 13.5).

Wheel-type knee control and extension bias aids are simple swing phase controls found on older style prostheses.

Combined swing and stance phase controls

These offer the closest possible approximation to natural gait. Examples are the C-Leg and CaTech hydraulic.

Microprocessor control. Application of high level technology to lower limb prosthetics ensures greater control, ease of use and reduction of effort by amputees during ambulation.

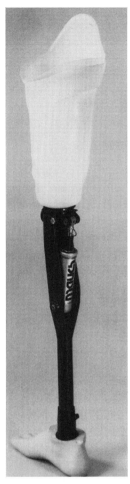

Figure 13.5 The Mauch Swing 'n Stance Knee unit on a trans-femoral prosthesis with an ischeal ramus containment socket. (Photograph by kind permission of C. A. Blatchford & Sons Ltd.)

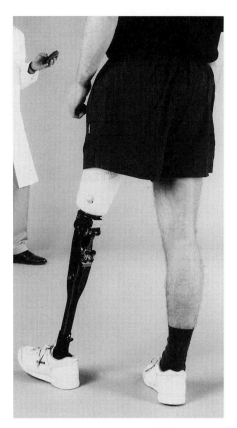

Figure 13.6 A microprocessor controlled knee component for a trans-femoral amputee being programmed by a prosthetist. (Photograph by kind permission of C.A. Blatchford and Sons Ltd.)

(swing phase control, see Fig. 13.6) and the C-Leg (swing and stance phase control).

FOOT COMPONENTS

For details of these see Chapter 8 (p. 105).

CHECK OF THE TRANS-FEMORAL PROSTHESIS

The prosthesis should be inspected by the therapist separately before putting it onto the amputee. A full understanding of the type of socket and the function of the joints and foot supplied is essential before being able to educate the amputee to don the prosthesis and achieve a good function from it. The cosmesis hides the

These designs employ electronic control of the hydraulic or pneumatic cylinder; on-board sensors collect real-time data to control movement and are designed to adjust automatically for different walking speeds. The finished prosthesis can be easily adjusted, and can be programmed while walking on any terrain outside a clinical environment, thus allowing for the most realistic conditions in the amputee's normal use.

These knees are expensive and consideration must be given to the need to change the batteries and attend the prosthetic centre for maintenance. Examples are the Intelligent Prosthesis Plus components, so should the prosthesis have been delivered without information, the prosthetist must be contacted to find out the prescription and properties of the components. The fit of the prosthesis should be checked by the therapist on the first attendance for gait re-education and subsequently at regular intervals. The amputee's ability to function with the prosthesis will depend upon a correct fit.

If there has been an interval of time between the delivery of the prosthesis and this first attendance, the amputee's body and residual limb may have changed in shape and size. The amputee should always be suitably undressed for this procedure.

Prosthetic sockets

Quadrilateral and H-type sockets

Ischial seating. To check that the ischial tuberosity is correctly placed on the socket, the amputee should stand with all weight on the remaining leg. The therapist locates the ischial tuberosity of the affected leg with the palmar aspect of two fingers and then asks the amputee to transfer their weight slowly onto the prosthesis. Full contact should be felt with the fingers between the amputee's ischial tuberosity and the seating area of the socket. If the ischial tuberosity slides down inside, the socket is too large. If the tuberosity is above the seating area, the socket is too small.

Socket too large: the therapist can add more stump socks of a variety of thicknesses.

Socket too small: the therapist can decrease the number and thickness of the socks. If the measures above do not correct the fit of the socket, the therapist should contact the prosthetist and request an appointment for adjustments to be made.

Adductor region. There should be no discomfort in this sensitive area. If the amputee reports discomfort.

- Check that the amputee is not 'sinking' into the socket and that there is correct weight-bearing through the ischial tuberosity.
- Check that the stump socks are well pulled up over the rim of the socket.

- Check for fixed flexion contractures in the affected hip and compare this with the set of the socket.
- Check the strength and function of the hip extensor muscles on the affected side.
- Observe the adductor flare of the socket with the amputee standing correctly. This may need adjustment by the prosthetist.

Distal end of the residual limb. No discomfort should be experienced in this area. If an area of redness appears on the anterior aspect of the distal end of the residual limb, the amputee may have a fixed contracture of the hip that is not adequately accommodated in the socket.

If oedema occurs in the distal end of the residual limb the amputee may need soft tissue support by means of a soft pad, or the socket may be too narrow causing interruption of lymphatic and venous return. For either of these problems the therapist should contact the prosthetist.

CAT–CAM and self-suspending sockets

These sockets can feel very hard to the amputee initially and the tissues of the residual limb have to become accustomed to them.

The problems that can occur are discomfort and a feeling of lack of suspension. This is because the interface between the residual limb and the socket is incorrect: the socket is too tight, too loose, or the method of application is incorrect.

The therapist can check the amputee's weight, general health and ability to don the prosthesis. The prosthetist then needs to be contacted if none of the problems mentioned above are contributing factors to the discomfort.

Length

To check the length of the prosthesis, the therapist stands behind the amputee, hands resting on the iliac crests. The amputee should be suitably undressed so that the whole spine can be observed for rotation and scoliosis. The iliac crests should be approximately level when standing with equal weight on both legs.

The more important check of the length of the

prosthesis is best observed in the dynamic situation when walking. There must be safe clearance of the foot from the floor without producing gait abnormalities.

If the prosthesis is too long the therapist should check that:

- the amputee is wearing two shoes that are a pair and of the original height for which the prosthesis was aligned
- the remaining knee is not held in flexion
- the socket is not too small so that the residual limb is being pushed up out of the socket.

If the prosthesis still appears to be too long, an adjustable sandal shoe raise (Fig. 13.7) can be used to assess accurately the discrepancy in length. A temporary shoe raise can then be applied to the shoe of the remaining leg.

If the prosthesis is too short the therapist should check that:

- the shoes are a pair
- the socket is not too large.

Again it is possible to use the adjustable sandal on the shoe of the prosthesis to assess any necessary raise required. In either case, it is advisable to contact the prosthetist for length adjustment.

Auxiliary suspension

TES belt

With the TES belt, the therapist should check that it has been passed above the opposing iliac

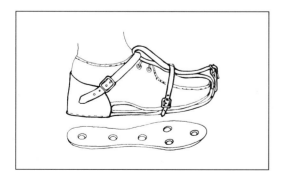

Figure 13.7 An adjustable sandal shoe raise. Extra insoles, like the one shown, may be added between the amputee's shoe and the sandal until the correct leg length is obtained.

crest and that it has been fastened with sufficient tension anteriorly.

Soft suspension

With the amputee suitably undressed, the therapist should check that the waist or Silesian belt is of the correct tension and the downstraps are correctly angled and also under correct tension when the patient is standing and walking.

Rigid pelvic band (RPB) suspension

This should fit snugly around the contours of the pelvis. If there is discomfort here, the therapist should:

- check the clothing that is worn between the RPB and the skin
- remove and re-apply the prosthesis.

However, if the discomfort persists, the set and position of the RPB will need to be adjusted, so contact the prosthetist. An incorrectly set RPB can also cause medial or lateral rotation of the prosthesis.

Shoulder strap (if used)

The tension of the shoulder strap must be checked with the amputee standing. If it is too tight it will tend to make the amputee stoop forwards. If it is too loose it will not contribute adequately to the suspension.

Knee components

The therapist should check the working of the knee components to ensure that it stabilises, flexes and (if a lock is present) locks and releases effectively. The amputees should fully understand the theory of the function of the knee components supplied.

Alignment

There are a variety of causes of malalignment observed during the gait cycle: the therapist and amputee are more likely to observe problems due to gait deviation. Therefore a period of trial walking in the parallel bars is needed before the prosthetist is alerted to any alignment problems, as the amputee needs time to increase confidence and become accustomed to the sensations transmitted by the new prosthesis.

The set of the socket must accommodate any hip flexion contracture present. This can be checked measuring the amputee in Thomas' position (see Fig. 2.3, p. 18) and the angle of the socket set checked against this measurement. The mobility of the individual's lumbar spine may be able to accommodate the hip flexion contracture, therefore the socket can be set in a more neutral alignment, making the prosthesis more cosmetically acceptable and the gait pattern improved.

If the fit of the socket is poor, or if the auxiliary suspension is not adequate, the alignment will be affected.

A problem with alignment is commonly observed at the knee joint level, but it should not be assumed that the problem can always be corrected here.

The set of the foot and the type of shoe used will also affect alignment. The prosthetist has to be contacted to correct alignment, but the therapist and amputee need to take a little time and practise before assuming something is wrong.

FUNCTIONAL RE-EDUCATION WITH THE TRANS-FEMORAL PROSTHESIS

The amputee should be given short, clear instructions at all stages of functional re-education. Competence in the use of the prosthesis is more quickly achieved if each stage is taken in turn.

Donning the prosthesis

Soft suspension

The prosthesis may be applied to the residual limb with the amputee sitting, but the fastening of the suspension can only be done when the amputee is standing. Standing balance is required without hand holds, but the amputee may find it easier to lean against a wall or sturdy furniture. The critical application of the angle

of the straps and the correct tension must be applied. If there are any problems the prosthetist should be contacted concerning the correct detail.

Self-suspending sockets

The amputee is first taught how to apply this type of socket by the prosthetist. It is difficult for the therapist to assist the amputee other than by encouraging the correct coordination of this procedure and providing time to practise.

In order to be successful in using their prosthesis, the amputee must have good coordination, standing balance and great patience, particularly during the first few weeks.

In carrying out the basic wrap method (see Fig. 13.8), the amputee is instructed to:

1. Stand up, with either a chair or the wall behind, and with the prosthesis resting close by.

2. Using a 15 cm wide Elset or crepe bandage, lightly bandage the residual limb with 2–3 turns (according to length of the residual limb) from medial to lateral, starting posteriorly and proximally (Fig. 13.8A)

3. Make a tuck with the long end of the bandage into the anterior dorsal twin turns, fixing the bandage to the residual limb and leaving a long portion free (Fig. 13.8B)

4. Feed the long end of the bandage inside the socket and pull it through the valve hole (Fig. 13.8C)

5. Place the residual limb inside the socket with the prosthesis in correct alignment.

6. Gradually withdraw the bandage through the valve hole, gently drawing the residual limb tissue down into the socket (Fig. 13.8D). During this procedure, gently ease the residual limb downward into the socket. Should the bandage become stuck at any stage, stop withdrawing the bandage: this allows time for the residual limb tissues to move. If possible, ease the residual limb away from the offending area, then resume withdrawing the bandage by pulling on each edge alternately.

7. The whole bandage should be pulled out through the valve hole. The residual limb should

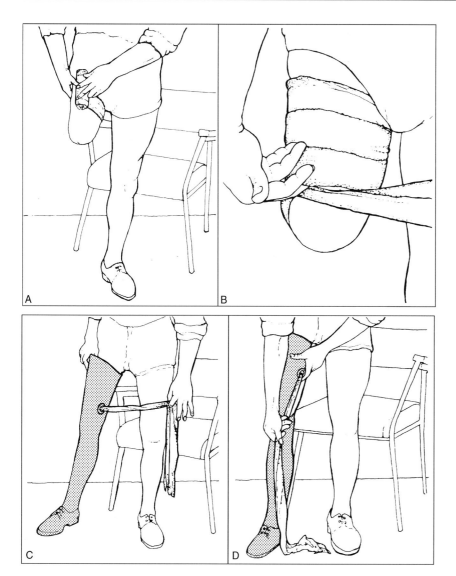

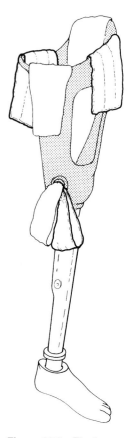

Figure 13.9 The two loop method showing the starting position of the two draped bandages.

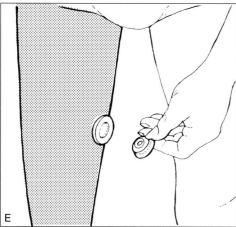

Figure 13.8 Donning the self suspending socket by the basic wrap method: (A) wrapping residual limb; (B) fixing bandage to residual limb; (C) pulling bandage through valve hole; (D) drawing bandage down the socket; (E) tightening valve.

be correctly positioned in the socket at this stage: there should be no space between the residual limb with the valve and the TSB socket, but there should be a small gap of approximately 2 cm with the suction socket.

8. Locate the valve in the valve hole and tighten (Fig. 13.8E).

The two-loop method

This is another method of application of the self-suspending socket (Fig. 13.9). Two 10 cm-wide Elset bandages are used in the positions shown. Four bandage ends are draped over the anterior, posterior, medial and lateral aspects of the brim of the socket: the length draped is determined by the amputee, but it should be at least as long as the residual limb. The amputee stands in narrow stride standing, with the remaining leg in front. The residual limb is pushed into the socket as far as it will go and then the bandage is drawn out equally through the valve hole, a little at a time. This will ease in each section of the residual limb at a time.

The wrap method will only ease the tissues in from the top of the circumference of the residual limb, whereas this method will ease in the buttock tissues as well and is the only method for the CAT–CAM socket. This method is also useful for amputees with fluctuating stump volume as it is a more rigorous method of drawing the tissues into the socket.

Some amputees may prefer to use a stump sock or a silk scarf instead of a bandage.

Rigid pelvic band (see Fig. 13.10)

This is the only suspension that can be applied easily while sitting down. The following instructions should be given to the amputee:

1. Sit on a firm bed, undressed apart from a vest.
2. Pull the stump sock smoothly over the residual limb (Fig. 13.10A).
3. With the knee joint of the prosthesis flexed and the foot in lateral rotation, slide the residual limb into the socket (Fig. 13.10B).

4 Fasten the RPB loosely over the vest (Fig. 13.10C).
5. Fasten the shoulder strap (if used) when sitting and adjust to the correct tension when standing (Fig. 13.10D).
6. Pull the stump sock up and over the rim of the socket to prevent wrinkling (Fig. 13.10E). This position can be maintained with a large safety pin securing the sock around the metal upright of the hip joint.
7. Stand and fasten the RPB securely. This will rotate the foot into the correct position.

Some amputees with good balance can slide the residual limb, with the sock on, into the socket of the prosthesis while they are standing. The knee joint should be locked and the prosthesis rotated laterally before the RPB is secured.

Dressing

The amputee should be instructed to:

1. Pull the underpants and trousers (if worn) up over the prosthesis before applying it to the residual limb.
2. Apply the prosthesis.
3. Slot the remaining leg into the underpants and trousers, then fasten over the suspension. If underwear is worn inside the suspension, use of the lavatory is impossible. Trouser legs, particularly jeans, may need to be widened with a triangular insert in the inside leg seam, as the socket may be broader than the thigh of the natural limb.
4. Check the shoe on the prosthesis, because the prosthetic foot is aligned for one height of heel. Also check that the matching shoe is on the remaining foot.
5. Dress the top half of the body in the normal way. The shoulder strap should be underneath the shirt/blouse.

Doffing the prosthesis

All amputees can do this seated, but those with excellent standing balance may prefer to remove the prosthesis while standing:

1. Unfasten the suspension, ease the socket off

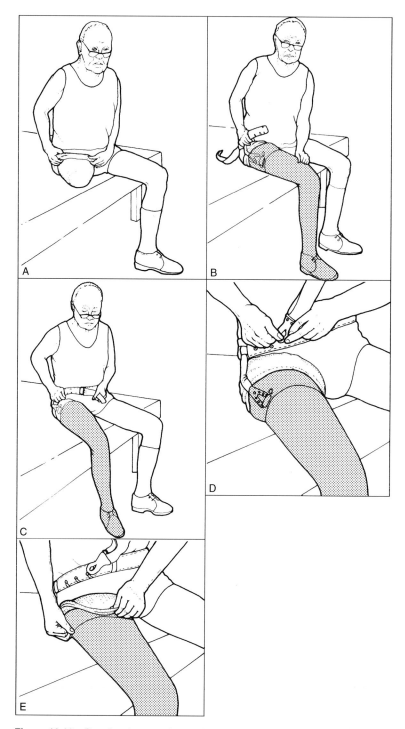

Figure 13.10 Donning the trans-femoral prosthesis with RPB.

the residual limb and remove the stump sock (if worn).

2. Inspect the residual limb for areas of redness, rubbing or spots; all amputees should be taught to do this. A mirror may be needed to view the posterior and medial aspects of the residual limb.

Using the toilet

1. A man can stand and urinate with few problems.

2. Good balance is necessary for the removal of clothing prior to sitting down: grab rails may be needed in the early stages of rehabilitation.

3. When sitting, amputees may prefer to abduct the hip to prevent soiling the stump sock and medial edge of the socket.

4. Some amputees may prefer to remove their prosthesis before using the toilet (particularly women).

GAIT RE-EDUCATION

The therapist must check the fit of the prosthesis before commencing gait re-education. The amputee should initially be in the parallel bars. It is important that regular strengthening and mobility exercises are maintained during this phase of rehabilitation.

The procedures for initial gait re-education and progression to walking aids are described in detail in Chapter 10. The trans-femoral amputee will take considerable time to achieve a reasonable gait pattern and to understand how to use the knee component to its full advantage. Trials are safest in the parallel bars. The age of the amputee, cause of amputation and presence of concurrent disease will have the greatest bearing on the intensity of the rehabilitation programme.

Walking on different surfaces

This must be practised both indoors and outside under the supervision of the therapist. Linoleum, shiny wood, stone floors, different thicknesses of carpet, pavement, grass, gravel and rough ground must all be attempted. The amputee must be confident on these surfaces both alone and when outside in crowded situations.

Different surfaces will transmit different sensations up through the socket to the residual limb. The amputee must learn to recognise these new feelings and adapt their gait pattern accordingly. The younger amputee can practise altering speed of reaction on a balance board or on a computerised balance performance monitor in the therapy facility.

Stairs

The amputee is first taught to climb stairs using two banisters. When ascending, the remaining leg leads; when descending, the prosthesis leads. Progress to using one stick and one banister is made. When descending, the amputee must place the stick down one stair before stepping down with the prosthesis.

Stairs must always be practised with the therapist, even if there are no stairs in the amputee's home environment. The amputee's life must not be limited by immediate surroundings. If the amputee walks with a frame, stairs can be managed with one stick and one banister. If this is difficult or unsafe, then the amputee faces the banister, grasps it with both hands, and ascends and descends sideways. Two walking frames are then provided: one to keep upstairs and one downstairs. Established users with a sophisticated hydraulic swing and stance control are able to descend stairs in a normal reciprocal pattern.

Step/kerb

Unless the amputee has practised negotiating steps or a kerb outside the therapy facility under supervision, it is unlikely that walking outside will be achieved with confidence.

The amputee should keep the feet as close to the kerb as possible, step up with the remaining leg first and step down with the prosthesis first.

Ramps hills

These are more difficult than stairs and may be accomplished with a greater degree of safety by proceeding sideways, ascending with the remaining leg first and descending with the prosthesis first.

On ascending in the forward direction, the amputee must lean forward, place the sticks well forward and lead with the remaining leg. The prosthesis should be brought level with the remaining foot.

On descending in the forward direction, the sticks are placed forward first, then the prosthesis. The remaining foot is brought forward parallel to the prosthetic foot, which is not completely in contact with the slope at this point.

When the gradient is steep, the hip extensor muscles of the residual limb must work hard to ensure balance on the prosthesis during the stance phase. If the gradient is excessively steep it is always safer to ascend and descend sideways. The more able and those with enabling knee components may achieve equal stride lengths on slopes.

Getting up from the floor

Teaching the amputee to fall down is both dangerous and unnecessary. It is the method of getting up that should be taught and practised. The amputee is always instructed to remain on the ground for a few moments after a fall to get over the shock and think out the method of recovering walking aids and getting up.

If a chair is available, the amputee should move across the floor to it either by rolling or by scooting on the buttocks, remembering to take the walking aids. The therapist should explain and demonstrate the three methods of getting up (listed later) to elderly amputees. Carers, relatives and friends are also shown these methods and are taught correct manual handling procedures. If able, they should practise these manoeuvres as part of their rehabilitation programme. All amputees are advised on how to ask for and direct help from a member of the public who has come to their aid: assertiveness on the part

of the amputee is essential for both their own and their voluntary assistant's safety.

Method 1 (Fig. 13.11)

1. Turn to face the seat.
2. Put both hands on the seat.
3. Kneel on remaining leg with prosthesis extended behind.
4. Push on hands and straighten up on remaining leg to stand.
5. Release grip on chair as balance is regained and use aids.

Method 2 (Fig. 13.12)

1. Sit close to chair with back touching the seat.
2. Put both hands on seat of chair.
3. Flex up the knee of the remaining leg.
4. Push up hard and slide both buttocks onto the seat.

Method 3 (Fig. 13.13)

(This method should be used if no seat is available.)

1. Gather walking aids.
2. Roll prone, leading with remaining leg.
3. Push up on forearms and flex remaining leg.
4. Start extending remaining leg, push up on one stick, regain balance and then push up on second stick.

If the amputee is unable to use any of these three methods, as they are unable to provide any help, their full weight must not be lifted by any assistant as this may cause physical harm to both the amputee and the assistant and is against the manual handling regulations (see Ch. 4, p. 49) – a mechanical method should be employed. For those who fall regularly or who are in residential accommodation, correct handling equipment, e.g. hoists and slings, must be available and all carers trained in their use.

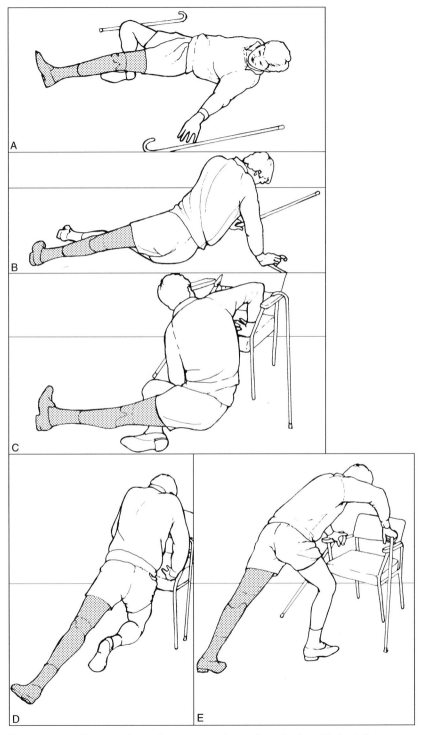

Figure 13.11   The trans-femoral amputee getting up from the floor (Method 1).

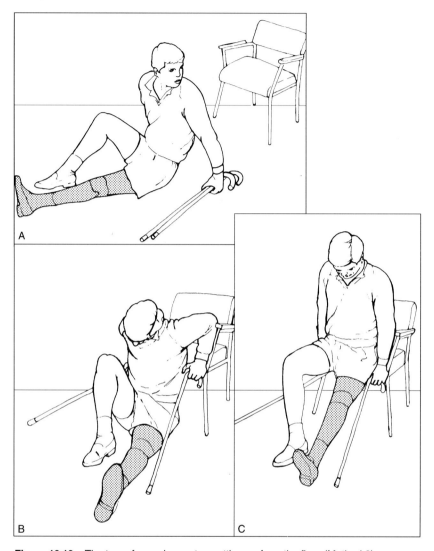

Figure 13.12 The trans-femoral amputee getting up from the floor (Method 2).

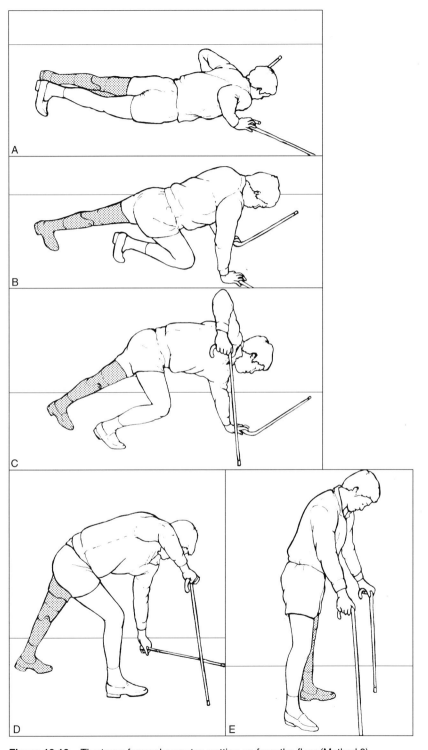

Figure 13.13   The trans-femoral amputee getting up from the floor (Method 3).

PROSTHETIC INFORMATION

Detailed information regarding prostheses available in the UK can be obtained from the manufacturers. The addresses are listed in Appendix 1.

BIBLIOGRAPHY FOR PREVIOUS EDITIONS

Gailey R, Newell C 1991 Metabolic cost of unilateral above-knee amputees walking: a comparison between the quadrilateral socket and the CAT-CAM socket. WCPT 11th International Congress Proceedings Book II:641–643

Judge G W, Fisher L 1981 A bouncy knee for above-knee amputees. Engineering in Medicine 10(1):27–31

Kristinsson O 1983 Flexible above-knee socket made from low density polyethylene suspended by a weight transmitting frame. Orthotics and Prosthetics 37(2):25–30

Radcliffe C W 1977 The Knud Jansen Lecture. Above-knee prosthetics. Prosthetics and Orthotics International 1(3):146–160

Redhead R G 1979 Total surface bearing self suspending above-knee sockets. Prosthetics and Orthotics International 3(3):126–136

Sabolich J 1985 Contoured adducted-trochanteric controlled alignment method (CAT-CAM): introduction and principles. Clinics in Prosthetics and Orthotics 9(4):15–26

Schuch C M 1988 Report from: International workshop on above-knee fitting and alignment techniques. Clinical Prosthetics and Orthotics 12(2):81–98

Simpson D 1980 Prosthetic replacement of knee function. Physiotherapy 66(8):262–265

Watts H G, Carideo J F, Marich M S 1982 Variable-volume sockets for above-knee amputees. Managing children following amputation for malignancy. Inter Clinic Information Bulletin 18(2):11–14

BIBLIOGRAPHY FOR THE THIRD EDITION

Boonstra A M, Schrama J M, Eisma W H, Hof A L, Fidler V 1996 Gait analysis of trans-femoral amputee patients using prostheses with two different knee joints. Archives of Physical Medicine and Rehabilitation 77:515–520

Farber B S, Jacobson J S 1995 An above-knee prosthesis with a system of energy recovery: a technical note. Journal of Rehabilitation Research and Development 32(4):337–348

Foerster S A, Bagley A M, Mote D, Skinner H B 1995 The prediction of metabolic energy expenditure during gait from mechanical energy of the limb: a preliminary study. Journal of Rehabilitation Research and Development 32(2):128–134

Jaegers S M H J, Vos L D W, Rispens P, Hof A L 1993 The relationship between comfortable and most metabolically efficient walking speed in persons with unilateral above-knee amputation. Archives of Physical Medicine and Rehabilitation 74:521–525

Jaegers S M H J, Arendzen J H, de Jongh H J 1995 Changes in hip muscles after above-knee amputation. Clinical Orthopaedics and Related Research 319:276–284

Lee V S P, Solomonidis S E, Spence W D 1997 Stump-socket interface pressure as an aid to socket design in prostheses for trans-femoral amputees – a preliminary study. Proceedings of the Institution of Mechanical Engineers 211(part H):167–180

14

Knee disarticulation and associated levels of amputation

There are four different levels of amputation about the knee joint:

1. Knee disarticulation
2. Gritti-Stokes
3. Transcondylar
4. Supracondylar.

Knee disarticulation

This is a disarticulation of the tibia from the femur. The patella is left in situ and the patellar tendon is sutured to the hamstring tendons and cruciate ligaments around the end of the femur. This residual limb has the capability to be fully end weightbearing and normal proprioception is maintained.

As all the muscles around the hip joint are intact, there is powerful control of the long lever of the residual limb, and its bulbous shape allows a self-suspending socket with rotational stability between socket and residual limb. Cosmesis is not always acceptable, particularly for women, as the socket with the knee component makes the knee joint line more distal than the natural knee. This is noticeable both when sitting down and the prosthesis protrudes, and when walking, as the shin appears short. However, lightweight endoskeletal prostheses and recent knee designs have greatly improved function and cosmesis.

It can be an ideal level for the elderly amputee and also for those who may become bilateral amputees. Full weightbearing is possible both on the residual limbs themselves and in prostheses.

Where prosthetic re-education is not possible, the long lever and endbearing properties of this level allow for good sitting balance in the wheelchair and the residual limb can be used as a prop when transferring.

It is also a good level for children as the distal femoral epiphysis is left intact ensuring normal growth. It can be used for the removal of a useless congenitally deficient lower limb.

This level is inadvisable if a hip flexion contracture is present. In this situation the prosthesis appears bulky and is cosmetically unacceptable. Furthermore, the weightbearing area may have to be transferred proximally to the ischium. This level thus becomes biomechanically the same as the above knee level, negating the endbearing properties of the residual limb.

Gritti–Stokes

The distal end of the femur is divided at the level of the adductor tubercle in the Gritti–Stokes level of amputation. The patella is retained, its articular surface is removed and it is sutured over the cut end of the femur. This is the classical Gritti-Stokes; however, it is rarely done.

Modified Gritti-Stokes/transcondylar

The distal end of the femur is divided at the level of the epicondyles. This is more commonly done than the classical Gritti-Stokes.

Supracondylar

The distal end of the femur is divided at about the level of the adductor tubercle. The medullary cavity is left open. This is treated as a very long trans-femoral amputation (see Ch. 13).

For positive confirmation of the Gritti-Stokes, transcondylar and supracondylar level of amputation, X-rays may be required. These three levels give a residual limb that is a long lever with powerful hip muscle control. The bulbous end of the residual limb is reduced so self-suspension of the socket is not always possible and some auxiliary suspension may be required. Proprioception is lost at these levels along with

some of the endbearing property of the residual limb, necessitating proximal weightbearing areas on the prosthesis. If the patella is retained, it frequently loosens and gives rise to pain when the amputee is walking.

CONSTRUCTION OF THE KNEE DISARTICULATION PROSTHESIS

Prosthetic sockets

Total contact

This is a total contact socket with a soft liner and an outer plastic hard shell. The Pelite liner (high-density foam material) is made on a cast taken of the residual limb, so that the fit is intimate. The liner has a small split made in it, so that on application it will open to allow the bulbous femoral condoyles to slide through the length of the liner. When the residual limb touches the distal end pad, the slit closes completely. It may also be made of leather or metal.

This type of socket is usually self-suspending with the amputee's weight taken totally on the distal end of the residual limb. If it is necessary to reduce endbearing, a proximal-bearing brim shape (e.g. quadrilateral or H-type) is incorporated as for a trans-femoral prosthesis. Occasionally the 'plug fit' socket is also used.

Conventional sockets

Blocked leather with lace-up front fastening or metal sockets are sometimes used with established limb wearers. Auxiliary suspension may also be required.

Auxiliary suspension

The three types of auxiliary suspension, namely rigid pelvic band, shoulder suspension and soft suspension are described in Chapter 13 and are occasionally used.

Knee components

The most usual knee component supplied is the polycentric design as it gives a better cosmetic

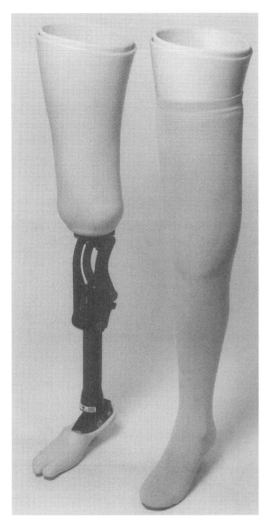

Figure 14.1 The Endolite prosthesis for the knee-disarticulation amputee. It has a four-bar linkage knee mechanism and a multiflex ankle mechanism. (Photograph by kind permission of C.A. Blatchford, & Sons Ltd.)

appearance. Other knee mechanisms as described in Chapter 13 may also be supplied (see Fig. 14.1).

CHECK OF THE KNEE DISARTICULATION PROSTHESIS

The fit of the prosthesis should be checked by the therapist on the first attendance for gait re-education and subsequently at regular intervals. The amputee's function will depend on the cor-

rect fit. The amputee should always be suitably undressed for this procedure.

Socket

The endbearing pad

The distal end of the residual limb must be supported by this pad to prevent distal oedema but the degree of weightbearing achieved will depend on the type of amputation and the stage of healing reached.

With plastic sockets it is important to check the fit of the liner on the residual limb, by palpating the residual limb through the liner; it should be a snug fit with no gaps.

If the amputee reports discomfort, too much weight may be taken distally. The reasons for this may be that:

- the socket is too large
- the stump sock has formed a wrinkle between the residual limb and end pad
- too much activity.

The therapist may remove the end pad and insert several layers of soft foam instead, thus reducing some of the distal pressure as a temporary measure.

Another reason for discomfort may be that too little weight is taken distally and there is proximal constriction. The therapist must teach the amputee to watch for a cold, blue and mottled end to the residual limb.

Socket too large

If the socket is too large, pistoning and rotation will occur and suspension and alignment will be lost. This happens commonly in the early stages of prosthetic re-education as the distal residual limb oedema subsides and the thigh muscles atrophy. It may also happen if the amputee's total weight drops by 4 kg or more.

Great care must be taken if adding more stump socks as too much pressure may be exerted over the distal condyles. The sock may be cut as a temporary measure to pad out the mid-thigh area only. Sometimes a sock added between the

Pelite liner and the hard plastic shell may create sufficient suspension as a temporary measure.

The prosthetist must be contacted for an assessment for a new liner, socket or both.

Socket too small

If the socket is too small, the residual limb will not slide down sufficiently to contact the end-bearing pad. Constriction of the distal residual limb occurs and it is unlikely that the amputee will function in this circumstance; 'ischaemic' residual limb pain may be reported. This will occur if the amputee gains a significant amount of weight.

The prosthetist must be contacted for a new liner, socket or both.

Length

Standing

A routine check of the length is made statically and dynamically (see Ch. 13).

Sitting

When the amputee sits down, with both knees flexed, the socket protrudes further than the natural knee. This is inevitable as the end pad and socket and knee joint components are distal to the natural knee joint line.

Auxiliary suspension

The suspension must be comfortable and secure if used (see Ch. 13).

Knee components

The therapist should check the working and function of the knee components supplied before the amputee uses the prosthesis for the first time. This will ensure that the correct method of use is taught. If there is any doubt, the therapist should contact the prosthetist to check the function of the components supplied.

Alignment

If a hip flexion contracture is present, it will cause a greater problem at the knee disarticulation than trans-femoral level of amputation as the residual limb is longer and there is no space. There is little scope for the prosthetist to accommodate flexion in the socket, so a cosmetically and functionally unacceptable prosthesis results. The therapist should do everything possible to treat and reduce such a contracture (see Ch. 5). For further details on alignment see Chapter 13.

FUNCTIONAL RE-EDUCATION WITH THE KNEE DISARTICULATION PROSTHESIS

The therapist should give short, clear instructions at all stages of functional re-education.

Donning the prosthesis (see Fig. 14.2)

The amputee should be instructed as follows:

1. Sit on a firm bed or chair and undress apart from a vest.
2. Pull the stump sock smoothly up over the residual limb (Fig. 14.2A).
3. Remove the Pelite liner from the plastic shell and pull it onto the residual limb (Fig. 14.2B). Sometimes this procedure is difficult because the liner is such a tight fit, but the distal end of the residual limb must be in contact with the foam end pad. A nylon sock is pulled over the Pelite liner (Fig. 14.2C)
4. Apply the plastic socket with the knee flexed, (Fig. 14.2D)
5. Fasten the auxiliary suspension (if present) over the vest.
6. Pull the stump sock up and out over the rim of the socket to prevent wrinkling.
7. Stand up with support, and re-adjust the suspension if necessary. (Fig. 14.2E).

Some amputees with good balance can apply the prosthesis while standing, but the knee joint of the prosthesis must be in extension. NB.:

- Donning the plug fit socket is the same as for the trans-femoral level of amputation.

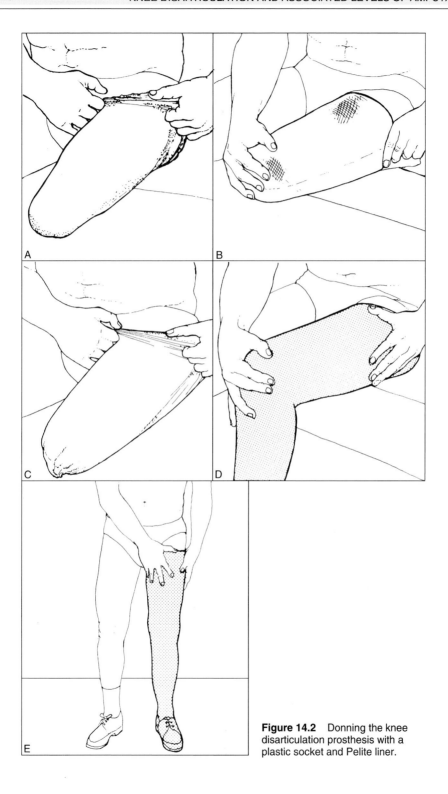

Figure 14.2 Donning the knee disarticulation prosthesis with a plastic socket and Pelite liner.

- Donning the blocked leather socket requires care in ensuring the residual limb is in close contact with the endbearing pad before fastening the socket securely.

Doffing

It is simpler to doff a prosthesis than to apply it and the less able amputee should attempt this first. The following instructions should be given:

1. Sit down on a firm bed or chair.
2. Undo the auxiliary suspension if present.
3. Ease the socket off the residual limb; the outer shell is removed first and then the Pelite liner.
4. Remove the stump sock.
5. Inspect the residual limb thoroughly, especially the femoral condyles, for any redness, rubbing or spots. A mirror should be used to check the distal and posterior aspects.

Dressing

The same procedure is employed for amputees with the knee disarticulation level of amputation as for those with the trans-femoral level (see Ch. 13). The width of the knee of the prosthesis may be greater than the natural knee, so alterations to trouser leg width may be required.

Using the toilet

Some patients prefer not to wear the prosthesis when sitting on the toilet seat in order to open their bowels.

GAIT RE-EDUCATION

Gait re-education is similar to that for the trans-femoral amputee. However, the main difference is that there is a long, powerful lever controlling the prosthesis. Smooth control of the knee mechanism and stride length using proprioception and cutaneous sensation is essential to avoid a long prosthetic stride and uneven gait pattern. Hip extensor exercises should be continued to control overactive hip flexion and resisted walking is a useful method of training.

The true knee disarticulation amputee is able to fully weightbear through the distal end of the residual limb. The amputee with the Gritti-Stokes level of amputation may also be able to fully weightbear distally at this stage. However, if the amputee complains of discomfort in the distal end of the residual limb, it may be that the patella has become detached from the femur and is moving as the amputee walks. In this instance, the therapist should contact the prosthetist or the surgeon.

Amputees with the modified Gritti-Stokes and supracondylar levels of amputation are never able to fully weightbear through the distal area of the residual limb and require ischial weightbearing sockets. Therefore, the function is similar to the trans-femoral amputee.

PROSTHETIC INFORMATION

Detailed information regarding prostheses available in the UK can be obtained from the manufacturers. The addresses are listed in Appendix 1.

BIBLIOGRAPHY FOR PREVIOUS EDITIONS

Baumgartner R F 1979 Knee disarticulation versus above-knee amputation. Prosthetics and Orthotics International 3(1):15–19
Baumgartner R F 1983 Failures in through-knee amputation. Prosthetics and Orthotics International 7:116–118
Houghton A, Allen A, Luff R, McColl I 1989 Rehabilitation after lower limb amputation: a comparative study of above-knee, through-knee and Gritti-Stokes amputations. British Journal of Surgery 76:622–624

Jendrzejczyk D J 1980 Prosthetic management for children with knee disarticulations. Inter Clinic Information Bulletin 17(7):9–16
Jensen J S 1983 Life expectancy and social consequences of through-knee amputations. Prosthetics and Orthotics International 7:113–115
Jensen J S, Poulsen T M, Krasnik M 1982 Through-knee amputation. Acta Orthopaedica Scandinavica 53:463–466

Martin P, Wickham J E A 1962 Gritti-Stokes amputation for atherosclerotic gangrene. Lancet ii:16–17

Mensch G 1983 Physiotherapy following through-knee amputation. Prosthetics and Orthotics International 7:79–87

Moran B J, Buttenshaw P, Mulcahy M, Robinson K P 1990 Through-knee amputation in high-risk patients with vascular disease: indications, complications and rehabilitation. British Journal of Surgery 77:1118–1120

Thyregod H C, Holstein P, Jensen J S 1983 The healing of through-knee amputations in relation to skin perfusion pressure. Prosthetics and Orthotics International 7:61–62

BIBLIOGRAPHY FOR THE THIRD EDITION

Ayoub M M, Solis M M, Rogers J J, Dalton M L 1993 Thru-knee amputation: the operation of choice for non-ambulatory patients. The American Surgeon 59:619–623

Hagberg E, Berlin Ö K, Renström P 1992 Function after through-knee compared with below-knee and above-knee amputation. Prosthetics and Orthotics International 16(3):168–173

Pinzur M S 1993 Gait analysis in peripheral vascular insufficiency through-knee amputation. Journal of Rehabilitation Research and Development 30(4):388–292

Yusuf S W, Makin G S, Baker D M, Hopkinson B R, Wenham P W 1997 Role of Gritti–Stokes amputation in peripheral vascular disease. Annals of the Royal College of Surgeons England 79:102–104

15

Trans-tibial level of amputation

Information from international sources indicates that almost all amputees will be successful prosthetic users at the trans-tibial level of amputation, irrespective of their age. The knee joint is preserved, enabling the amputee to gain as near normal a gait as is possible.

Amputees of this level consume less energy than those with higher levels of amputation, as there is a long lever controlling the prosthetic foot and ankle. It is possible to prosthetically re-educate the vast majority of trans-tibial amputees, provided that the correct surgical technique preserves muscle bulk, creates a good residual limb shape and scar position and that the prosthesis fits correctly and is comfortable. The patellar tendon bearing-type prosthesis supplied for trans-tibial amputees is cosmetically very acceptable and deviations from the normal gait pattern are usually undetectable. The suitable length for a trans-tibial residual limb varies. The residual limb is measured from the joint line to the distal end of the residual limb, with the knee flexed to 90°. Prosthetic fitting can be achieved with almost any length, from just below the knee joint to the musculo-tendinous junction of the calf muscles, but the length has some effect on the control of the prosthesis and symmetry of gait.

For children, a trans-tibial amputation does not affect the upper epiphyseal plate of the tibia, and therefore the residual limb grows with the child, unlike the trans-femoral residual limb.

It must be noted that in dysvascular cases, the residual limb may be slow to heal; amputees may have to wait some time before prosthetic re-education can commence and they may become frustrated. The continued use, however, of exercise and the early walking aid (see Chs 5 & 6) helps to maintain the function and mobility during this slow healing stage.

The literature indicates that approximately 30% of dysvascular primary amputees lose their remaining leg within 2–3 years and if only one of these amputations is trans-tibial, a significant level of function and mobility may be obtained.

There are, however, a few *contraindications* to selecting this level of amputation:

1. Hemiplegic patients requiring an amputation on the affected side should never have this level selected, as however minimal the abnormal reflex neurological patterns may appear prior to surgery, a flexor pattern will emerge or increase following surgery, making prosthetic rehabilitation impossible. This type of patient is most suited to a knee disarticulation or trans-femoral amputation.

2. Any patient assessed as unfit for prosthetic re-education may encounter the following problems with a trans-tibial residual limb that may lead to surgical revision at a higher level:
- muscle imbalance resulting in knee flexion contracture
- severe damage and tissue breakdown of the residual limb caused by knocking furniture while manoeuvring the wheelchair.

3. The condition of the knee joint prior to surgery must be carefully assessed. A grossly unstable, painful or flexed joint will not control a prosthesis easily. Conditions such as rheumatoid arthritis, severe osteoarthrosis and ligamentous instability may initially appear stable enough to control this level of amputation, but it must be remembered that these can deteriorate with time. Patients with little range of movement, or an arthrodesed knee are unlikely to benefit from this level of amputation.

Many other conditions, such as wasted muscles in the lower leg, adherent scars, uneven bone contours, skin grafts and poor sensation, can be prosthetically accommodated and the amputee rehabilitated with success at this trans-tibial level. This is dependent on whether the surgeon is adept and imaginative when fashioning the residual limb and expert prosthetic services are available offering a range of the newer materials.

PATELLAR TENDON BEARING (PTB) PROSTHESIS

There is a wide range of different socket designs that come under this generic heading. They all allow the amputee to walk with a natural free knee gait from the outset of prosthetic re-education. They are suitable for amputees with a residual limb with minimal oedema.

The advantages are that they are easy to don, easy to use and cosmetically acceptable. The disadvantage is that the fit has to be intimate and this is difficult to achieve in amputees where residual limb volume fluctuates, e.g. those with diabetes or cardiac pathology, those taking diuretics and those receiving renal replacement therapy. The amputee must learn to add and subtract socks of different thickenesses as necessary to maintain the correct fit.

Maintenance of an intimate fit means that frequent adjustments to the socket may be required. This can be a problem where there are either transport difficulties or the amputee is geographically distant from the prosthetist. The amputee cannot continue with prosthetic re-education if skin problems are caused by the socket. Alternative means of mobility (e.g. wheelchair or crutches) must be used. This can interrupt the amputee's functional independence at home.

Close liaison is required between the therapist and the prosthetist in the early stages of gait re-education with a PTB-type prosthesis. There is a wide variety of interchangeable socket designs and auxiliary suspension available for the residual limb with fitting or skin problems. Great skill and imagination are required of both professions to overcome difficulties, and reassurance must be given to the amputee that a correct fit may take a little time and effort to achieve if the residual limb is not 'ideal'.

Prosthetic sockets

There is a variety of socket designs, some self-suspending and some requiring auxiliary suspension; however, most are designed to accommodate pressure-tolerant and pressure-sensitive areas of the trans-tibial residual limb.

The following weightbearing areas are emphasised (see Fig. 15.1A):

- patellar tendon area
- medial flare of the tibia and tibial condyle (and to a lesser extent the lateral flare)
- posterior muscle bulk.

Weightbearing is relieved in the following areas (Fig. 15.1B):

- distal end of the tibia
- crest of the tibia and tibial tubercle
- head and distal end of the fibula
- hamstring tendon insertions, both medial and lateral.

PTB socket

This socket is intimately fitting with minimal relief over the pressure-sensitive areas. There is a patella tendon bar filling the space between the inferior pole of the patella and the tibial tubercle. The socket fits closely under the medial tibial condyle and there is good support to the popliteal surface of the residual limb and a flare to accommodate the hamstring tendons (see Fig. 15.2).

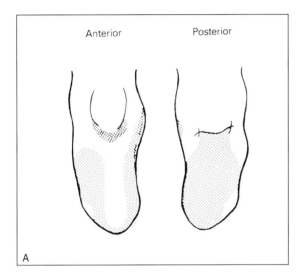

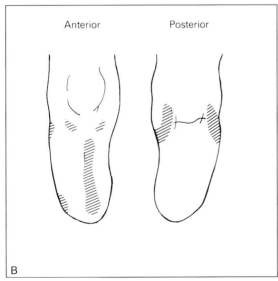

Figure 15.1   The pressure tolerant (A) and pressure-sensitive (B) areas of the trans-tibial residual limb.

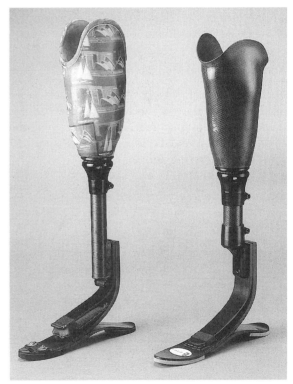

Figure 15.2   Trans-tibial sports prostheses. The PTB supracondylar socket is on the left; the standard PTB socket on the right. Note the dynamic response feet (Flexfoot). (Photograph by kind permission of C.A. Blatchford and Sons Ltd.)

PTB supracondylar socket

This socket is basically the same as the PTB socket, but the medial and lateral walls are high enough and suitably shaped to enclose the medial and lateral femoral condyles, thus increasing the suspension particularly for short residual limbs and for preventing hyperextension in knees with ligamentous laxity (see Fig. 15.2).

Prosthèse tibiale supracondylienne (PTS) socket

This is as the PTB/supracondylar socket, but the anterior wall of the socket is raised and suitably shaped to encompass the patella further increasing the suspension.

It should be noted that in most instances, these sockets are set in a slight degree of flexion and adduction to ensure correct weightbearing, particularly on the patella tendon, which is emphasised by the counterforce of the upper part of the posterior wall.

Köndylen bettung Munster (KBM) socket

With this socket, weight is taken much more on the medial flare of the tibia and the patellar tendon bar is not so marked. It is a dynamic casting method and is done with the amputee standing in a casting jig.

Silicone sockets (e.g. Iceross)

These are made of a pliable silicone material in the shape of a closed-end sleeve. Suspension is achieved by adhesion between skin and silicone and the elasticity of the sleeve enables it to follow the contours and movement of the skin of the residual limb. They are roll-on sleeves used to improve both comfort and suspension (see Fig. 15.3). The silicone sleeve attaches to a hard shell (PTB shape) by either a lanyard or a ratchet lock mechanism. They may or may not be used with a Pelite liner. Care is needed not to damage the sleeve with long fingernails or sharp objects. Contraindications for this type of socket include ulceration of the residual limb, unhealed scars, poor patient hygiene and inability to handle the

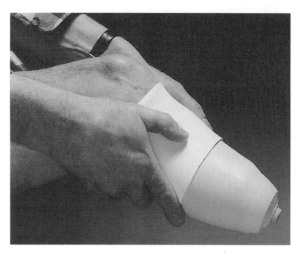

Figure 15.3   The Iceross silicone sleeve applied to a trans-tibial residual limb. (Photograph by kind permission of Ossür UK.)

delicate material or understand the concept of its application.

These sockets are also used for other levels of amputation (see Ch. 8).

Icex

This is a fabrication method with combined casting, fabricating and fitting of a prosthetic socket in one session. The prosthesis is a silicone sleeve with a hard carbon braid outer shell; this outer shell is formed directly on the amputee using Icecast apparatus. It is a total surface bearing socket (see Fig. 15.4).

Socket liners

Pelite liner

This is a liner made on a cast taken of the residual limb; it is a high density foam material. The residual limb will have either a stump sock or other liner applied before the Pelite liner, and then the hard outer shell socket comes over all of these.

TEC liner

The interface of the TEC liner is made of a urethane material that has the ability to ease

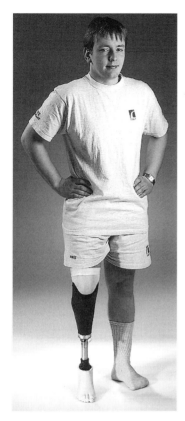

Figure 15.4   The Icex prosthesis. (Photograph by kind permission of Ossür UK.)

the pressure-sensitive areas of the residual limb. It is custom made and is especially useful over adherent scars and skin grafts. It may or may not be used with a Pelite liner.

Alpha liner

The inner liner of this is composed of a mineral oil-based gel and it provides extra padding and comfort. There are two types: (1) a cushion liner alone; and (2) a cushion liner plus a locking mechanism (as that described for the silicone socket). It may or may not be used with a Pelite liner.

Auxiliary suspension

Leather cuff

This passes immediately above the patella, fits snugly around the femoral condyles and fastens firmly posterolaterally, usually with a buckle. Angled side straps attach the cuff to the socket (see Fig. 15.8E). The actual design of the supracondylar cuff can vary. Some have an elasticated middle portion, which is particularly useful for amputees with ill-defined contours about the knee.

Silicone socket or neoprene-impregnated gel liner

These are both described as sockets and as suspension techniques.

Elastic sleeve suspension

Fits over the distal femur and the proximal socket. It may be made of elastic stocking material, e.g. Juzo suspension sleeve, or Neoprene. Amputees require strong hands with maximal dexterity to apply these sleeves.

Elastic stocking

The female amputee can suspend the prosthesis with a specially made elastic stocking attached to a suspender belt.

Pick-up strap

Added to the cuff suspension and attached to a waist belt; may be required if the contour of the amputee's knee is ill-defined or the residual limb is short (see Fig. 15.5).

Articulating supracondylar prosthesis

Here there is a firm, wide supracondylar cuff to augment the suspension provided by the socket (see Fig. 15.6).

Check of the PTB-type prosthesis

A full explanation of the correct weightbearing areas must be given to the amputee by the therapist. This must be fully comprehended because the fit of this prosthesis is intimate. It is essential

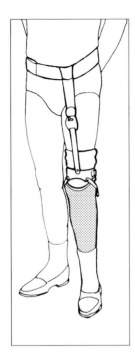

Figure 15.5 A pick-up strap attached to the supracondylar cuff of the PTB prosthesis improves suspension.

that the skin is checked regularly during the day, *at least every 5 minutes* to begin with; skin checking is the amputee's responsibility. If any redness or soreness is noted they must stop walking and remove the prosthesis immediately. The most satisfactory method of checking the fit of the socket can be achieved when the therapist applies the prosthesis onto the residual limb.

Sitting

The amputee should be sitting, the affected leg suitably undressed and the residual limb held in about 40° flexion at the knee.

The stump sock (if used) should be eased over the residual limb ensuring no creases are present and that the shape is correctly aligned to the individual.

The liner of the socket should then be eased on:

* if made of Pelite it is possible to feel the correct position, i.e. the weightbearing bar of the socket is in direct contact with the patella tendon of the amputee. The residual limb

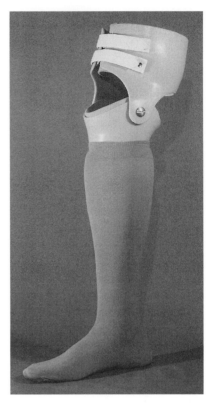

Figure 15.6 Articulating supracondylar prosthesis. (Photograph by kind permission of Rehabilitation Services Ltd).

should be fully supported by this liner, i.e. there should be total surface bearing with no obvious gaps, either distally or around the rim of the liner and condyles. It may be necessary to fill the end of the liner with pieces of cut foam or unravelled wool (e.g. from an old stump sock) to ensure distal tissue support.
* if a silicone, TEC or Alpha sleeve is used, the therapist should roll it onto the residual limb, noting the ease of application; if difficulties arise, a lubricant or talc can be used if this is recommended by the manufacturer. It should fit with total surface bearing.

The outer hard socket should then be applied over the liner:

* if a Pelite liner is used, the therapist should slide it into the hard socket and the fit between the two should be perfect.

- if a silicone, TEC or Alpha sleeve is used, the hard outer socket is then applied and the locking mechanism (if present) checked.

In all cases, the amputee should be able to flex the knee to 90° and the therapist should check that there is adequate flaring of the posterior brim to accommodate the hamstring tendons. There should not be excessive bulging of tissue in the popliteal area.

Auxiliary suspension (if used) is then fastened:

- the position of the supracondylar cuff should be such that it traps the patella between the cuff and the anterior brim of the socket. It must be firmly fastened but with enough space to allow two fingers to pass underneath it; the tourniquet effect must be avoided. The amputee should be sufficiently dextrous to fasten the cuff correctly. If a buckle is unmanageable or unsightly, Velcro can be used. The therapist should make sure that the side straps are firm when the knee is in extension and a little looser when the knee is flexed.
- if an elastic sleeve, elastic stocking or pick-up straps are used, the amputee must be able to fasten them correctly and the therapist should check that suspension is maintained.

If the socket is difficult to apply, the following remedies can be tried:

1. The therapist may decrease the number and thickness of the stump socks. It is possible to use a PTB socket while wearing only a nylon sock, providing a careful check of the skin is kept by both the therapist and amputee. It is often necessary to experiment with different types of socks for several days until the residual limb has settled down and the oedema has reduced.

2. Sometimes the liner fits, but the hard outer socket appears too tight, i.e. it is either very difficult or impossible to ease over the liner. This may occur if the shape of the residual limb is bulbous distally. If a nylon sock (and/or talcum powder) is applied between the liner and the outer socket it will ease donning and doffing.

3. If the residual limb is grossly oedematous and the prosthesis is impossible to apply it may

be possible to reduce the oedema by the following methods:

a. Place the amputee supine, with the residual limb in high elevation and apply a stump bandage or shrinker sock (see Ch. 4). Leave the residual limb in this position for 1 hour, instructing the amputee to perform muscle contractions in the residual limb before trying to apply the prosthesis again.

b. If available, a variable air pressure machine (e.g. Flowtron, Jobst, etc.) should be used with the residual limb elevated (see Ch. 4).

4. There may be other reasons for the tightness of the socket and the therapist should always investigate the persistently oedematous residual limb. If the remaining leg also shows oedema, the amputee may have poorly controlled congestive cardiac failure or diabetes. They may also have put on weight, and a weight variation of more than 2.5 kg can affect residual limb volume. A medical opinion may be necessary.

5. If the socket is too loose, the therapist must increase the number and type of stump socks worn between the skin and the Pelite liner; the preferred maximum number of socks is three thick socks. In the case of prosthetic sockets with silicone 'liners' such as Iceross, Alpha and TEC, socks can be added between the liner and hard outer socket. If these adjustments do not work, the therapist must contact the prosthetist as adjustments to the prosthesis or a new socket will be needed.

Standing

The amputee then stands supported and partially weightbears through the prosthesis, and a further check of the prosthesis is made. The therapist should check that the shoe worn has a heel of equal height and diameter to that for which the prosthesis was aligned and that the amputee is wearing a matching pair of shoes.

If a Pelite liner is worn, about 0.5 cm of the liner should be visible above the rim of the socket and the anterior brim should extend to the middle of the patella. If a locking silicone or other type of sleeve is worn, the therapist should check that the locking mechanism is working.

If the amputee reports discomfort when standing, has reduced sensation in the residual limb or is unable to report reliably, the therapist must check that there is sufficient tissue contact between the distal end of the residual limb and the liner, but not undue pressure. This may be determined by inserting a piece of Blu-Tac or Plasticine inside the Pelite liner prior to application of the prosthesis. After the amputee has been standing for a few minutes, the prosthesis is removed and the Blu-Tac or Plasticine examined for marks of indentation from the stump sock. 'Touch' pressure for tissue support must be present. If it is not, cut pieces of shaped foam or unravelled wool (e.g. from an old stump sock) should be inserted into the liner to produce this tissue support. This is necessary to prevent terminal oedema and undue stress on a scar line, which is often directly over the cut end of the tibia.

If the indentations on the Blu-Tac are heavy, the residual limb has sunk too far down into the socket. This usually occurs if the socket is too large, in which case the therapist should:

- Add socks without losing the shape of the residual limb relative to the socket; a sock can also be added between the liner and the hard outer socket
- Check the suspension
- Check to see if the set of the socket in flexion is sufficient to maintain correct weightbearing on the appropriate areas
- Add a popliteal pad between the liner and the hard outer socket in order to push the residual limb forwards onto the patella tendon bar.

Walking

When walking in the parallel bars, a dynamic check of the fit is made. There should be no obvious discomfort in any part of the residual limb and minimal pistoning between the residual limb and the prosthesis. A line drawn on the sock or sleeve along the posterior brim is a useful guide to check pistoning when the amputee is observed from behind. This should be no more than 1 cm. The socket (and auxiliary suspension if used) should maintain adequate suspension throughout the gait cycle. If it does not, either adjustments to the auxiliary suspension must be made or the design of the socket and/or auxiliary suspension and materials used must be changed.

All trans-tibial amputees will report pressure over the correct weightbearing areas during the early stages of PTB-type prosthetic rehabilitation. It takes time for the skin to harden to pressure and the amputee must be reassured that discomfort should subside with time. Those wearing PTB/supracondylar, PTS or KBM sockets may report redness and/or soreness over the femoral condyles and the inferior and lateral borders of the patella. The skill is in developing a balance between an acceptable level of 'new soreness' (as a good suspension of these sockets is dependent on a snug fit) and an actual pressure sore. The following measures may be used to improve comfort:

- To reduce friction, a nylon sock may be worn between the residual limb skin and the other stump sock. Alternatively, a special gel impregnated or another 'comfort' sock may be used instead. It may be possible to apply an ordinary wool or cotton sock on the outside of the comfort sock if extra 'padding-out' is needed.
- To protect the skin, a small, smooth dressing can be applied over the patella tendon, which is removed after gait re-education sessions.
- To prevent any skin breakdown occurring, the therapist and amputee must constantly check the condition of the skin of the residual limb. Gait re-education may have to be limited to short periods of time during the initial phases. Skin abrasions are a disaster, particularly for those with diabetes and marked peripheral vascular disease.

When checking the PTB-type prosthesis, the therapist should be aware that amputees with peripheral vascular disease may be experiencing ischaemic pain in the residual limb. This will not be helped by alterations to the fit of prosthesis. Ischaemia may be detected by:

- A blue/red mottled colour to the skin of the residual limb, which is cold to the touch and blanches on elevation

- The reporting of intense pain
- An indolent wound in which slough is present.

It should be realised that in some cases further surgery may be required and therefore relevant medical investigations should be obtained. A full progress report should be sent from the therapist to the surgeon.

Alignment

The socket, suspension and set of the foot are visually checked to maximise the perfection of the gait cycle.

Functional re-education with the PTB-type prosthesis

Donning the prosthesis

With sock and Pelite liner (see Fig. 15.7)

1. The amputee should be sitting down, the amputated side undressed apart from underwear.

2. The stump sock should be pulled up smoothly over the residual limb. If more than one sock is used, they must be applied separately (Fig. 15.7A)

3. The Pelite liner should be eased onto the residual limb with the knee held in about 40° flexion (Fig. 15.7B & C)

4. If used, the supracondylar cuff should be folded forward over the anterior aspect of the hard socket before the prosthesis is applied over the liner.

5. The hard socket is pulled on, with the knee in flexion. It may be necessary to exert downward pressure through the residual limb, by pressing the heel of the prosthesis onto the floor, in order to slide the residual limb right down into the socket (Fig. 15.7D).

6. If used, the cuff is pulled up over the knee and must be fastened securely (Fig. 15.7E).

7. The stump sock should be pulled up firmly (some amputees prefer to fold the sock back down over the cuff).

8. If an elasticated sleeve or stocking is used, the amputee must be able to stand to fasten securely.

PTB/supracondylar and PTS sockets. The amputee should slide the residual limb into these sockets before 'climbing in' over the posterior brim so that the residual limb is not caught by the supracondylar flares. The knee joint can be in near extension and the socket should be at a forward-tilted angle of 45° to the residual limb.

KBM socket. The stump sock is applied, then a tubular stocking is put over the sock and residual limb. The residual limb is drawn down into the liner by pulling the tubular stockinette out through an opening in the bottom of the liner. The stockinette is then folded back over the liner and the hard outer socket is applied.

The prosthetist will determine the exact method for donning the KBM socket and it is essential that the therapist is made aware of the chosen method.

It should be noted that this pull-in technique can be used to draw a fleshy residual limb into any PTB-type liner if it is a tight fit. Care should be taken not to pinch the tissues in the split in the Pelite liner to accommodate the large circumference being pulled through it.

Silicone sleeve (see Fig. 15.3). The silicone sleeve must be turned inside out before application. A small amount of talcum powder or water is then put into the sleeve (i.e. onto the outer wall) to assist donning the hard socket. The distal end of the residual limb is then placed against the distal end of the sleeve and this is then rolled onto the limb. It may take a little while for the amputee to manage this with ease. No talcum powder or water should be applied to the inside wall of the sleeve that touches the skin of the residual limb.

The coupling device, consisting of a pin attached to the silicone sleeve, slots and locks audibly into a receptacle within the outer socket. This is done either with the amputee sitting and applying pressure through the heel of the prosthesis with the knee at about 60° flexion (assisted if necessary by downward hand pressure through the knee) or by standing and applying pressure through the prosthesis.

If using a lanyard, it must be pulled firmly at the same time as the amputee pushes the residual

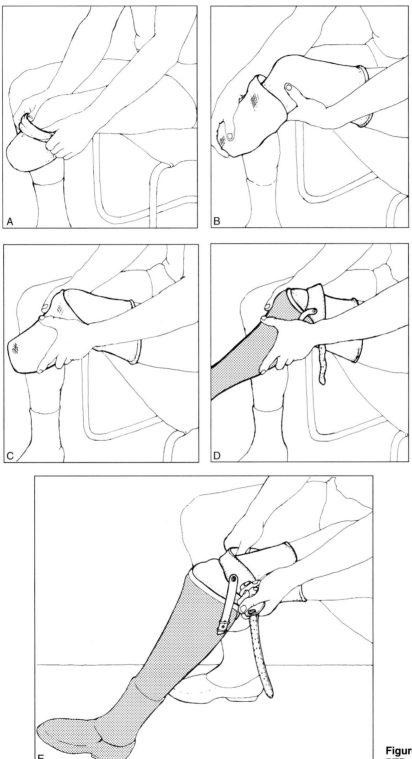

Figure 15.7 Donning the PTB prosthesis.

limb down into the hard socket. Once the liner is completely pulled in, the thumb wheel that traps the lanyard must be tightened. The cord is then either wound around the prosthesis or over the thumb wheel. After a few steps, the therapist and amputee should check whether the lanyard needs to be tightened.

TEC liner. To don this liner, a lubricant is applied to the residual limb and the liner is pulled on. Sometimes it may be necessary to invaginate the liner and roll it over the residual limb. Stump socks are not normally worn with the TEC interface system. Once the liner is in place any remaining air trapped between the liner and limb is massaged away. The liner is then fitted into the hard outer socket.

Alpha liner. This liner has two colours indicating thicker and thinner walls; the thicker part is worn anteriorly and the thinner posteriorly to allow for flexion of the knee. The liner is rolled down on itself into a doughnut shape and the distal end placed directly against the residual limb. It is rolled up over the limb and the top trimmed to length for each amputee. A Pelite liner may also be applied and then the hard outer socket. If a locking pin is present, the outer socket is applied as for the silicone sleeve.

Doffing the prosthesis

1. The amputee should sit down and undo any auxiliary suspension.

2. With the knee held in 30–40° flexion, the residual limb should be eased out of the prosthesis. If there is no locking pin present, the socket, liner and sock usually all come off together. If there is a locking mechanism for the sleeve, the release knob should be pressed (or the lanyard unsecured) while withdrawing the residual limb from the hard outer socket, then the sleeve should be gently turned back on itself (i.e. the reverse of donning) and eased off the skin.

3. The skin of the residual limb should be inspected using a mirror if necessary. The correct weightbearing areas for the design of prosthesis may be red: this is normal. However, the weight-relieved areas should not be red or rubbed – if they are, alterations to the prosthesis may be

necessary if this persists. No terminal oedema should be present.

Dressing

If a skirt is worn, there will be no difficulty in applying this type of prosthesis either before or after dressing. If tight trousers or jeans are worn it is better to dress the PTB before donning it.

In the early stages of gait re-education, when frequent examination of the skin of the residual limb has to be made, it is better if shorts or track suit trousers are worn.

Gait re-education with the PTB-type prosthesis

The main consideration that the therapist has to take into account here is the time spent wearing the PTB prosthesis, which is limited initially by the tolerance of the skin of the residual limb. It is the therapist's responsibility to remind the amputee to constantly check the residual limb and decide when activity must be interrupted for an interval to allow the skin to recover. Frequently, those who are enthusiastic wish to continue walking for too long and must be persuaded to rest. As a general rule, gait re-education should initially not be longer than 1 hour per morning and afternoon. It must be made clear to the amputee that walking is not permitted at home until skin tolerance of the weightbearing areas is satisfactory and independence has been achieved with a suitable walking aid in the therapy facility.

The aim of gait re-education with this prosthesis is to achieve a normal gait pattern and it should start in the parallel bars. Most of these amputees will have used an early walking aid (EWA), and if this was a Ppam aid, they will be accustomed to hip hitching and walking with a stiff knee; smooth hip and knee flexion prior to toe off must be practised. At heel strike, controlled knee flexion is required in order to prevent either hyperextension or sudden knee flexion and sometimes a different type of shoe with a softer heel is needed to facilitate this control.

An even stride length and rhythm should be encouraged. A mirror and video are very helpful visual aids. The therapist should observe the gait pattern from in front, at the sides and behind.

When a near-normal gait pattern has been achieved in the parallel bars, progression to walking aids can be made. Although the majority progress to walking sticks very quickly, elderly and frail amputees may need the full support and confidence given by a walking frame or tetrapods.

In the early stages it may not be possible to use a normal gait pattern on stairs or ramps, but as knee control, skin tolerance and muscle strength improve, ability increases. Later on, most will climb stairs normally with the exception of the elderly and those with concurrent pathology.

There are no special methods for getting up after a fall. However, before getting up it is important that the amputee remains seated on the floor for a short time to overcome shock and retrieve walking aids.

THIG CORSET PROSTHESIS
(see Fig. 15.8)

This type of prosthesis continues to be supplied to those amputees accustomed to the design who do not wish to change, or when there are contraindications to any type of PTB design.

Examples of conditions in which the thigh corset may be used are:

- an unstable knee joint. This may be stabilised by the side steels of this design, which act as a caliper
- A knee flexion contracture of more than 25°
- Malformation of the patella or knee joint area, e.g. congenital abnormality of the patella, occasionally patellectomy, or deformities caused by fractures
- An amputee whose occupation or hobbies involve heavy work, e.g. farming, mountaineering, oil rig workers, etc. – these people may need a thigh corset design for work, but can be supplied with a PTB-type prosthesis for social activities.

Those amputees who then need to change from a thigh corset to a PTB-type prosthesis will need to be well motivated, have time to adapt and be prepared to commit themselves to a muscle strengthening, gait and function retraining programme with a therapist. In later life, an amputee may suffer from peripheral vascular disease and the thigh corset will restrict arterial blood flow to the residual limb with consequent claudication discomfort.

Construction of the thigh corset prosthesis

Thigh corset

This is made of blocked leather with a front fastening and may be ischial or buttock weight-bearing; some weight is taken through the length of the corset itself.

Knee joint

Articulated side steels extend either side of the thigh corset down to the lower leg. Very occasionally a locking mechanism may be supplied.

Socket

The trans-tibial residual limb is contained in the shank, which is made of either metal, wood or plastic. The socket is usually proximally weight-bearing and made to fit around the upper half of the residual limb approximately 3 cm from the lower pole of the patella.

With a metal shank, a blocked leather slip socket is always present (see Fig. 15.8), which is made on a plaster cast taken of the residual limb. The slip socket is placed into the shank in such a way that it allows both it and the residual limb to move when the amputee is sitting, thus protecting the residual limb from knocking against the shank. Sometimes elastic straps are attached from the thigh corset to the slip socket in order to maintain firm contact with the residual limb while walking and sitting.

Backstrap

A leather backstrap attaches the thigh corset to the shank posteriorly to prevent hyperextension of the knee.

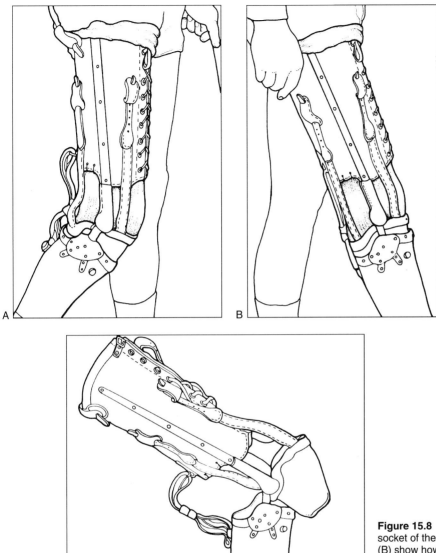

Figure 15.8   The blocked leather slip socket of the thigh corset prosthesis. (A) and (B) show how it moves with the trans-tibial residual limb during walking. (C) shows the slip socket lifted out of the metal shank.

Suspension

This type of prosthesis may be self-suspending, although the following auxiliary suspension may be used:

• a waist belt suspension with one anterior strap extending to below the knee, which aids swing through, and one posterior downstrap attaching to the corset

• a shoulder strap that crosses over the opposite shoulder from the amputated side and fastens with anterior and posterior straps.

Check of the thigh corset prosthesis

The therapist should check that the amputee is wearing nothing under the stump sock.

Standing

The amputee must be standing with the knee fully extended and weight evenly distributed. If the prosthesis is ischial weightbearing, the therapist should carry out the check in exactly the same way as for the trans-femoral prosthesis (see Ch. 13). The thigh corset should be fastened correctly. It must not be fastened too tightly as circulatory embarrassment can occur. The length of the prosthesis is checked in the same way as for the trans-femoral prosthesis (see Ch. 13).

The slip socket must be correctly positioned so that some weight is taken on the patella tendon area and upper part of the residual limb. If this seems too loose, a short stump sock can be added.

The auxiliary suspension should be firm when the amputee stands erect and it should maintain the correct position of the prosthesis throughout the gait cycle.

Sitting

The prosthetic knee joint must be aligned with the natural knee joint line. If there is a slip socket present, the therapist should check that it moves with the residual limb when the amputee sits down. The buckles on the elastic straps attaching the slip socket to the thigh corset can be adjusted if necessary.

If there is no slip socket present and the amputee experiences discomfort in the residual limb while sitting with the knee flexed to 90°, the therapist should contact the prosthetist for alterations.

If discomfort persists when the amputee is sitting, the therapist should remove and reapply the prosthesis to check for correct positioning and fastening of the thigh corset. Amputees can 'fasten' themselves either 'in' or 'out' of the prosthesis.

Walking

The blocked leather thigh corset will soften slightly with body heat; re-fastening after about an hour of gait re-education may be necessary.

However, the amputee should not fasten it too tightly as this produces a tourniquet effect.

Pistoning can be checked by observing the gait from behind. After checking the fastening of the thigh corset and auxiliary suspension, and the number and thickness of the stump socks, the therapist may decide to contact the prosthetist for further suspension.

The adductor region at the groin must be comfortable. The therapist must check that the prosthesis has been applied at the correct angle, that the stump socks are well pulled up out over the brim of the corset and that the amputee is using hip extensor muscles maximally at heel strike. If there is a flexion contracture at the knee joint it is possible that a hip flexion contracture is also present, which may not have been accommodated in the set of the thigh corset. If adjustments are necessary, the prosthetist should be contacted.

The therapist should check and if necessary re-educate the knee joint function to prevent hyperextension at heel strike. If it persists, the backstrap can be tightened. The alignment of the prosthesis should be observed throughout the gait cycle and if obvious abnormality is present, the prosthetist must be contacted.

Functional re-education with the thigh corset prosthesis

Donning the prosthesis

The amputee must sit down in order to ease on the prosthesis, but then must be able to stand up to put downward pressure through the foot before fastening the corset. Considerable dexterity and balance are required. The auxiliary suspension must be fastened while sitting, but adjusted to the correct tension while standing.

If the amputee is unable to manage the lacing of the thigh corset it can be changed to straps and buckles or Velcro. This is particularly important for amputees who may have diminished sensation in the fingers and visual impairment.

Gait re-education

The hip muscles will be used more than the knee muscles to control the prosthesis and this can produce a rather uneven gait with an energetic swing phase and pronounced heel strike. The therapist should use a mirror or video as an adjunct to feedback for the amputee to gain a smoother gait.

Progress to walking aids is made as for the PTB-type prosthesis.

It should be noted that the thigh muscles of a user of this type of prosthesis will atrophy in time through disuse.

PROSTHETIC INFORMATION

Detailed information regarding prostheses available in the UK can be obtained from the manufacturers. The addresses are listed in Appendix 1.

BIBLIOGRAPHY FOR PREVIOUS EDITIONS

Boldingh E J K, Van Pijkeren T, Wijkmans D W 1985 A study on the value of the modified KBM prothesis compared with other types of prosthesis. Prosthetics and Orthotics International 9:79–82

Donn J M, Porter D, Roberts V C 1989 The effect of footwear mass on gait patterns of unilateral below-knee amputees. Prosthetics and Orthotics International 10:139–141

Enoka R M, Miller D I, Burgess E M 1982 Below-knee amputee running gait. American Journal of Physical Medicine 61(2):66–84

Fleurant F W, Alexander J 1980 Below knee amputation and rehabilitation of amputees. Surgery, Gynaecology and Obstetrics 151:41–44

Isakov E, Mizrahi J, Susak Z, Onna I 1992 A Swedish knee cage for stabilising short below-knee stumps. Prosthetics and Orthotics International 16:114–117

Kegel B, Burgess E M, Starr T W, Daly W K 1981 Effects of isometric muscle training on residual limb volume, strength, and gait of below-knee amputees. Physical Therapy 61(10):1419–1426

Renstrom P, Grinby G, Larsson E 1983 Thigh muscle strength in below-knee amputees. Scandinavian Journal of

Rehabilitation 9:163–173

Robinson K P 1972 Long-posterior-flap myoplastic below-knee amputation in ischaemic disease. Lancet Jan 22:193–195

Robinson K P, Hoile R, Coddington T 1982 Skew flap myoplastic below-knee amputation: a preliminary report. British Journal of Surgery 69(9):554–557

Saadah E S M 1988. Bilateral below-knee amputee 107 years old and still wearing artificial limbs. Prosthetics and Orthotics International 12:105–106

Vittas D, Larsen T K, Jansen E C 1986 Body sway in below-knee amputees. Prosthetics and Orthotics International 10:139–141

Weiss J, Middleton L, Gonzalez E, Lovelace R E 1983 The thigh corset: its effect on the quadriceps muscle and its role in prosthetic suspension. Orthotics and Prosthetics 37(3):58–62

Wilson A B 1979 Lightweight prostheses. Prosthetics and Orthotics International 3:150–151

Wirta R W et al 1990 Analysis of below-knee suspension systems: effect on gait. Journal of Rehabilitation Research and Development 27(4):385–396

BIBLIOGRAPHY FOR THE THIRD EDITION

Anderson S P 1995 Dysvascular amputees: what can we expect? Journal of Prosthetics and Orthotics 7(2):43–50

Blumentritt S 1997 A new biomechanical method for determination of static prosthetic alignment. Prosthetics and Orthotics International 21(2):107–113

Boonstra A M, van Duin W, Eisma W 1996 International forum. Silicone suction socket (3S) versus supracondylar PTB prosthesis with pelite liner: trans-tibial amputees' preferences. Journal of Prosthetics and Orthotics 8(3):96–99

Cortés A, Viosca E, Hoyos J V, Prat J, Sánchez-Lacuesta J 1997 Optimisation of the prescription for trans-tibial (TT) amputees. Prosthetics and Orthotics International 21(3):168–174

Dasgupta A K, McCluskie P J A, Patel V S, Robins L 1997 The performance of the ICEROSS prostheses amongst trans-tibial amputees with a special reference to the

workplace – a preliminary study. Occupational Medicine 47(4):228–236

Gailey R S, Nash M S, Atchley T A et al 1997 The effects of prosthesis mass on metabolic cost of ambulation in non-vascular trans-tibial amputees. Prosthetics and Orthotics International 21:9–16

Humzah M D, Gilbert P M 1997 Fasciocutaneous blood supply in below-knee amputation. The Journal of Bone and Joint Surgery 79B(3):441–443

Isakov E, Burger H, Gregoric M, Marincek C 1996 Stump length as related to atrophy and strength of the thigh muscles in trans-tibial amputees. Prosthetics and Orthotics International 20:96–100

Johnson V J, Kondziela S, Gottschalk F 1995 Pre and post-amputation mobility of trans-tibial amputees: correlation to medical problems, age and mortality. Prosthetics and Orthotics International 19:159–164

Johnson W C, Watkins M T, Hamilton J, Baldwin D 1997 Transcutaneous partial oxygen pressure changes following skew flap and Burgess-type below-knee amputations. Archives of Surgery 132:261–263

Kaufman J L 1995 Alternative methods for below-knee amputation: reappraisal of the Kendrick procedure. Journal of the American College of Surgeons 181:511–516

Liao K I, Skinner H B 1995 Knee joint proprioception in below-knee amputees. The American Journal of Knee Surgery 8(3):105–109

Pinzur M S, Cox W, Kaiser J, Morris T, Patwardhan A, Vrbos L 1995 The effect of prosthetic alignment on relative limb loading in persons with trans-tibial amputation: a preliminary report. Journal of Rehabilitation Research and Development 32(4):373–378

Powers C M, Boyd L A, Torburn L, Perry J 1997 Stair ambulation in persons with trans-tibial amputation: an analysis of the Seattle Lightfoot. Journal of Rehabilitation Research and Development 34(1):9–18

Saleh M, Datta D, Eastaugh-Waring S J 1995 Long posteromedial myocutaneous flap below-knee amputation. Annals of the Royal College of Surgeons England 77:141–144

Smith D G, Horn P, Malchow D, Boone D A, Reiber G E, Hansen S T 1995 Prosthetic history, prosthetic charges, and functional outcome of the isolated, traumatic below-knee amputee. The Journal of Trauma: Injury, Infection and Critical Care 38(1):44–47

16

Symes and partial foot levels of amputation

SYMES AMPUTATION

This was first performed by James Syme of Edinburgh in 1842. The amputation is a disarticulation of the ankle: the os calcis is removed and the tibia is sectioned just proximal to its distal articular surface, with the removal of the medial malleolus. The lateral malleolus is removed at the same level. The heel pad and tough skin overlying it are retained and swung forward to cover the ends of the tibia and fibula. The suture line is anterior. It is essential postoperatively that the dressings maintain the heel pad in position, so that a firm contact is established between it and the bone ends. The heel pad should not slip posteriorly. A frequent cause of failure of this level of amputation is related to the position, fixation or viability of the heel pad. The ideal residual limb should be capable of total endbearing, with or without a prosthesis, and should be short enough to allow a prosthetic foot to be fitted to a normal shoe, i.e. there should be a ground clearance of the residual limb of at least 4 cm. If the residual limb cannot fully endbear, a patelar tendon bearing (PTB) brim is needed at the proximal end of the socket.

This residual limb has similar attributes to those of knee disarticulation, i.e. it is a long, endbearing residual limb with proprioceptive properties. The indications for this procedure are:

1. trauma
2. congenital shortening of the leg
3. chronic infection of the foot.

Trauma

Severe trauma to the forefoot, provided that the plantar heel pad is intact, can be treated with this level of amputation. Cold trauma, i.e. frosbite, is another reason for this amputation.

Congenital shortening of the leg

The foot may be normal in appearance but useless functionally in this situation. Prosthetic management with extension prostheses (see Ch. 21) can be facilitated by removal of the foot.

Chronic infections of the foot

Patients with perforating ulcers, possibly diabetic in origin, or infections secondary to a neuropathy (diabetes, leprosy and spina bifida) may benefit from this level of amputation, providing there is adequate sensation in the heel pad. In countries where sophisticated drugs are less readily available, this level of amputation may be the first choice of treatment for these conditions.

Very occasionally, this level may be selected where there is distal diabetic vascular disease, but it is rarely successful in atherosclerosis.

SYMES PROSTHESIS

Depending on the speed of wound healing, the amputee can mobilise very early, in a prosthesis. The materials used for the construction of the socket are blocked leather and thermoplastics.

Enclosed metal Symes prosthesis

This prosthesis is cosmetically acceptable and some women with this level of amputation favour it. There is a leather socket, with a posterior flap opening, which fits inside the metal shin and attaches to it. The foot is uniaxial or low profile SACH (see p. 106).

All plastic Symes prosthesis
(see Figs 16.1 and 16.2)

This prosthesis has improved cosmesis, with a smooth outline and reduced ankle width. There

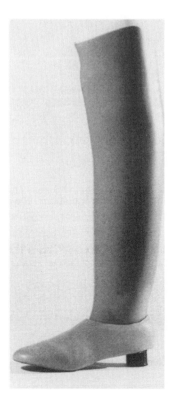

Figure 16.1 The all plastic Symes prosthesis.

is a Pelite liner, which fits into the hard plastic outer socket. There is no access panel and it is described as a 'push fit'. This is similar to the knee disarticulation plastic socket (see Ch. 14). However, the Canadian window-type Symes prosthesis has a posterior or medial access panel held in place by Velcro straps or elastic cuffs. The foot is as for the enclosed metal Symes with the addition of the Quantum foot, or carbon fibre blade, e.g. the Spring Lite foot or Low Profile Symes from Flex-Foot (see Ch. 8, p. 106).

CHECK OF THE SYMES PROSTHESIS

The therapist should check that the weightbearing areas of the residual limb for which the prosthesis is constructed are being utilised correctly.

Total endbearing prosthesis

As stated previously, some residual limbs can be totally endbearing and some require the weight

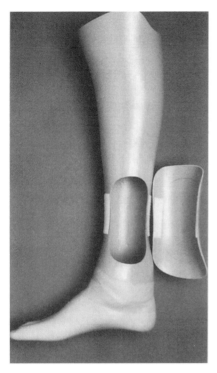

Figure 16.2   The Canadian window-type Symes prosthesis. (Photograph From Redhead et al.)

to be distributed proximally. The heel pad should not become red or sore during walking. The scar line must be watched carefully during the early stages of prosthetic use.

Amputees who have a hyposensitive residual limb should have gait re-education within the level of their skin tolerance. The therapist must frequently remove the prosthesis and examine the residual limb for areas of redness, rubbing or spots. The amputee must be taught to examine the residual limb, using a mirror to check the heel pad. If a totally endbearing prosthesis is used and the amputee complains of discomfort on the heel pad, the reasons may be that:

- The stump sock has not been pulled up over the residual limb correctly and has possibly formed wrinkles over the weightbearing areas.
- A different type of stump sock may be needed, e.g. the thick terry-cotton sock.
- The socket is too loose, which allows excessive movement of the residual limb.

- The socket is too tight, causing constriction of circulation.
- The socket is ill-fitting around the bony contours of the residual limb.
- The set of the prosthetic foot may need adjustment in order to prevent excessive shear forces, particularly at heel strike and toe off.

The therapist can alter the endbearing pad with pieces of foam, change the type and thickness of the stump sock and check that the prosthesis has been applied correctly.

Partial endbearing prosthesis

Some amputees need to distribute the weight between the following areas: the distal end of the residual limb, the length of the residual limb, the medial tibial condyle and the patellar tendon. However, some are totally proximally weighbearing.

Prosthetic re-education in the early stages must be limited to short sessions to allow for progressive hardening of the skin over the proximal weightbearing areas (see Ch. 15).

It must be remembered that if the therapist is unable to solve a fitting problem the prosthetist must be contacted for any necessary alterations to be made.

The position of the heel pad over the bone ends can slip after a period of prosthetic use. Discomfort will be reported in this area and no amount of alteration to the prosthesis will help. The hospital surgeon must be contacted with a view to revision of the residual limb.

PARTIAL FOOT AMPUTATION

Mid-tarsal amputation (Chopart)

This is a disarticulation between the talus and calcaneus proximally and the navicular and cuboid distally.

Tarsometatarsal amputation (Lisfranc)

This is a disarticulation of the forefoot at the tarsometatarsal line. These amputations are rarely carried out, the only indications being severe crush injury of the forefoot and frostbite. Occasionally they are carried out for infection of the forefoot. The disadvantages of these levels of amputation are that the residual limb tends to be pulled into equinus by the unbalanced pull of the Achilles tendon and into inversion by tibialis anterior. Also, even after the wound has healed, the skin that remains over the antero-inferior aspect of the residual limb tends to develop callosities and corns with prosthetic wear. These can become painful and troublesome.

Therapy is required pre-operatively and immediately postoperatively in order to maintain ankle joint mobility and the length of the Achilles tendon, thus avoiding the equinus deformity.

Shoe fillers

Therapists, chiropodists or an orthotist can make temporary weightbearing bootees using the thermoplastic material, or a Drushoe can be used (see Fig. 2.4, p. 20).

When using shoe fillers the skin of the residual limb should be checked regularly by the therapist and amputee.

Partial foot prostheses

There are several prostheses for this level of amputation, three of which are described here:

1. A short leather ankle corset attached to a wooden foot, which may be worn inside a normal shoe. The amputee takes weight through the heel pad and the corset must be securely fastened to prevent a sliding movement of the residual limb. Full ankle range is maintained.
2. A custom-made silicone socket/slipper is a very cosmetically acceptable alternative (see Fig. 16.3). The advantage of this type of prosthesis is that they may be worn with or without a shoe. The disadvantages are that they are rather sweaty, heavy and the forefoot lever may be insufficiently rigid. This design is very popular with partial foot amputees. Care must be taken when applying silicone feet as the material can be torn.

3. A simple shoe filler made of leather-covered Ortholene, which fits inside a normal shoe.

It should be noted that the design of the prostheses for the Chopart and Lisfranc amputations will be dictated by the weightbearing properties and shape of the individual residual limbs.

FUNCTIONAL RE-EDUCATION OF THE SYMES AND PARTIAL FOOT LEVELS OF AMPUTATION
Donning the prosthesis

The Symes and most Chopart levels of amputation have a stump sock that must be pulled up smoothly to ensure that there are no wrinkles over the weightbearing areas.

With partial foot prostheses, an ordinary ankle sock can be worn. No specific instruction is required for the donning of these prostheses.

All partial foot amputees will need to obtain shoes that fit over the prosthesis and some effort may be required in finding a suitable pair.

Gait re-education

Amputees with these distal levels of amputation often experience a greater sense of functional loss than those with more proximal levels of amputation.

Balance training is the most important consideration, particularly for the forefoot and first toe amputees. Initially, rhythmic stabilisation in standing and a balance board can be used, and the therapist must encourage the amputee to walk outside over different surfaces such as gravel, rough ground, hills, etc. It is on these surfaces particularly that amputees will notice their altered balance reactions.

Loss of push off is progressively more noticeable, the more distal the amputation. Seemingly minor amputations may produce a very uneven gait pattern.

Although one of the benefits of the Symes and Chopart levels is that they are endbearing, enabling the amputee to walk without wearing a prosthesis, it should be realised that as the initial cause of amputation is often neuropathic,

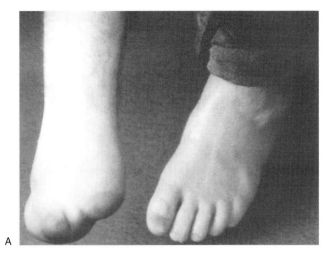

A

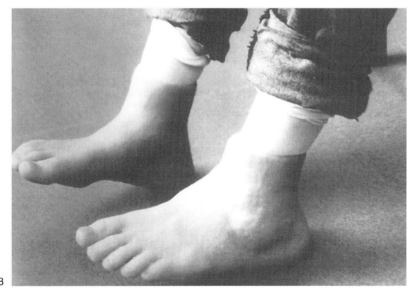

B

Figure 16.3   A bilateral foot amputee. (A) Shows the extent of amputation; (B) shows the cosmetic silicone partial foot prostheses. (Photograph by kind permission of Hugh Steeper Ltd.)

sensation of the residual limb is diminished. Damage may therefore occur, which may not be perceived immediately when the amputee walks about the home without the prosthesis. If an open area occurs and becomes infected, re-amputation may be necessary. The therapist should test the sensation of the residual limb in all distal levels of amputation. The danger of damage and the simple measures that can be taken to avoid this must be fully explained to the amputee. A home visit is necessary to check out the floor coverings, the presence of loose carpet, tacks, etc.

TRANS-METATARSAL AND TOE AMPUTATIONS

The trans-metatarsal level involves amputation of the toes proximal to the metatarsal heads. The indications are:

• Trauma

- Slowly progressive localised gangrene precipitated by minor injury. A high proportion of these patients are diabetic
- After major reconstruction of large vessels for peripheral vascular disease, the distal part of the foot may not be revascularised and may require amputation
- Deformity.

Amputation of all the toes is indicated either for extensive trauma, frostbite or multiple deformities, e.g. rheumatoid arthritis.

Amputation of an individual toe with its corresponding metatarsal is called a 'ray' amputation.

Wherever amputation of the toes is thought to be indicated, due consideration must be given to the stability, biomechanics and viability of the remaining foot. For example, if the first ray is amputated (the most stable ray), weight is then transferred onto the lateral border of the foot, which frequently ulcerates and breaks down, particularly if toes four and five are in a poor state. However, if the second ray is removed, a stable situation exists and the foot is more likely to survive.

The full biomechanical assessment that can be made by a chiropodist/podiatrist using force plat-forms is advisable with these levels of amputation.

Prostheses for distal amputations

Therapists are often asked to make insoles and/or shoes. This is possible using thermoplastic materials, or alternatively by adapting the amputee's own shoes as a temporary measure. It must be remembered when making these shoes that sufficient depth should be allowed in order to accommodate the increased depth of the foot and allow sufficient room for extra cushioning needed for the redistribution of weight.

The hospital appliance/orthotic department and the chiropody service are able to make more permanent and suitable footwear. Custom-made insoles or toe blocks can be made by them and advice given regarding firms that make shoes to measure. In the case of the first toe amputation, an insole with a toe block is needed to prevent friction over the first metatarsal head as this ulcerates easily. For amputation of individual toes, a single toe block is required to prevent further distortion of foot shape. This can be made of silicone rubber.

PROSTHETIC INFORMATION

Detailed information regarding prostheses available in the UK can be obtained from the manufacturers. The addresses are listed in Appendix 1.

BIBLIOGRAPHY FOR PREVIOUS EDITIONS

Anderson L, Westin G W, Oppenheim W L 1984 Syme amputation in children: indications, results and long-term follow-up. Journal of Pediatric Orthopaedics 4:550–554

Bahler A 1986 The biomechanics of the foot. Clinical Prosthetics and Orthotics 10(1):8–14

Baker W H, Barnes R W 1977 Minor forefoot amputation in patients with low ankle pressure. American Journal of Surgery 133:331–332

Hayhurst D J 1978 Prosthetic management of a partial-foot amputee. Inter Clinic Information Bulletin 17(1):11–15

Lange T A, Nasca R J 1984 Traumatic partial foot amputation. Clinical Orthopaedics 185:137–141

Millstein S G, McCowan S A, Hunter G A 1988 Traumatic partial foot amputations in adults: a long-term review. Journal of Bone and Joint Surgery 70B:251–254

Mustapha N M, McCard F, Brand A T 1980 Case note – a combined end-bearing and patellar-tendon-bearing prosthesis for Chopart's amputation. Prosthetics and Orthotics International 4(3):156–158

Oppenheim W L 1991 Fibular deficiency and the indications for Syme's amputation. Prosthetics and Orthotics International 15:131–136

Pearl M, Johnson R J 1983 An air-ventilated Syme's leg prosthesis. Inter Clinic Information Bulletin 18(5):5–6

Rubin G 1984 The partial foot amputation. Journal of the American Podiatry Association 74(10):518–522

Sarmiento A 1972 A modified surgical-prosthetic approach to the Syme's amputation. Clinical Orthopaedics June 85:11–15

Wagner F W Jr 1977 Amputation of the foot and ankle – current status. Clinical Orthopaedics 122:62

BIBLIOGRAPHY FOR THE THIRD EDITION

Balkin S W 1995 Lower limb amputation and the diabetic foot. Journal of the American Medical Association 273(3):185

Chang B B, Bock D E M, Jacobs R L, Darling III R C, Leather R P, Shah D M 1994 Increased limb salvage by the use of unconventional foot amputations. Journal of Vasular Surgery 19(2):341–349

Chang B B, Jacobs R L, Darling III R C, Leather R P, Shah D M 1995 Foot amputations. Surgical Clinics of North America 75(4):773–782

Choudury S N, Kitaoka H B 1997 Amputations of the foot and ankle: a review of techniques and results. Orthopedics 20(5):446–457

Giurini J M, Rosenblum B I 1995 The role of foot surgery in patients with diabetes. Clinics in Podiatric Medicine and Surgery 12(1):119–127

Habershaw G M, Gibbons G W, Rosenblum B I 1993 A historical look at the transmetatarsal amputation and its changing indications. Journal of the American Podiatric Medical Association 83(2):79–80

Heim M 1994 A new orthotic device for Chopart amputees. Orthopaedic Review March:249–252

Lieberman J R, Jacobs R L, Goldstock L, Durham J, Fuchs M D 1993 Chopart amputation with percutaneous heel cord lengthening. Clinical Orthopaedics and Related Surgery 296:86–91

Mueller M J, Allen B T, Sinacore D R 1995 Incidence of skin breakdown and higher amputation after transmetatarsal amputation: implications for rehabilitation. Archives of Physical Medicine and Rehabilitation 76:50–54

Mueller M J, Salsich G B, Strube M J 1997 Functional limitations in patients with diabetes and transmetatarsal amputations. Physical Therapy 77(9):937–943

Mueller M J, Strube M J, Allen B T 1997 Therapeutic footwear can reduce plantar pressures in patients with diabetes and transmetatarsal amputation. Diabetes Care 20(4):637–641

Pinzur M S, Izquierdo R 1997 Reconstruction of the heel pad in ankle disarticulation with a free muscle transfer. The American Journal of Orthopedics July:491–493

Santi M D, Thoma B J, Chambers R B 1993 Survivorship of healed partial foot amputations in dysvascular patients. Clinical Orthopaedics and Related Research 292:245–249

Stuck R M, Sage R, Pinzur M, Osterman H 1995 Amputations in the diabetic foot. Clinics in Podiatric Medicine and Surgery 12(1):141–155

Vitti M J, Robinson D V, Hauer-Jensen M et al 1994 Wound healing in forefoot amputations: the predictive value of toe pressure. Annals of Vascular Surgery 8(1):99–106

Vowden K, 1997 Diabetic foot complications. Journal of Wound Care 6(1):4–8

Wagner F W 1994 Letter to the Editor. Clinical Orthopaedics and Related Research 313:293–294

17

Bilateral lower limb amputation

The rehabilitation potential of the bilateral lower limb levels of amputation depends on the underlying pathology, the extent of any other disease process present, and the individual's adjustment to the situation. The ablation of both lower limbs is a devastating experience and great tact and sympathy of approach is needed from the whole team, both when treating the amputee and when talking to the relatives and carers.

Acceptance of the situation by the patient can take time, and may require the specialist help of a clinical psychologist or counsellor (see Ch. 3) which in turn may slow down physical rehabilitation. This period of adjustment is vital. While recovery and adjustment are taking place, the team must be planning ahead for the amputee's future management.

It is known that 30% of unilateral amputees suffering from peripheral vascular disease (PVD) will become bilateral amputees within 3 years. Those unilateral amputees who have walked well until a few weeks before the second amputation have a good chance of successful prosthetic rehabilitation. Unilateral amputees who have become chairfast because of pain in the remaining leg, will be less generally fit and will always take longer to rehabilitate. There is also a small group of amputees with PVD who have both legs amputated simultaneously. Apart from experiencing the obvious psychological shock, the individual is also systemically ill and recovery may take many weeks. Rehabilitation for this group of amputees will take longer.

Those who become bilateral amputees because

of gross trauma are few in number. They encounter the same problems as the vascular group, the systemic problems of progressive disease are not present although concurrent injuries can present their own problems. Once recovery and rehabilitation are complete, the amputee's potential is much greater since there is likely to be no limitation from cardiorespiratory dysfunction. A very few patients have both legs amputated simultaneously due to gross infection such as meningococcal septicaemia. This devastating condition is covered in Chapter 21.

PRE-OPERATIVE TREATMENT

Unilateral amputees suffering from PVD and admitted to hospital for further vascular or diabetic investigation should be monitored by the ward therapist. Their physical condition may well have deteriorated markedly since they were last seen by a therapist, and joint contractures, muscle weakness and deterioration in the condition of the remaining foot may present a problem. In order to maintain patients as unilateral amputees for as long as possible, it may be necessary to start an exercise programme for those confined to bed, or to assess patients for general mobility and possibly make specialist footwear (e.g. a Plastazote shoe), provide walking aids or alter the prosthetic fit.

If it becomes apparent that a second amputation is likely, a further assessment is required. The most important factor here is the home situation. This has to be considered in a different manner from the assessment for the unilateral amputee. Is the home suitable or adaptable for a wheelchair and is help at hand in the house? The most effective way of initially assessing this is to carry out a home visit taking just the wheelchair: the amputee does not need to attend at this stage. The social worker/care manager may need to be contacted immediately with regard to finding a suitable care package for future placement or rehousing and involving relatives if difficulties are apparent.

Relevant goal setting in a realistic time frame is the key to managing the bilateral amputee. Many are unlikely to be able to walk with any degree of functional independence and false hopes must be avoided. Rehabilitation takes a long time, often many months, and involves a large team of professionals, carers and relatives. It may be more realistic to transfer the amputee after surgery to a specialist centre, which is able to provide this time and resource.

All bilateral amputees will require a wheelchair, (see Ch.6), irrespective of their age, condition and level of amputation as it is the only safe alternative without prostheses. This wheelchair must have the rear wheels set back 7.5 cm to compensate for the alteration of weight distribution of the amputee in the chair, owing to the loss of both lower limbs. If the amputee already possesses a wheelchair that does not conform to these requirements, it must be changed. (see Ch. 6).

Therapy techniques employed at this stage involve the teaching of independent transfers, (see Figs 4.12, p. 50 and 4.13, p. 51), strengthening of upper limbs and trunk within the limits of the amputee's medical condition, pain tolerance and functional activity.

POSTOPERATIVE TREATMENT

In the first few postoperative days, it is difficult for the bilateral amputee to move about in bed. The standard high/low bed should have been prepared pre-operatively with cot sides, monkey pole and pressure area relief aids (see Ch. 2). The essential activities that need to be taught by the therapist from the *first postoperative day* are:

1. Sitting up in bed
2. Balance
3. Bed mobility
4. Transfers.

Sitting up in bed

This must be achieved by the amputee pushing down on the bed with the arms one at a time and rotating the trunk a quarter turn to one side then a quarter turn to the other (see Fig. 4.4, p. 44).

The monkey pole is only useful for bilateral amputees for lifting up onto bedpans and for pressure area care.

Balance

It is very common for bilateral amputees (particularly those with higher levels of amputations) to overbalance backwards. Rhythmic stabilisations in unsupported sitting are the most useful exercises. Manual resistance should initially be applied to the trunk; when balance is achieved in this manner, the resistance is then applied distally to the amputee's outstretched arms.

Bed mobility

This is best achieved by hip hitching in upright sitting, and moving each buttock alternately. Forwards, backwards and sideways 'walking' on the buttocks is practised. Most bilateral amputees require push-up blocks (see Fig. 5.2, p. 60) in order to achieve this mobility, particularly if they have short arms or are on a soft surface.

Transfers

Backwards transfer off the bed into a suitable wheelchair is taught (see Fig. 4.12, p. 50).

Success in these early activities and future potential for independent mobility will be based on four physical considerations:

1. *Muscle strength*: good upper limb and trunk strength, as well as balance, will determine ease of mobility.
2. *Trunk mobility*: a full range of movement in the joints and general flexibility is needed.
3. *Body proportions*: those amputees with a long trunk and short arms, and those with large abdomens, will find mobility difficult.
4. *Medical condition*: cardiovascular status, level of cerebral function and rate of deterioration in progressive conditions will also affect mobility.

Exercise programme

Progression is made to an exercise programme in the therapy facility as outlined in Chapter 5, as it is much easier to assess and treat using a firm wide plinth. At this stage the amputee should be dressed. Dressing practice is a crucial activity, particularly for the lower half of the body and clothing adaptations may be necessary. The ability to dress will be a strong indicator of the amputee's ability to don the prostheses. It may take up to 5 weeks for the amputee to independently dress the lower half of their body.

Rolling is an excellent activity for both function and exercise. Once strength and confidence have been gained, further exercise can be done on a mat on the floor (Fig. 17.1). Here, for the fitter, more active amputee, free active exercise can be

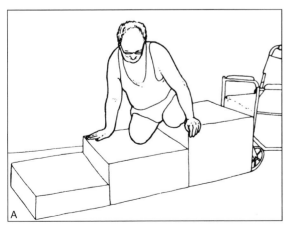
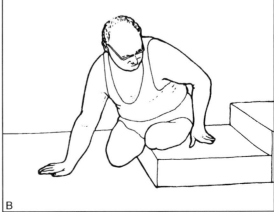

Figure 17.1 A bilateral trans-femoral amputee transferring from a wheelchair to the floor using graded box heights.

carried out quickly and energetically, without the fear of falling. This is usually more popular with those with more outgoing personalities who are used to exercise. Games can be made fun and competitive: adapted badminton, hockey, netball, etc. are all of value. Hydrotherapy is also a useful therapeutic activity.

Unilateral trans-tibial amputees who were competent prosthetic users may be able to use the existing prosthesis after becoming bilateral amputees, for transfers and limited mobility. Some can regard this as their 'normal' leg, managing standing pivot transfers (see Ch. 4). A unilateral knee disarticulation or trans-femoral amputee who was competent on a prosthesis before becoming a bilateral amputee will not be able to use the existing prosthesis for mobility owing to the loss of their own knee joint. They may use this prosthesis for comfort, cosmesis and psychological reassurance when sitting in the wheelchair.

Great caution must be observed in the use of early walking aids (EWAs) with bilateral amputees. If the first amputation was at the trans-tibial level and the amputee was a good prosthetic user, an EWA on the second residual limb can be used along with the existing prosthesis. Standing and walking should only be attempted within the exercise tolerance of the amputee in the parallel bars under the close supervision of the therapist. If walking is unsuccessful, it may be that the amputee is too tall, making leverage difficult. EWAs are more useful as additional assessment tools for the bilateral amputee, rather than for oedema control, pre-prosthetic preparation of the stump and walking. Two Ppam aids should never be used at one time, because of lack of stability, pistoning and possible damage to the wounds. Lack of success using the Ppam aid, however, does not necessarily mean that the amputee is unsuitable for prostheses. Femuretts, provide more support and may be more suitable for assessment of prosthetic capability. The general considerations outlined in Chapter 7, regarding suitability for prosthetic rehabilitation should be referred to; however, it must be remembered that this decision can be changed at any time if the amputee's condition or circumstances alter.

Prosthetic rehabilitation procedure

After full assessment by the hospital rehabilitation team (see Ch. 7), bilateral amputees may be referred on to the local prosthetic service; this will be a familiar procedure for some, as they will have already attended as unilateral amputees. For others, this first visit may be quite challenging.

A detailed medical, rehabilitation and social assessment, including a home visit report, should accompany the amputee in order for the team at the prosthetic service to understand the individual's situation.

Prostheses supplied to bilateral amputees are generally reduced in height to lower the patient's centre of gravity so that the ability to balance is retained. Careful explanation of this must be given.

Considerable time is needed to rehabilitate amputees using two prostheses, and regular sessions in a therapy facility are required. It is preferable that bilateral amputees attend a rehabilitation unit with a prosthetist in attendance because often many small adjustments to the sockets need to be made.

Prosthetic rehabilitation may take many months. If, after a month of regular attendances, there is little sign of improvement, the therapist, doctor and amputee must seriously consider whether it is worth continuing gait training. Many bilateral amputees, especially those with the higher levels of amputation, are unrealistic about their future capabilities using prostheses. It may be important that they have the opportunity to try, but, if they are unsuccessful, the team and the amputee must decide when they should stop. It may then be appropriate to supply cosmetic prostheses for wheelchair use (see Fig. 7.1, p. 92) and other rehabilitation goals are explored. Independence and activity do not solely depend on the use of prostheses.

BILATERAL TRANS-FEMORAL AMPUTEE

Early walking aids (EWAs)

Bilateral trans-femoral amputees usually commence walking using shortened femuretts, to lower

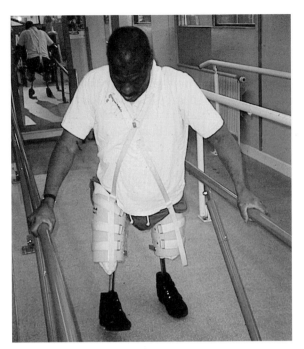

Figure 17.2   A bilateral trans-femoral amputee using two shortened Femuretts. (Photograph by kind permission of the prosthetic physiotherapy service, Oxford.)

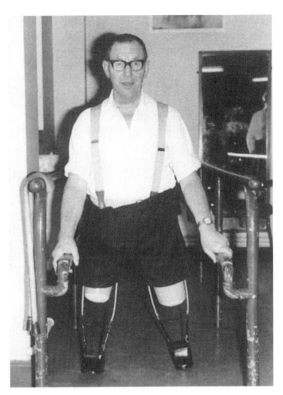

Figure 17.3   A bilateral trans-femoral amputee wearing short rocker pylons. Note the height of parallel bar required.

the centre of gravity and thus increase stability (see Fig. 17.2). These are not articulated and the amputee's weight is taken through the ischial tuberosity. Suspension consists of shoulder straps and may be augmented by TES belts. The Femuretts are fitted with SACH feet, so normal footwear can be worn. The Femurett is used initially as an assessment tool and may then proceed to be used for early gait training prior to prosthetic supply.

In some centres, short rocker pylons (SRPs) are used (see Fig. 17.3). The sockets are individually made, are ischial weightbearing, the suspension consists of two rigid pelvic bands (RPBs); and they have backward facing rocker bases.

The supply of prostheses will depend upon the amputee's ability and mobility with these EWAs.

Donning of EWAs and prostheses

It takes time to learn how to don and doff prostheses, and the bilateral amputee must be able to carry this out independently at home. If this is too difficult and tiring, the amputee will become disenchanted with the whole process of using prostheses and will probably give up. The suspension may be provided by a TES belt, or alternatively by two RPBs that have fastenings anteriorly and posteriorly that can be augmented by shoulder straps.

The following instructions should be given (see Fig. 17.4):

1. Transfer forwards onto a large solid bed the same height as the wheelchair seat, e.g. a Bobath plinth. Do not use a narrow high bed, as it is both dangerous and frightening. (Later on the amputee must also repeat this activity on a bed similar to that at home before discharge from rehabilitation.)
2. Undress so that only a long vest is worn. (Men prefer to keep their underpants on. Women will either have to put their

underwear on over the prostheses, or not wear underwear, in order that they can use the toilet.)

3. Pull on stump socks (see Fig. 17.4A)
4. Position the prostheses on the bed within arm's reach. The shoulder straps and the RPBs should be fastened posteriorly, if used.
5. Gradually ease the residual limbs into the socket, at the same time pulling the TES belt or RPBs back up over the buttocks onto the hips. This may be carried out by the amputee rolling from buttock to buttock pulling alternately on the TES belt/RPBs (Fig. 17.4B and C). Or the amputee may prefer to push up on the hands and lift the trunk up over the fastened TES belt/RPBs and then pull belts up over the buttocks to the hip level (Fig. 17.4D).
6. Once the TES belt or RPBs are in the correct position, the anterior fastening should be secured (Fig. 17.4E).
7. The stump socks should be pulled up and turned down over the rim of the sockets (Fig. 17.4F). It may be necessary to secure the stump sock around the upright of the hip joint using a safety pin, or tuck it into the thigh section of the TES belt.
8. The shoulder straps should be fastened at the front (see Fig. 17.4G). These should be crossed at the back and adjusted when standing so that the correct tension is achieved (see Ch. 13).
9. Transfer backwards into the wheelchair, as it is easier to stand up from a chair with arms than from the bed.

After the first few attempts at donning the prostheses, the amputee is then taught to dress the prostheses with trousers first (if worn). Once the prostheses are on the amputee, it is exceptionally difficult to thread them into trouser legs.

Some bilateral amputees who are rotund find it impossible to don the prostheses with the RPBs fastened posteriorly. In these cases, it is necessary to put on each prosthesis separately and then fasten the RPBs at the back afterwards. This is only possible if there is a Velcro and D-ring, or a large buckle fastening, and even then it may

be impossible to fasten this independently. For correct alignment of the prostheses, the posterior fastening must be secured in exactly the same position each time.

Sometimes, amputees at the short femurett and rocker pylon stage can don them by sitting in a chair or on a bed and sliding down into the standing sockets. This usually means that another person has to hold the prostheses steady for this procedure. This is not a very safe method and the amputee does not learn how to apply the prostheses independently. Furthermore, this method is impossible in the later stages with longer prostheses.

For comfort, some men may need to wear a scrotal support as the medial brims of the sockets may be close together.

Check of the EWAs and prostheses

This is first carried out with the bilateral amputee seated. The TES belt or RPBs must be comfortable, and the anterior brim of the socket must not impinge upon the soft tissues of the abdomen. The amputee then stands supported by parallel bars. The fit of the sockets, the suspension, the alignment and the correct length is checked (see Ch. 13). Rotation of the feet or rocker bases is determined by adjusting the application of the sockets or the RPB fastenings.

It is often worth waiting for several sessions before attempting many adjustments, or telephoning the prosthetist for assistance, as it takes several days for the new bilateral amputee to become used to wearing two hard sockets. Several treatment sessions are often required for the amputee to learn to stand up straight, and this may have a direct bearing on the therapist's opinion concerning the correct length of the prostheses. Incorrect leg length may be made apparent by the amputee who is unable to initiate swing phase; this can be confused by amputees who have an inability to hip hitch.

Gait re-education

Walking must always commence in the parallel bars at whatever stage of prosthetic fitting.

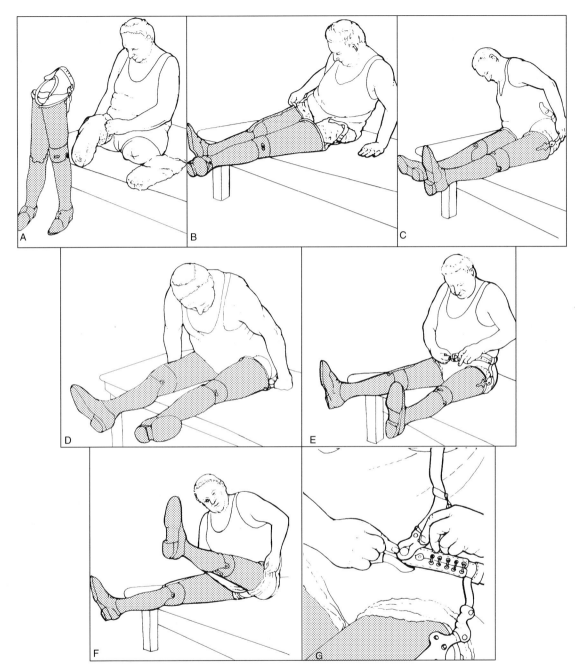

Figure 17.4 Donning bilateral trans-femoral prostheses.

Special low bars may be required for those using SRPs (see Fig. 17.3). At first, the therapist should stand behind amputees and gently rock them backwards and forwards, so that they become used to the rocking motion in standing. The amputee is then encouraged to stand as straight as possible during this exercise. When using two femuretts or prostheses, the therapist must be inside the parallel bars with the amputee, and if sitting on a stool with wheels, the therapist can comfortably and safely control the amputee's balance and direct weightbearing exercises. The amputee is encouraged to rock from side to side, gradually learning to hitch the non-weight-bearing prosthesis up each time. They can then progress to stepping forwards. After that, walking starts: the pattern is wide based, giving the amputee greater stability. A common habit, observed with all bilateral amputees, is forward flexion at the hips. This should be corrected as much as possible by teaching the amputee to extend the hip and lower trunk when weight-bearing. However much both the amputee and the therapist try to correct this, it often remains, and the amputee tends to walk using a flexed action, relying heavily on walking aids for support. This is a balance and mobility problem, and in many cases it is not related to hip flexion contractures.

During the stages of prosthetic rehabilitation, the bilateral trans-femoral amputee may initially walk with a stiff knee gait pattern. This involves alternate hip hitching and is often slow and laborious with a wide base. A degree of circumduction is inevitable.

The gait pattern at the later stage will depend very much upon the ability of the amputee and the prescription of the knee components supplied.

Progression to walking aids

As soon as the amputee is mobile and balanced within the parallel bars, progression is made to suitable walking aids; either walking sticks or tetrapods should be used. Those who have a good sense of balance and are reasonably mobile can progress to using two sticks. Those who are flexed and find walking rather laborious, require two tetrapods. Occasionally, amputees manage with one stick and one tetrarapod; if at all possible this is preferable as it reduces the space required to manoeuvre.

It is extremely inadvisable for any bilateral trans-femoral amputee to use a walking frame. The action of lifting the frame up and moving it forwards alters the centre of gravity and disturbs their sense of balance; consequently, they tend to fall backwards. The width of the frame restricts the walking base, and the rocking action of the amputee often tips the frame sideways, and although the frames are supportive they can be dangerous if the amputee falls.

Standing from a chair

The choice of chair is important. It must have strong arms that extend to the edge of the seat and be of sufficient height to enable the amputee to push into standing. Care must be taken to ensure that the chair will not slide backwards as they push on it to stand up. The bilateral trans-femoral amputee's own wheelchair is often the most suitable as it has the advantages of brakes and stability. It must also be wide enough to enable the amputee to stand up without catching the suspension or sockets on the arms of the chair. In some cases, if the amputee is obese, it may be necessary to order an extra-wide chair, or outset the front fixing slot of the arm rests to accommodate this problem. The height of the chair may have to change if the length of the prostheses alters.

With short femuretts or rocker pylons

The following instructions should be given:

1. Ease bottom forward until the posterior edges of the feet or rocker bases are touching the floor.
2. Push up on the arms of the chair, extending the elbows; at the same time pull or walk the bases backwards, until they are in total contact with the floor. (At this stage the amputee's bottom should be off the seat of the chair.)
3. Continue pushing on the arms of the chair, rocking onto the bases, until an upright position is achieved. Note: At the moment of push up from the chair the amputee must transfer their weight from the arms of the chair onto walking aids. This action may be carried out forwards from the chair, or at an angle. The amputee may well feel very unsafe at this moment.

If the bilateral trans-femoral amputee is using walking sticks, these must be held in each hand

BILATERAL LOWER LIMB AMPUTATION

at the beginning of this pushing up movement. Those amputees using tetrapods find it easier to stand up, as the aids are free-standing and can be grasped once in the upright position.

With prostheses (see Fig. 17.5)

1. Straighten one knee.
2. Twist the trunk on the seat of the chair towards the flexed knee (Fig. 17.5A).

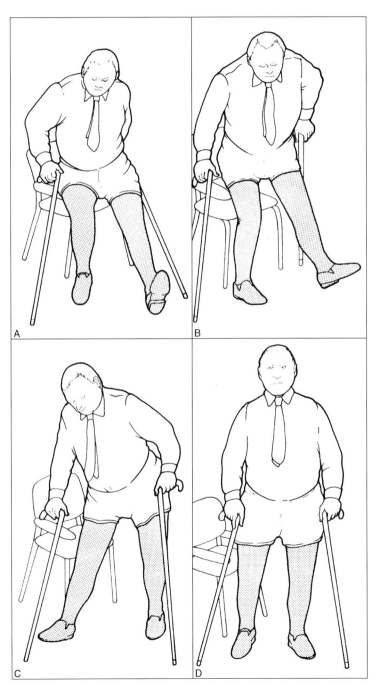

Figure 17.5 A bilateral trans-femoral amputee rising from a chair using one stiff and one flexed knee.

3. Ease the body forward so that the foot of the prosthesis with the flexed knee is in total contact with the floor.
4. Push up on hands on the arms of the chair, extending the elbows; the body is still slightly towards one side, and the bottom should be off the chair seat (Fig. 17.5B).
5. At this stage extend the residual limb with the flexed knee. The hand on the side of the extended knee must push off from the arm of the chair and come forwards using the stick for support (Fig. 17.5C).
6. As soon as balance is achieved, remove the second hand from the chair and take weight through the second stick. Stand fully upright (Fig. 17.5D).

This is a more difficult method, but it has to be utilised if the prostheses are too long for the amputee to push up into a standing position while facing forwards.

Success with either of these procedures depends on the length of the prostheses and how this relates to the length of the amputee's arms and trunk. If the amputee cannot carry out either method, the therapist must decide if the prostheses are too long. Often the height and length of chair arms must be altered or it will be necessary to contact the prosthetist so that the prostheses can be shortened.

Unless standing up from a chair can be achieved independently with ease and safety, a bilateral amputee is unlikely to walk.

Sitting down

The methods described above apply here but in reverse order. The most important aspect is that the amputee aligns their body with the chair correctly. Many try to sit down at an angle, grabbing one arm rest; this invariably tips the chair, making the whole procedure unsafe. Many position themselves so closely to the seat of the chair that they become wedged, with the bases or feet jammed on the floor and the trunk jammed against the seat. This is very uncomfortable, and the amputee has to be taught how to gauge the distance correctly.

Using the toilet

Bilateral trans-femoral amputees need to organise their bladder and bowel habits; using the toilet whilst wearing the prostheses may be difficult, unhygienic and uncomfortable.

Men like to stand to urinate and many are able to use their prostheses for this, but for a bowel motion it is preferable not to wear prostheses. Women generally prefer not to use the prostheses for either bladder or bowel motion, and for some women this inconvenience may determine whether they continue to use prostheses at all.

Independence in the application of the prostheses, standing up from a chair, walking and using the toilet are the basic goals that the bilateral trans-femoral amputee must achieve if prosthetic use is to be possible. In many cases this is all that the therapist and amputee can hope to achieve, even with great effort, determination and hard work on all sides.

The following activities will only be achieved by the younger, fitter, more agile and determined patient.

Stairs

Although two methods are illustrated here (Figs 17.6 and 17.7), variations may need to be worked out for different individuals, depending on their ability and the type of stairs they have at home.

Initially, a method is taught using two bannisters until strength and safety have been achieved. Progress to one stick and one bannister may be possible, but walking upstairs using two sticks is usually difficult for the bilateral trans-femoral amputee. The safety of any bannisters to be used, either in a therapy facility or at home, must be checked, as the force and leverage exerted on them is considerable.

Slopes

These are much more difficult than stairs. A very wide-based gait is used (Fig. 17.8). Ideally, a very gentle incline should be commenced, with progression to steeper inclines later in the rehabilitation programme.

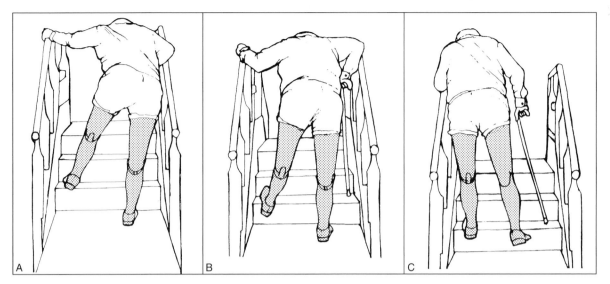

Figure 17.6   A bilateral trans-femoral amputee ascending the stairs using one bannister and one stick. Note the wide arc of movement of the pelvis and trunk.

Step/kerb

This is the most difficult obstacle for the bilateral trans-femoral amputee. The correct starting position is vital; the amputee should stand as close as possible to the step (see Figs 17.9 and 17.10). Coordination, weight transference, balance and arm strength are all necessary. The ability to climb up a step also depends on the height of the step, the length of the prostheses and the type of knee components present.

Progression to a kerb outside in the street is not easy, as the camber of the gutter, any drain covers, road markings (as these are raised and slippery), as well as the worry of passing traffic and other pedestrians, make the kerb more difficult to negotiate.

Getting up from the floor

The method illustrated (Fig. 17.11) can only be used by the exceptionally fit bilateral trans-femoral amputee. Those unable to succeed with this method must either enlist the help of two people with manual handling equipment, one carer with a hoist or other mechanical lifting equipment, or remove the prostheses and try to

get up using arm strength and items of furniture in stages.

BILATERAL KNEE – DISARTICULATION AMPUTEE

Hip flexion contractures are disastrous for these individuals and may preclude prosthetic use (see Ch. 13).

The method of application of the prostheses is similar to that for the bilateral trans-femoral level of amputation, but obviously the sockets and suspension may be different (see Ch. 14). Rehabilitation follows the same pattern as that described for the bilateral trans-femoral level of amputation.

It is possible for a bilateral knee-disarticulation amputee to walk directly on the weightbearing residual limbs, fitted with thermoplastic 'booties'. It is recommended that these are made by a prosthetist. It is important that the wounds have healed well and that the residual limbs can tolerate pressure before the amputee commences walking directly on the residual limbs. This enables the amputee to walk in the home, permitting access to the toilet and bathroom and spaces

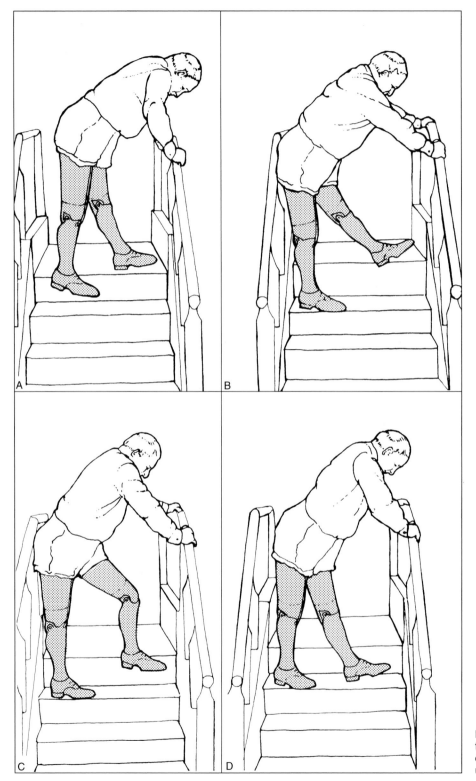

Figure 17.7 A bilateral trans-femoral amputee descending the stairs using one bannister.

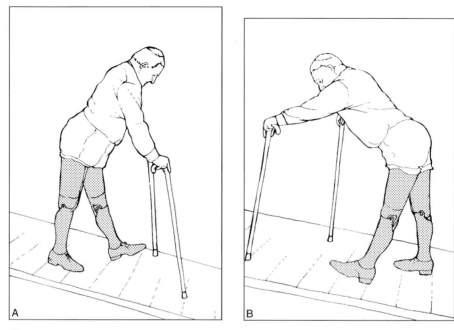

Figure 17.8 A bilateral trans-femoral amputee descending (A) and ascending (B) a slope. Note the amount of forward flexion required in B.

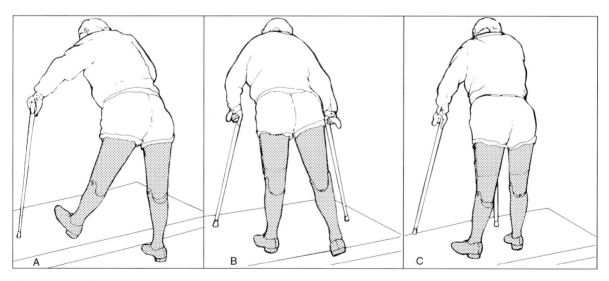

Figure 17.9 A bilateral trans-femoral amputee ascending a step using two stiff knees. This method is only possible for low steps.

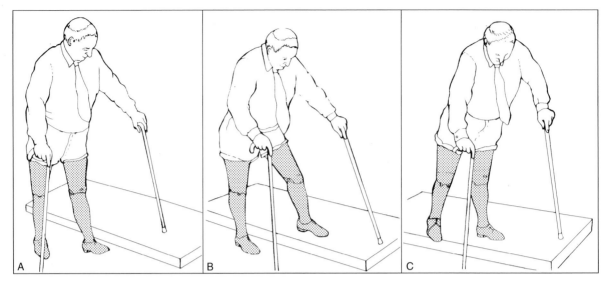

Figure 17.10 A bilateral trans-femoral amputee ascending a step sideways.

too small for the wheelchair to negotiate. The amputee can also walk outside with these boots in order to transfer into a car.

TRANS-TIBIAL AND KNEE – DISARTICULATION OR TRANS-FEMORAL COMBINATION

The presence of one natural knee joint can speed up and facilitate rehabilitation, enabling the bilateral amputee to achieve greater levels of activity and mobility. However, if there is a problem with the natural knee joint, or if the residual limb is unhealed, or breaks down as a result of forces exerted on it, it will be a hindrance.

Pre-prosthetically, balance and movement in the bed can be as difficult for these amputees as for other bilateral amputees. The trans-tibial residual limb tends to be pushed hard into the mattress and soreness or wound breakdown can result.

The speed of rehabilitation depends on whether the trans-tibial amputation was performed first or second. If it was performed first, and prosthetic rehabilitation had been achieved, progression is easier. If it was performed second, then the trans-tibial residual limb is more liable to

serious damage, as it will tend to be used more than the contralateral side, both pre- and post-prosthetically.

The amputee learns to apply the prostheses using a wide plinth the same height as the wheelchair seat, but each prosthesis is applied separately.

For prosthetic rehabilitation, the trans-tibial side may be regarded as a normal leg; this gives the patient a greater chance of being able to manage steps, stairs, slopes and rough ground. These activities will cause considerable stress to the tissues of the trans-tibial residual limb, particularly during the early stages. The therapist and amputee must frequently check the skin for redness, soreness or abrasions (see Ch. 11 and 15).

Even with one natural knee joint present, the amputee's height may be reduced to improve balance.

BILATERAL TRANS-TIBIAL AMPUTEE

Nearly all bilateral trans-tibial amputees are supplied with prostheses, and they can expect to be able to walk and become independent, within their capabilities. Despite this, a wheelchair is always necessary for toileting and washing,

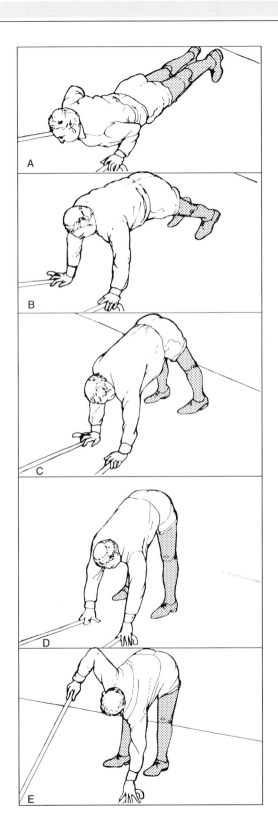

Figure 17.11 A bilateral trans-femoral amputee getting up from the floor. Note the amount of trunk and hip mobility required.

morning and evening, and for travelling longer distances. Initially, the skin of the residual limbs will not tolerate long walking distances and a slow and gradual build up of tissue tolerance to weightbearing must be allowed. Occasionally, the overall height of the bilateral trans-tibial amputee will be reduced to facilitate balance and function and to minimise energy expenditure while walking.

During gait re-education, frequent checks must be made on the skin (see Ch. 15). Although the amputee gains independence quickly and may be capable of walking with sticks at an early stage, attention to skin problems must be uppermost in the amputee's and therapist's minds. Initially, treatment sessions may be very short, with frequent rests. Frank breakdown of the skin or opening of the wound is a disaster and can happen within a very short time, possibly 1 hour, if care is not taken.

Application of the prostheses is not difficult, provided there is sufficient manual dexterity, cognition and vision, the methods are described in Chapter 15. It is advisable that the amputee learns to apply the prostheses on a bed, as well as in the chair.

The walking aids most commonly used for this level of amputation are a pair of walking sticks, and many amputees progress to using one stick once the residual limbs have matured. Obstacles such as stairs, slopes, steps and rough ground can be negotiated by most, including the elderly. It is advisable for the amputee to use a chair with arm rests, which will assist push-up to standing. Getting up after a fall, or from the floor, can be managed by kneeling before standing.

BILATERAL HIP-DISARTICULATION AMPUTEE

This extremely severe and mutilating level of amputation is rarely seen. The two most important rehabilitative goals for the patient to achieve are sitting balance and transfers. A sitting 'shell' or a postural management system may be useful for balance and to prevent pressure sores and can be ordered through the local wheelchair clinic. Cosmetic prostheses can be attached to this seat so that normal body image is maintained.

If the amputee wishes to walk and the team assessment is such that this is possible, pros-

theses are supplied, which provide a swing-through gait with locked knees (similar to a paraplegic gait). The amputee must have very strong arms and trunk muscles, good balance, a mobile lumbar spine and great determination.

It is difficult for the amputee to don the prostheses at this level and almost impossible to stand up from a chair independently.

PROSTHETICS INFORMATION

Detailed information regarding prostheses available in the UK can be obtained from the manufacturers. The addresses are listed in Appendix 1.

BIBLIOGRAPHY FOR PREVIOUS EDITIONS

DuBow L L, Witt P L, Kadaba M P, Reynes R, Cochran G V B 1983 Oxygen consumption of elderly persons with bilateral knee amputations: ambulation vs wheelchair propulsion. Archives of Physical Medicine and Rehabilitation 64:255–259

Kerstein M D, Zimmer H, Dugdale F E, Lerner 1975 Associated diagnoses which complicate rehabilitation of the patient with bilateral lower extremity amputations. Surgery, Gynaecology and Obstetrics 140:875–876

McCollough N C 1972 The bilateral lower extremity amputee. Orthopedic Clinics of North America 3(2):373–382

McCollough N C, Jennings J J, Sarmiento A 1972 Bilateral below-the-knee amputation in patients over fifty years of age. Journal of Bone and Joint Surgery 54A(6):1217–1223

Moverly L 1990 Discovering water's redeeming features. Therapy Weekly 17(7):4

Muthu S 1983 Limb fitting and survival in the dysvascular double above-knee amputee. Journal of the Royal College of Surgeons of Edinburgh 28(3):157–159

Svetz W R 1983 A novel concept in fitting bilateral above-knee amputees: a case history. Orthotics and Prosthetics 37(3):63–66

Van de Ven C M C 1973 A pilot survey of elderly bilateral lower-limb amputees. Physiotherapy 59(10):316–320

Van de Ven C M C 1981 An investigation into the management of bilateral leg amputees. British Medical Journal 283:707

Volpicelli L J, Chambers R B, Wagner F W 1983 Ambulation levels of bilateral lower-extremity amputees. Journal of Bone and Joint Surgery 65A(5):599–604

Wolf E et al 1989 Prosthetic rehabilitation of elderly bilateral amputees. International Journal of Rehabilitation Research 12(3):271–278

BIBLIOGRAPHY FOR THE THIRD EDITION

De Fretes A, Boonstra A M, Vos L D W 1994 Functional outcome of rehabilitated bilateral lower limb amputees. Prosthetics and Orthotics International 18(1):18–24

18

Sports and leisure activities

Most amputees are discharged from therapy as soon as they are walking adequately; however, a fuller lifestyle depends on far more than this. In order to increase amputees' functional capabilities a link should always be maintained between amputees and a therapy facility, the community service or the therapist and prosthetist at the local prosthetic service.

It should also be remembered that the psychological aspect of picking up the pieces of life again will take differing amounts of time for each individual, and the therapist's approach to increasing activity should be very sensitive. Going out of the house for the first time can be daunting, and participation in other activities or sport is only possible when the individual feels confident in himself and his own abilities.

Participation in sports has given many disabled people a new sense of achievement and there are many facilities available. The amputee is able to enjoy a very wide range of activities. Taking part in some form of regular leisure activity provides important social contact and the thrill of achievement and possibility of competition. The challenge of sport may be the only personal challenge experienced by some individuals, particularly in these days of increased unemployment.

OUTDOOR MOBILITY

The lower limb amputee should already have practised negotiating kerbs, ramps and rough ground, usually in the controlled situation in the therapy facility or on a very quiet street.

Coping in a busy street with bustling pedestrians, uneven pavements, irregular-height kerbs and gutters with a steep camber, requires greater concentration. Those who have acquired their amputation as a result of pedestrian or motor vehicle accidents may find crossing roads very anxiety provoking. Crossing a road can be hazardous: it requires forethought, mobility and speed. Drivers may be unaware that the amputee requires more time: even if the amputee is young and mobile, it is advisable, when outside, to carry a walking stick so that the general public are aware of a disability requiring consideration.

It may be necessary for trans-femoral and knee-disarticulation amputees to learn to move quickly for a very short distance to avoid cars and other fast moving hazards. Normal running is impossible but the following method should be used for speed: a stride is taken with the prosthesis; this is followed by a stride, then a hop on the sound leg; this double stance phase allows sufficient time for the prosthesis to swing through and land in full extension; a stride is taken again with the prosthesis (step – step – hop – step). It is best to attempt this first by holding onto one parallel bar. Then the therapist should practise this with the amputee around the safe confines of the facility. Trans-tibial amputees can practise running once the residual limb has matured and a treadmill is useful equipment for a safe start for this.

Amputees who live in a hilly area require special help from the therapist. Descending a steep incline is difficult and unnerving, and the amputee must practise this often by walking sideways with frequent changes of direction. Wet leaves, muddy surfaces, high winds and icy conditions are all hazards, and the amputee must be constantly aware of these potential dangers. Suitable footwear can assist balance, and a variety of ferrules are available to stabilise the walking aid.

Escalators present a problem to most lower limb amputees (see Fig. 18.1). They should be advised to step both on and off leading with the unaffected leg and keeping a free hand to hold the handrail.

Stepping off an escalator is more difficult as

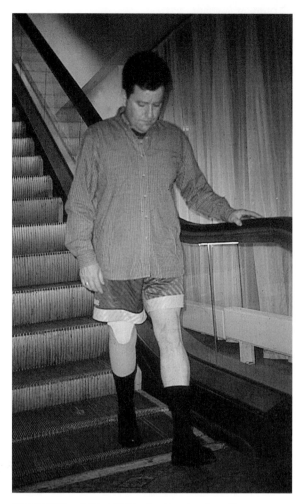

Figure 18.1 A trans-tibial amputee stepping off an escalator with the unaffected leg leading. (Photograph by kind permission of the prosthetic physiotherapy service, Oxford.)

the momentum gained tends to push the trunk forward too fast for the legs. A helper should be in front to clear a space so that the amputee can step on and off with safety.

TRANSPORT

Car

The therapist should be aware of the legal requirements for the vehicle licensing authority and their insurance company to be notified of any changes in a person's medical condition.

If amputees are able to drive without having a car adapted, they often do not realise that they are driving illegally if they have not contacted the licensing authority.

All amputees should have been shown how to transfer in and out of a car before discharge from their initial rehabilitation programme (see Fig. 18.2). Those who would like to drive must consider certain factors before attempting to drive their own car, or purchasing a new one. Some large driving instruction schools have a 're-learning' programme for those with physical disabilities. Driving assessment and advice can be obtained from a local member of the Forum of Mobility Centres. Information concerning these units is available from the local prosthetic service. The therapist should advise even the experienced driver to use one of these re-learning programmes, or to begin driving again as if a novice, and explain that, after a period of hospitalisation, speed of reaction is slowed and the amputee's proprioception is altered.

Upper limb amputees should seek advice on car adaptations from their therapist at the specialist prosthetic centre.

There are various motoring organisations who can supply more details concerning the law, car adaptations, etc. to the amputee (see Appendix 1).

Bicycle

Those amputees who were regular cyclists will need to practise on a static bike in the therapy facility in order to evaluate whether the prosthesis permits active use of the pedals, and to check mounting and dismounting procedures. (see Fig. 18.3).

Amputees with hip disarticulation or high trans-femoral levels of amputation who wish to cycle may have the prosthetic side pedal fixed in the down position and pedal entirely with the remaining leg using toe clips. This is hard work and initially stabilisers may be needed on the bicycle.

Motorcycle

The choice of model used will depend on the side of the kick-starting mechanism, or the presence of an electric starter, and on the height and location of the pedals, as knee flexion may have to be greater than 90°. The amputee must first practise off public roads to achieve proficiency in manoeuvring the machine.

Train and bus

In order to cope with these forms of transport the amputee needs quick, long strides, either up steps or across gaps. To gain confidence, the amputee will often prefer to practise at a quiet time of day with a therapist, before trying it alone or with a friend or relative. If the amputee has a certain route that must be travelled in the rush hour, advice is given to practise the route first at a quiet time of day.

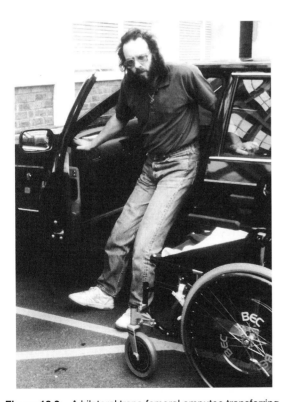

Figure 18.2 A bilateral trans-femoral amputee transferring into a car. Note the upper limb strength required. (Photograph by kind permission of Richmond, Twickenham and Roehampton Healthcare NHS Trust).

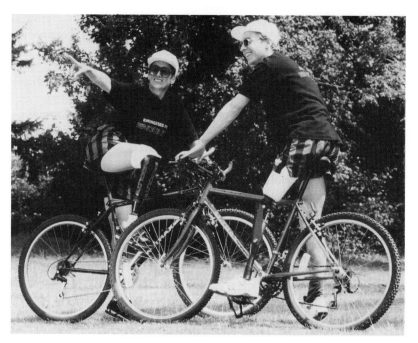

Figure 18.3 A trans-tibial and a trans-femoral amputee enjoying bicycling. (Photograph by kind permission of C.A. Blatchford and Sons Ltd.)

Aeroplane

The majority of amputees must plan the air journey well in advance to check access to the plane and to the lavatories: an aisle seat is recommended. Even if the amputee is quite mobile it is advisable to ask the airline for a wheelchair to be provided, as airport corridors can be very long. Security staff should be informed that an artificial limb is worn. Dysvascular amputees may have problems due to reduced oxygen levels present in the aircraft should they have an unviable segment in the remaining limb. The residual limb volume of all amputees may alter because of changes in air pressure in the cabin, causing fitting difficulties with the prosthesis. Therefore it is advisable not to remove the prosthesis as it may be impossible to don when leaving the aircraft for the onward journey.

Boats

Travel by sea must also be pre-planned. Wet deck surfaces can be dangerous and the amputee must have good balance to cope with the swell. Stairways can be steep and the location of seats should be ascertained in advance.

LEISURE ACTIVITIES

During the latter stages of learning functional prosthetic activity, the primary amputee will have discussed with the therapist (and possibly with other amputees) the sort of leisure and social activities they have enjoyed in the past, or wish to enjoy in the future (see Ch. 10). Once proficiency and confidence has been gained in outdoor mobility and use of transport, a wider range of choices is available to the individual. Getting out to socialise in a club, pub or religious centre, or pursuing more intellectual pastimes offered by colleges of further education, University of the Third Age etc., are all possible, particularly if help and encouragement is given by friends and carers (see Fig. 18.4).

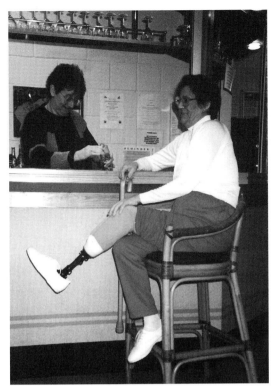

Figure 18.4 A trans-tibial amputee enjoying a drink at her club. (Photograph by kind permssion of Richmond, Twickenham and Roehampton Healthcare NHS Trust).

SPORT

Participating in sport, where the amputee may have to undress or change shoes, may initially make them feel extremely self-conscious and embarrassed; these feelings must be understood, if not overcome, before amputees can move forward into more fulfilling pursuits. Speaking to another amputee who understands these fears and anxieties is often helpful and self-help organisations such as the Limbless Association and British Amputee and Les Autres Sports Association can provide this support, as well as the professional support available from the members of the treatment team at the local facility.

The therapist can suggest sport and leisure activities, but must give realistic advice and understand the limitations involved. Young amputees, in particular, are anxious to know, often very soon postoperatively, what their capabilities

will be regarding their favourite sport. It will take some time before this advanced function can be achieved, possibly as much as 1 year following the amputation. (see Appendix 1 for addresses of organisations that can supply advice).

The main physical considerations before starting a sporting activity are:

- A well-healed, mature residual limb that can tolerate increased activity
- General and specific muscle strength, balance and coordination
- Good stamina
- An intimately fitting socket.

These are the same considerations as for any individual who is considering starting a sport, and the same training rules apply:

- The technique of the sport must be properly learned
- A correct training programme must be followed (see Figs 18.5 & 18.6).
- The amputee must have adequate supervision in the early stages.

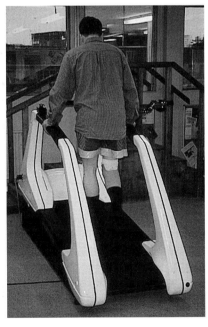

Figure 18.5 A trans-tibial amputee working out on a treadmill. (Photograph by kind permission of the prosthetic physiotherapy service, Oxford.)

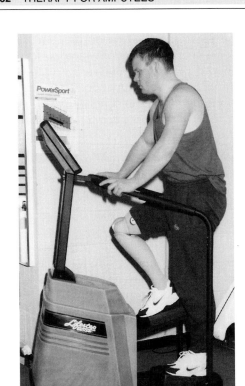

Figure 18.6 A trans-femoral amputee training on a step machine. (Photograph by kind permission or Richmond, Twickenham and Roehampton Healthcare NHS Trust).

If the amputee was proficient at a certain sport before the amputation, it may be easier to return to that same sport rather than learn a new activity. Returning to such an activity can be very distressing for some people as they are unable to achieve the same level of performance as before and it is frustrating to have to compromise their personal standards. Sometimes finding a new challenge is more effective.

For those who were not active in sports prior to amputation, but who would like to have a go, the therapist can advise suitable sports and organisations that can give specific help (see Appendix). Amputee and disabled peoples' sports groups are good starting points as they have facilities nationally. The limited competition here may be too restricting for some individuals and they may wish to join local sports and leisure

centres or clubs. The therapist or prosthetist may be able to introduce one amputee to another who is interested in a particular sport and can often give the initial help, practical advice and psychological support needed.

It is important that the amputees themselves are determined to try and participate, because then they will find a way of succeeding, providing it is within their capabilities. Sport is to be enjoyed: amputees should not be pressurised by others into trying even if they were actively involved prior to amputation. There is a period of psychological adaptation to their condition that must not be rushed and some individuals take longer than others.

Amputees using prostheses who enjoy sports may require special adaptations, but these must be discussed with the rehabilitation doctor and prosthetist. It may be necessary to fabricate a prosthesis for the special individual requirements of the amputee and the sport.

The following lists contain examples of possible sporting activities available to amputees. The lists are not comprehensive.

Sports for the less active individual, the more sedentary and elderly people

Darts. This can be enjoyed by the amputee either seated or standing, and supported by one walking aid if necessary.

Bowls. Indoors or outdoors; either from a wheelchair or using a prosthesis. The amputee must be able to bend down to the ground.

Fishing. Access and toilet facilities must be considered. It can be enjoyed from a wheelchair, seated, or standing. A latex cover is needed for a lower limb prosthesis if the amputee intends to wade in the water.

Billiards, snooker, pool. These slow precision games require only enough balance by the amputee to manage while leaning on the table, but there should be good upper trunk mobility.

Table tennis. Fast reactions are required, but it may be enjoyed from a wheelchair.

Archery. Although usually performed standing, this sport can be performed from a wheelchair but requires a strong trunk and arms. (see Fig. 18.7).

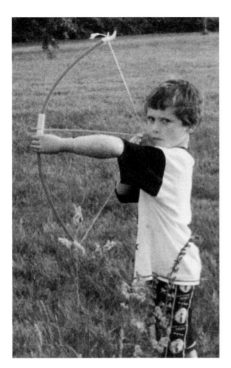

Figure 18.7   A child with a trans-radial amputation enjoying archery using a myoelectric prosthesis. (Photograph by kind permission of Mrs Holdsworth and Reach.)

Adapted terminal devices are available for upper limb amputees, the appropriateness of each depending on the hand dominance.

Sport for the more active amputee, irrespective of age

Swimming (Fig. 18.8). Access to the pool or the sea and availability of helpers must be considered. A lot of advice and direction is needed about getting from the changing room to the pool and vice versa. Local councils have lists of pools that hold special swimming groups for swimmers with restricted ability where help is available for those who feel they need it. Water activity prostheses are available and may afford safer access to the pool (see Fig. 18.9).

Croquet. The amputee must be able to balance and walk short distances without a walking aid.

Horse riding. There is a possibility here of discomfort between the residual limb and socket, particularly for the trans-femoral amputee who may be more comfortable using a cavalry or Western saddle rather than an English one. They may need an adapted prosthesis or ride side-saddle (see Fig. 18.10).

Bicycling. Again the saddle is important: a

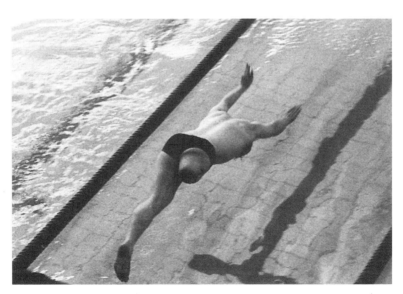

Figure 18.8   A trans-femoral amputee diving into a swimming pool. (Photograph by kind permission of Mr D. Breakwell.)

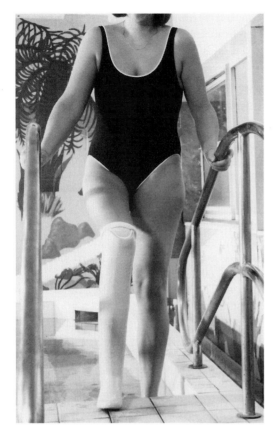

Figure 18.9 A trans-tibial amputee wearing a water activity prosthesis. (Photograph by kind permission of C.A. Blatchford and Sons Ltd.)

leather touring design is more comfortable. Toe clips should not be used as they can be dangerous if the amputee falls off. A good gripping material on the sole of the shoe will ensure a good hold on the pedals, e.g. good quality sports shoes (Fig. 18.3). Upper limb amputees should use a tandem brake, i.e. one with both cables going to one brake lever. Discussing problems with a good bicycle shop can be helpful in finding solutions.

Boating/Canoeing/Sailing. The skills required include launching the boat, carrying and loading the equipment, and getting on and off, often from steep, slippery and rocky banks. Therefore most amputees will require a prosthesis with a waterproof latex covering. Some sailing associations have facilities for those in wheelchairs who must have able-bodied helpers present. Some amputees may prefer not to wear their prosthesis in a yacht or canoe for ease of movement. (See Fig. 18.11)

Golf. All amputees who can stand can play golf, irrespective of the level of amputation (see Fig. 18.12). A torque absorber may need to be fitted to the prosthesis to reduce rotational sheer forces on the residual limb. A motorised golf 'buggy' can be used for those with limited walking distance.

There are special terminal devices for arm amputees wanting to play golf.

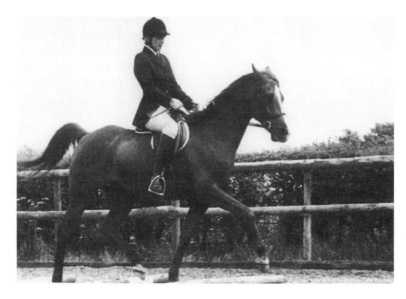

Figure 18.10 A trans-tibial amputee horse riding, with an adapted-boot. (Photograph by kind permission of Mrs. P. Upton.)

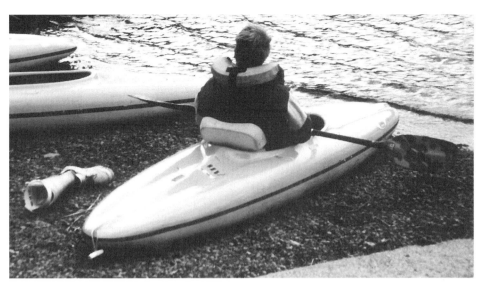

Figure 18.11   A trans-tibial amputee who finds it easier to canoe without his prosthesis. (Photograph by kind permission of the prosthetic physiotherapy service, Roehampton.)

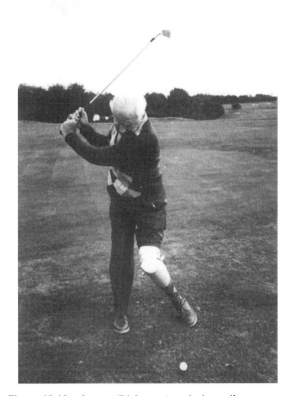

Figure 18.12   A trans-tibial amputee playing golf. (Photograph by kind permission of Mr P. Everett.)

Dancing. Disco, ballroom, old time: this can be enjoyed by all, and leaning on one's partner is acceptable!

Shooting. Clay-pigeon shooting is suitable for those who cannot walk far, but excellent standing balance with rotation is required. Rough-shooting is for the more active walker but a peg leg may be more useful for mobility in the undergrowth for higher levels of amputation.

Exercise classes. These are available for all levels of activity and stamina; the therapist should help the amputee to seek one they would both enjoy and be successful in, with a qualified instructor able to adapt movements for the individual's ability (see Fig. 18.13).

Sports for the very active, vigorous and determined amputee

Skiing. Amputees with trans-femoral and knee disarticulation levels of amputation should start learning without wearing their special prosthesis. There are special poles with elbow-crutch tops and outrigger bases to aid balance (Fig. 18.14). Good skiers at these levels can use their prosthesis once basic skills have been mastered, but it does slow them down. A stabilised knee must be

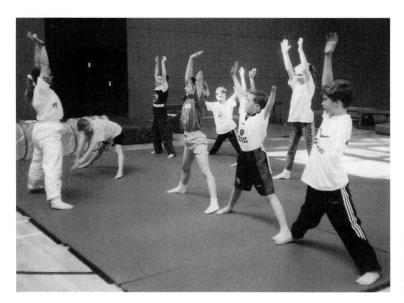

Figure 18.13 A mixed exercise class of children, some able bodied and some with upper limb deficiency. (Photograph by kind permission of Mr K. McCowan and Reach).

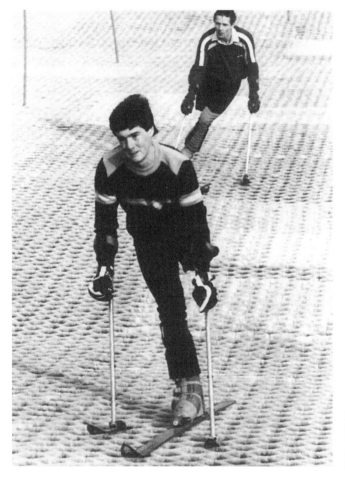

Figure 18.14 A young trans-femoral amputee learning to ski on a dry ski slope with an instructor, Mr. M. Hammond, who is also an amputee. Note the adapted ski poles with outriggers. (Photograph by kind permission of the Harlow Gazette.)

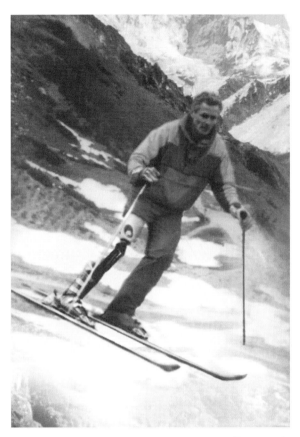

Figure 18.15 A trans-femoral amputee skiing. (Photograph by kind permission of C.A. Blatchford and Sons Ltd.)

set to lock only on very forceful impact (Fig. 18.15). Amputees with trans-tibial and Symes levels of amputation should wear their prosthesis to learn the sport and may need a thigh corset adding to a patelar tendon bearing (PTB) design to improve suspension for downhill skiing. Very good skiers can achieve higher speeds and skills on one leg. It can be useful to attempt this sport first on a dry slope (Fig. 18.14). One of the major problems for those not wearing their prosthesis is access to the slope, lift and snack bar on one leg. Hopping in a ski boot is almost impossible. Bilateral lower limb amputees can enjoy skiing using a ski seat.

Protection for the residual limb is vital if a prosthesis is not worn, as injury from cold or trauma must be avoided.

Tobogganing and other snow sports that do not put as much strain on the residual limb are also possible.

Water skiing. Learning this sport should be attempted on one leg without a prosthesis (Fig. 18.16). The trans-tibial amputee who wishes to use a prosthesis requires a special waterproof design with an extra grip material on the sole. For those on mono-skis, rising up out of the water should be achieved on the unaffected leg and the prosthesis slotted into place once upright. For those wishing to use two skis, rising up from the crouch position may be limited by dorsiflexion

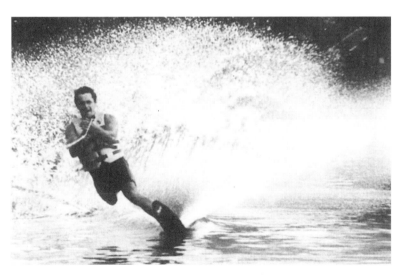

Figure 18.16 A trans-femoral amputee water skiing. (Photograph by kind permission of Mr. M. Hammond.)

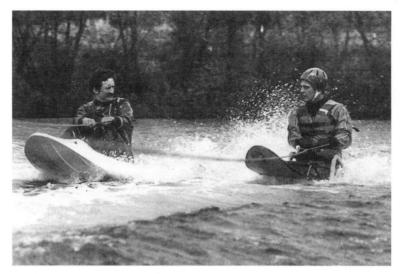

Figure 18.17   A bilateral amputee (on the right) water skiing with an instructor. (Photograph by kind permission of Mr Berkeley and Mr I. D. Hassall.)

of the prosthetic ankle. It is possible for bilateral amputees to enjoy this sport seated (Fig. 18.17).

Wind surfing. A non-slip sole on the prosthesis is essential as it is difficult to maintain control on one leg. The trans-femoral and knee-disarticulated amputees require a special peg leg; the trans-tibial amputee requires a 'water activity leg'.

Surfing. Most amputees do not use a prosthesis but the trans-tibial amputee can manage with a 'water activity leg'. Prone lying or kneeling positions on the board achieve the best balance.

Scuba diving. A 'fin-leg' may be specially made, but many manage without a prosthesis (Fig. 18.18). All those participating in watersport activities using a prosthesis must have a water activity leg, an exoskeletal prosthesis (see Ch. 8) made with full waterproof or specialised materials and stable suspension. For swimming there is a special design of prosthesis, which is vented so that water flows in and out of the casing (see Fig. 18.19), this is to prevent excessive buoyancy, which may cause the dangerous, unexpected, whole-body movement of 'turning turtle'. Upper limb amputees need a prosthesis with neutral buoyancy. A flotation buoy must be attached to the prosthesis, so that it does not sink and is able to be retrieved should it fall off the amputee.

Initially, it is advisable for all amputees who wish to try water sports wearing special prostheses to practise walking, wading, floating and swimming in a shallow, guarded swimming pool such as a hydrotherapy pool within a rehabilitation facility with a therapist present. This is to test buoyancy and balance.

Hang gliding and parachuting. Highly dangerous for anyone!

Climbing. A prosthesis with very secure suspension should be used. Initially, practise on an indoor climbing wall with an instructor and safety harness is recommended to allow the residual limb to become accustomed to the severe angular pressures and the climber to retrain the fine balance reactions needed. Frequent changes of sock or liner are needed to avoid damage to the skin of the residual limb (see Fig. 18.20).

Hiking and fell walking. Footwear must be suitable. The prosthesis must be very comfortable and well fitting. Extra stump socks should be carried so that changes can be made when necessary. This activity is not for the amputee liable to claudication (see Fig. 18.21).

Motorcycle scrambling. Much practice is needed to achieve the correct balance for this activity.

Squash/volleyball/badminton/tennis. Although am-

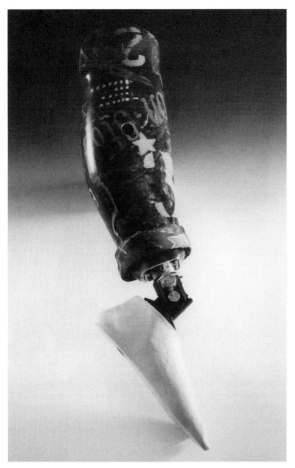

Figure 18.18 A trans-tibial swimming prosthesis with a hinged ankle enabling transition from walking to swimming. (A flipper can be attached to the foot.) (Photograph by kind permission of Ortho Europe.)

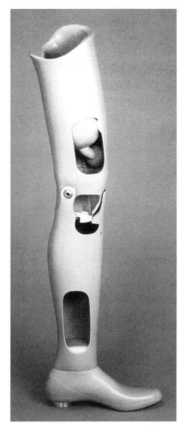

Figure 18.19 A saggital section of a trans-femoral water activity prosthesis. (Photograph by kind permission of Otto Bock UK Ltd.)

putees must be agile to attempt these sports, they learn to adapt their game to reduce the need to run about too much. Skilled placing of shots enables them to be competitive (Fig. 18.22).

Wheelchair basketball. A vigorous team sport gaining popularity in the UK with a national league and some television coverage. Suitable for highly motivated amputees who will accept a wheelchair sport or who cannot cope with a sport requiring a prosthesis.

Athletics. Running is one activity that will show the greatest difference between the trans-femoral and trans-tibial levels of amputation (see Fig. 18.23):

the latter can run normally, albeit slower. Amputees with trans-femoral and knee disarticulation levels have a markedly abnormal running gait which is much slower, appears ungainly and many will not participate in track and field sports because of this. There are prosthetic knee and foot components available which permit a normal running pattern and some very fit amputees can succeed in this. Bilateral amputees and high level unilateral amputees can compete in throwing events using a special throwing frame to assist balance.

Contact sport (football, hockey, lacrosse, etc.). The usual rules of fitness for contact sport apply. The prosthetist, however, must be made aware that the amputee is using the prosthesis for these activities (Fig. 18.24).

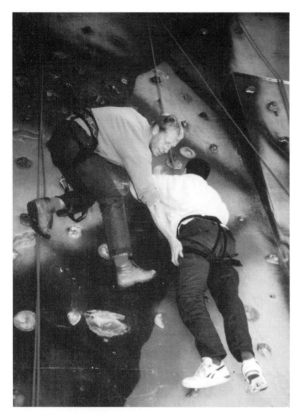

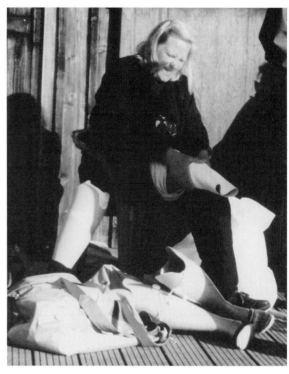

Figure 18.20 An amputee with a hip disarticulation prosthesis being instructed on an indoor climbing wall. (Photograph by kind permission of the prosthetic physiotherapy service, Roehampton and the Calvert Trust.)

Figure 18.21 An active trans-tibial amputee who takes several prosthess and liners out with her during walking holidays to ensure comfort of the residual limb. (Photograph by kind permission of the prosthetic physiotherapy service, Roehampton.)

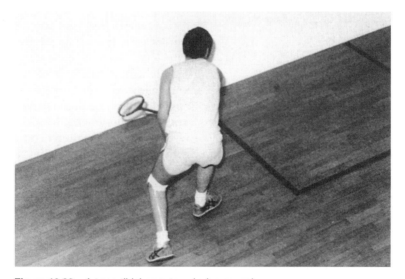

Figure 18.22 A trans-tibial amputee playing squash.

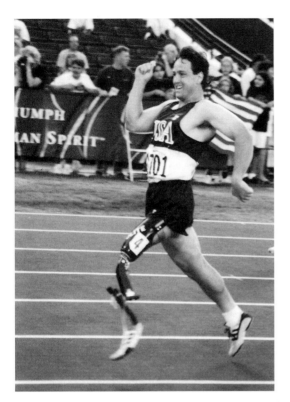

Figure 18.23   Todd Schaffauser (a trans-femoral amputee) winning the bronze medal for the 100 m at the 1996 Paralympic Games. He is using an Endolite Hi-Activity prosthesis with CaTech hydraulic knee control. (Photograph by kind permission of C.A. Blatchford and Sons Ltd.)

Competition

At elite level competitive events, e.g. the para-lympics, there will be an attendant prosthetist and sports physiotherapist to help with any problems the amputee may encounter in the performance of their sport.

SPECIALISED PROSTHETIC COMPONENTS

The established amputee who has achieved full independence on the first prosthesis may require the next prosthesis to be fitted with specialised components to enable even more active mobility. The components supplied will vary with the individual needs demonstrated by the amputee, with regard to either work, sport or leisure activities. Those who enjoy high activity often dispense with the cosmetic cover in order to be able to make frequent adjustments to the foot and ankle components (see Fig. 8.15, p. 108).

The availability of specialised components should first be discussed between the amputee and the prosthetist. Some amputees, once they have become interested in a certain activity, will find out about those components that may help mobility for that activity from a fellow amputee.

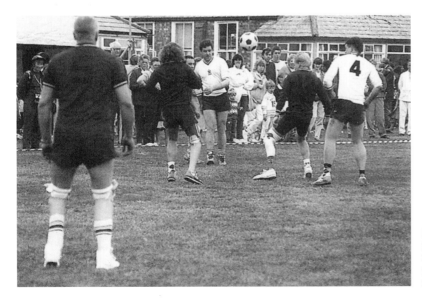

Figure 18.24   A demonstration football match at the Queen Mary's University Hospital annual garden party. (Photograph by kind permission of Ms. J. Jackson.)

The amputee must then write to the prosthetic centre doctor stating the case for a specialised order. Therapists must be prepared to be a strong advocate for those amputees who would benefit from sophisticated (therefore expensive) prosthetic devices.

BIBLIOGRAPHY FOR PREVIOUS EDITIONS

Burgess E M, Hittenberger D A, Forsgren S M, Lindh D V 1983 The Seattle Prosthetic Foot – A design for active sports: preliminary studies. Orthotics and Prosthetics 37(1):25–31

Gailey R 1992 Recreational pursuits for elders with amputation. Topics in Geriatric Rehabilitation 8(1):39–58

Gailey R, Stinson D 1991 Analysis of above-knee running gait. Proceedings, World Confederation of Physical Therapy 11th International Congress

Hittenberger D A 1982 Extra-ambulatory activities and the amputee. Clinical Prosthetics and Orthotics 6(4):1–4

Kegel B 1986 Journal of Rehabilitation Research and Development: Clinical Supplement No 1. Veterans Administration USA

Kegel B, Carpenter M L, Burgess E M 1978 Functional capabilities of lower extremity amputees. Archives of Physical Medicine and Rehabilitation 59:109–119

Levesque C, Gautier-Gagnon C 1987 An above-knee prosthesis for rock climbing. Orthotics and Prosthetics 40(1):41–45

Rubin G, Fleiss D 1983 Devices to enable persons with amputation to participate in sports. Archives of Physical Medicine and Rehabilitation 64:37–40

Sports Activities 1978 Physiotherapy 64(10):290–301, (11):324–329

BIBLIOGRAPHY FOR THE THIRD EDITION

Buckley M, Heath G 1995 Technical note. Design and manufacture of a high performance water-ski seating system for use by an individual with bilateral trans-femoral amputations. Prosthetics and Orthotics International 19:120–123

Clinical Interest group in Prosthetics, Orthotics and Wheelchairs, College of Occupational Therapy and Forum of Mobility Centres 1998 Driving after amputation, 3rd edn. British Limbless Ex-Servicemen's Association, Romford, Essex

Mital A, Scheer S J, Plunkett J M, Pennathur A, Govindaraju M 1996 Enhancing physical fitness levels of paraplegics and lower extremity amputees: a critical need. Critical Reviews in Physical and Rehabilitation Medicine 8(3):221–234

Pasek P B, Schkade J K 1996 Effects of a skiing experience on adolescents with limb deficiencies: an occupational adaptation perspective. American Journal of Occupational Therapy 50(1):24–31

Saadah E S 1992 Swimming devices for below-knee amputees. Prosthetics and Orthotics International 16(2):140–141

St Jean C, Goyette C 1996 Case report forum. Observations of ice-skating prostheses developed for a 7-year-old trans-tibial amputee. Journal of Prosthetics and Orthotics 8(1):21–23

Sanderson D J, Marton P E 1996 Joint kinetics in unilateral below-knee amputee patients during running. Archives of Physical Medicine and Rehabilitation 77(12):1279–1285

19

Upper limb amputation and congenital limb deficiency

Fiona Carnegie

The ratio of upper to lower limb amputation in the UK is very low (approximately 1:24). The number of primary upper limb amputees and limb-deficient children registered annually in the UK is approximately 330, which accounts for about 6% of all primary amputees. It is not surprising, therefore, that few cases are seen in any one hospital. However, it is important that any hospital department is able to carry out the initial treatment required before the patient moves on to the prosthetic stage attending a prosthetic service with comprehensive and specialist occupational therapy rehabilitation available.

There are two distinct groups of clients requiring upper limb prostheses: those with an acquired amputation, and those with congenital upper limb deficiency. There are major differences in the management of these two groups because of the nature of the disabilities and age disparities (see Table 1.2, p. 4).

Acquired amputation

Trauma

In the UK and the developed countries, this is usually the result of a road traffic accident, industrial injury, a severe domestic accident, explosion or gunshot wounds. Amputation for trauma is most frequently seen in the adolescent and adult working population where exposure to trauma is more likely to occur. The incidence is greater in men than women. The number of traumatic arm amputations has reduced over the past 20 years as health and safety legislation in the UK has resulted in workplaces becoming safer; sociological, technological and economic changes mean that fewer people are working in industrial environments and more are working in less hazardous office-based jobs. For those who do have traumatic hand injuries, microsurgical techniques have improved, resulting in the hand sometimes being saved. Trauma that results in the totally avulsed brachial plexus leaves a flail arm with no sensation. Sometimes repair is possible but often the arm remains flail and insensate. If after 2 years there is no improvement, the patient may choose to have the arm amputated. This should be carried out at mid-humeral level and, if the patient wishes to use a prosthesis, the shoulder joint should be arthrodesed in 10° abduction and 10° flexion. Traumatic amputation of the upper limb may also occur in children and the elderly, but this is much less common.

Disease

Malignancy, septicaemia, thrombosis/embolism and leprosy (Hansen's disease) fall into this category. It can occur at any age and may be of slow or sudden onset. General vascular insufficiency such as peripheral vascular disease very rarely causes upper limb amputation, but occasionally, severe Raynaud's or Buerger's disease may result in upper limb amputation.

Changes in treatment of oncological disease have resulted in fewer amputations and improved prognosis; early prosthetic intervention is strongly recommended. Patients with amputations following septicaemia often have multiple amputations, involving both upper and lower limbs. They may also have damage to other tissues. They are often young adults and usually the disease is of sudden onset. Patients with thromboses or emboli can be of any age, usually only one limb is affected. The onset is often very sudden.

Leprosy patients have problems with neurological damage so particular attention is required with care of the residual limb (for more details see Ch. 21).

Congenital limb deficiency

This is rare within the whole amputee popu-

lation, but forms 40% of all primary upper limb referrals per year. Specialised treatment techniques are required, with constant review, particularly throughout growth and development in childhood and adolescence.

The reasons for most congenital limb deficiencies remain unknown. Apart from the thalidomide tragedy in the early 1960s, the number of children born each year with limb deficiencies remains relatively constant at 1:10 000 live births.

There are two main types of limb deficiency: transverse and longitudinal, as defined by international standard ISO 8548-1 (see Bibliography).

Transverse. The limb develops normally up to a defined point when growth is arrested. For example, a middle-third forearm transverse arrest is similar to a trans-radial amputation. Finger buds are often present. It is thought that this is most likely to be caused by an interruption in the blood supply to the developing limb. In rare cases, amniotic bands constrict a limb and lead to its amputation in utero. In such cases, there will be no finger buds and there are often constrictions on other parts of the child's limbs.

Longitudinal. In these deficiencies all or part of the long bone is absent, but some of the distal parts may remain intact. In describing these longitudinal deficiencies the absent parts are named, e.g. a radial club hand will be described as: 'longitudinal arrest, radius partial, carpals partial, ray 1 total'. This child is unlikely to require a prosthesis.

However, a child with two fingers remaining at shoulder level may well benefit from prosthetic provision. It is this group of children who are most likely to have genetic reasons for the limb deficiency and it is advisable for these families to have genetic counselling.

The treatment procedures for those two distinct groups of patients will be divided into two sections for clarity: acquired amputation and congenital deficiencies.

ACQUIRED AMPUTATION

Pre-operative assessment (See Ch. 2)

Most upper limb amputations result from trauma so there is rarely an opportunity for a pre-amputation consultation with a rehabilitation doctor, therapist or prosthetist experienced in upper limb rehabilitation. However, when there is the opportunity, the patient can be informed about prosthetic options and future management. In some cases, there may be an element of choice for the patient, e.g. when surgical intervention following trauma has been unable to create a functional hand (many years following a brachial plexus injury). The choice may be either to have the arm removed or fashion a residual limb on which a functional prosthesis would give benefit. It is also helpful when surgeons can be advised on appropriate levels of amputation.

General assessment will be the same as for the lower limb amputee (see Ch. 2). Specific areas to note are:

Range of movement of cervical and thoracic spine, shoulder girdle, shoulder joint, elbow, forearm, wrist and hand of affected and unaffected arms.

Muscle power controlling these joints. If a patient has no active flexion, a trans-humeral amputation will be required. If no active shoulder movement is possible, a shoulder arthrodesis may be indicated.

Pain control. Experience has shown that there is a link between pain in the arm in the pre-amputation phase and phantom pain occurring postoperatively; therefore pain relief prior to surgery is essential. Amputation should not be performed to relieve pain: other treatment modalities should be explored (see Ch. 20).

Scar tissue. If a patient has extensive surgical or burn scars, the condition of the skin may dictate the level of amputation both for healing of the residual limb and for subsequent prosthetic provision.

Home situation and family support. Information will indicate the level of assistance the patient will need in the early post-operative period and after discharge – both physical help and psychological support. Where possible the patient's family should be included in aspects of pre-amputation consultation; they may require psychological support and information on practical issues.

Employment. The type of employment should be considered carefully. If the injury occurred at work, aspects of compensation may need to be discussed. Some employers may offer alternative work if the previous job is no longer possible for the amputee.

Leisure pursuits. The activities in which the patient was involved prior to amputation should be discussed. They may choose or be advised to start a new hobby, rather than struggle to return to one in which they were very accomplished. However, such decisions should not be made hastily.

Psychological aspects of upper limb amputation (see also Ch. 3)

Whatever the cause of the amputation, the loss of an arm has serious psychological implications. The upper limb, and in particular the hand, play an important part in self-image, in personality development and in manipulative skills. As stated by Crosthwaite Eyre:

'Arms and particularly hands are an integral part of personality development and are an extremely complex mechanical part of our bodies. They are a means of expression through affection, sexual identity, manual dexterity, sometimes speech and importantly as a means of providing for the family as tools of work. Very often the initial shock of losing an upper limb affects the patient's attitude towards his total body image, subjecting him to feelings of inadequacy and incapacity. These factors are augmented when the dominant side is affected. The realisation that present technology is so far unable to provide a replacement with perfect or near-perfect function, or sensation, and can only offer a partial degree of cosmetic acceptability, causes additional concern. Therefore these individuals need a great deal of psychological support and encouragement which must continue until they return to their normal lifestyle.'

This psychological disturbance after limb loss must be handled sensitively and realistically. It is frequently the therapists within the multidisciplinary team who can provide much of the help that is required, reassuring the amputee by planning treatment programmes directed towards ultimate independence with or without the use of a prosthesis.

Hand dominance

A prosthesis replaces the non-dominant function of stabilising something while the remaining hand carries out the manipulative task. This is because of the lack of dexterity and sensory feedback available in the prosthesis. If the patient loses the dominant hand, time must be spent training the remaining hand to take on the dominant role. For some this is extremely difficult and very frustrating. For others, not all functions of the dominant hand can be taken over by the remaining hand due to cultural and religious reasons.

All tasks carried out will be part of this learning process, but it may be beneficial to encourage playing peg games or one-handed computer games to promote fine finger work and hand/eye coordination.

Writing should be encouraged from an early stage. A few upper limb amputees achieve adequate writing with their prosthesis but most eventually write better with their remaining hand. Practice should start with basic pencil skills, using a large felt-tip pen, drawing large patterns and shapes first, and maintaining a relaxed grip. The bilateral amputee will probably write better with the longest residual limb, but all possibilities should be pursued: initially they may write with both residual limbs together. They may benefit from a leather gauntlet with an appropriately angled pocket for a pen.

Pre-prosthetic treatment

The aims of treatment are:

- Maintain and increase joint mobility and muscle strength
- Control of oedema
- Functional activity
- Desensitising the residual limb
- Care of the residual limb
- Psychological adaptation.

Maintain and increase joint mobility and muscle strength

Early active movements of all joints above the level of amputation, including the whole of the shoulder girdle and neck, should be commenced with the therapist on the first postoperative day.

Resisted active exercises can commence as pain permits.

These exercises should concentrate particularly on all movements of the shoulder joint and shoulder girdle: elevation, depression, protraction and retraction. Ability to retain the smooth gliding movement of the scapula on the chest wall in protraction is essential. This movement, coupled with flexion of the shoulder joint, is the main power force for working a body-powered prosthesis, particularly for the trans-humeral amputee. The shoulder joint can be exercised with manually resisted techniques, such as proprioceptive neuromuscular facilitation, or by mechanical resistance, such as Cliniband or a pulley system; a leather gauntlet may be required to attach the resistance to the residual limb (Fig. 19.1). Bilateral activities are particularly useful. If the elbow joint is present, a full range of movement must be achieved daily to prevent any flexion contractures. The forearm support prone position is useful for performing resisted head and neck patterns. This encourages shoulder girdle movement and biceps and triceps activity, as well as accustoming the residual limb to pressure.

The general posture of the neck and upper trunk must be corrected and trunk rotation during walking must be maintained. Single arm amputees tend to flex towards the affected side. The trunk may become rather rigid during walking, as loss of arm swing and trunk rotation may lead to a feeling of imbalance. Retraining of postural reactions, by use of manually resisted exercises and balance boards, either in lying, sitting or standing, must start early in the exercise programme. The arm amputee must also be encouraged to try different paces of gait, i.e. jogging, running, etc., as these activities will initially feel very different. An elderly amputee may find balance affected, especially when turning. Sport and leisure pursuits should be discussed with the amputee and attempted at an appropriate time in the rehabilitation programme.

Control of oedema

Elevation of the upper limb is difficult to achieve. The residual limb can be elevated on a pillow

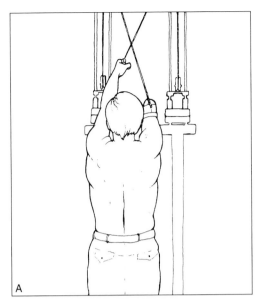

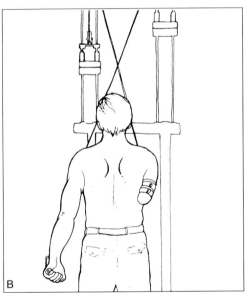

Figure 19.1 A trans-humeral amputee mobilising and strengthening the shoulder girdle and shoulder joint using a Westminster pulley system. Note the scapula excursion between (A) and (B).

when the amputee is in bed. Some amputees find a sling helpful, but caution in the use of the sling is needed as it encourages elbow flexion and internal rotation of the shoulder joint; it may however be helpful in the first few postoperative days.

Active contraction of the residual limb muscles will reduce oedema and should be encouraged at regular intervals. Generals use of the residual limb in everyday activity will also help reduce oedema.

Stump bandaging should not be used until the wound is healed and sutures are removed. Care should be taken to ensure that the joints above the level of amputation can move freely and that pressure is exerted on the distal end of the residual limb with diagonal turns (see Fig. 19.2). A poorly applied bandage can be damaging; at no time should a tourniquet effect be allowed to happen. These principles are the same as for the lower limb amputees (see Ch. 4). Pressure garments may also be used, giving a more consistent degree of pressure.

Functional activity

In order to maintain normal movement patterns, use of the residual limb should be encouraged as soon as possible. All amputees should be encouraged to feed themselves at an early stage; a plate guard to assist loading the fork may prevent frustration, a rocker knife may be helpful to assist in cutting up food and a non-slip mat can help stabilise the plate. Sensitivity in the choice of food perhaps with the help of the dietician will also maximise ability. Once the residual limb can tolerate it (around days 2–3), a leather gauntlet or webbing strap can be made and cutlery placed in it to be a pusher for two-handed feeding. A bilateral amputee may require a thermoplastic gauntlet into which cutlery can be fitted, or may use both residual limbs to hold cutlery.

Many arm amputees find dressing very difficult, especially buttons, zips and pulling up clothes on the lower half of the body. Wearing easy clothing such as tracksuits should be encouraged initially and major clothing adaptations should be delayed. Most unilateral amputees can manage to do up buttons after a few weeks, bilateral trans-radial amputees may require a button hook. Managing a trouser zip is easier if thread or a split ring is attached to the zipper.

Balance may be difficult initially, and missing a hand to hold on with can make getting in and

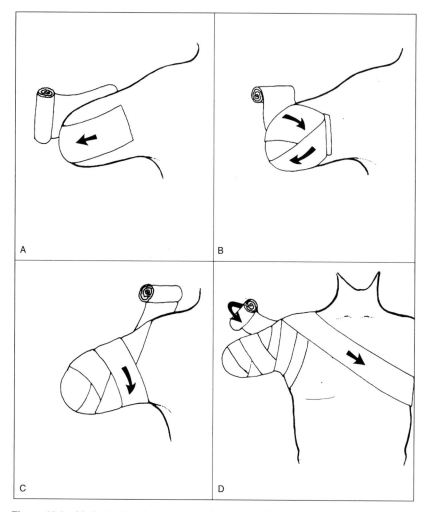

Figure 19.2 Method of bandaging a trans-humeral residual limb.

out of the bath or shower difficult. A non-slip mat will make this safer and some older amputees will require rails.

Reaching to wash the whole body with one hand is hard. Washing the unaffected hand and arm is difficult until the residual limb is healed and can be used; before then the hand and arm can be rubbed between the knees. Washing requires the amputee to have a very agile spine and legs. A washing mitt or long handled sponge may be helpful.

Writing, as previously discussed, should be encouraged, holding the paper still with the residual limb is possible. Reading can also encourage the use of the residual limb by holding the book, magazine or newspaper.

A leather gauntlet (Fig. 19.3) can be applied over the wound dressing to which simple devices can be attached and the amputee encouraged to carry out tasks using the residual limb. Care must be taken to keep these activities realistic and practical. This is more easily achieved with the trans-radial amputee. Typing with a simple peg attached to the gauntlet helps retrain proprioception. Painting with a paint brush at an easel or table encourages control of the residual limb in finer precision activity; in addition, it helps to develop control in differing shoulder girdle

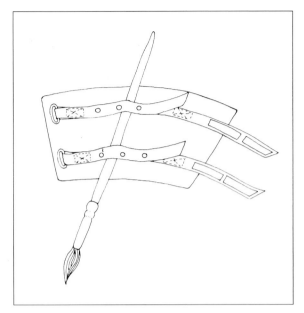

Figure 19.3 A leather gauntlet with paintbrush attached. (Reproduced by kind permission of Baillière Tindall, from Robertson E 1978 Rehabilitation of arm amputees and limb deficient children.)

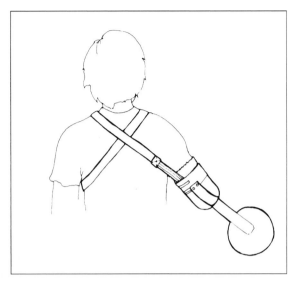

Figure 19.4 A leather gauntlet with extended table tennis bat attached. (Reproduced by kind permission of Baillière Tindall, from Robertson E 1978 Rehabilitation of arm amputees and limb deficient children.)

ranges of movement. Because of very unequal arm lengths, activities for the trans-humeral amputee are more difficult to plan. However, an extended table tennis bat attached to the gauntlet with a figure-of-eight strap around the opposite axilla can be used to encourage forward shoulder flexion in remedial games (Fig. 19.4).

Desensitising the residual limb

The amputee should be encouraged to touch the residual limb as soon as possible, at first over the dressing and later, directly on the skin. If this is not achieved in the first few days it may become more difficult and the residual limb may become hypersensitive.

The residual limb should be gently massaged and gradually handled more vigorously, and to enable the amputee to become accustomed to pressure, leaning on the residual limb in preparation for prosthetic wearing.

Phantom sensation should be discussed to relieve anxiety. If the sensation is painful or unpleasant, methods to resolve it should be

pursued and medication may be required (see Ch. 20).

Psychological adaptation

The amputee needs to adapt to the new body image. Some find it hard to look in a mirror or to look at the residual limb. If these difficulties persist, rehabilitation progress will be affected. However, it is important to take cues from the amputee as sometimes it is detrimental to push them too fast. Helping them regain independence in normal activities will increase self-esteem and help adjustment. Some may benefit from early referral to a clinical psychologist or counsellor (see Ch. 3).

Care of the residual limb

It is important for the amputee to be aware of the need to wash the residual limb. Use of moisturising cream prevents dryness and encourages a supple skin. Regular inspection of the skin of the residual limb is vital, especially if sensation is reduced, using a mirror if necessary; this must continue when a prosthesis is used.

PROSTHESES

A prosthesis replaces the body part that is absent. The arm is primarily present to position the hand so that it can fulfil a particular task: to manipulate an object, to express a feeling, to explore the environment.

No prosthesis is able to replace all functions satisfactorily. It is essential that the arm amputee has a good understanding of prosthetic options available so they can have a realistic idea as to how their requirements can best be met. The therapist must appreciate the amputee's functional, social and psychological needs at that time so the correct prosthetic prescription can be made.

A prosthesis may be cosmetic, functional or a combination of both. As soon as the amputee's health permits, referral to a prosthetic centre should be made so they can be informed about all the prosthetic hardware and learn of the prosthetic rehabilitation process (see Ch. 8 for further details on prosthetic construction).

Types of prostheses and control systems

Cosmetic

No control system is required. This is the simplest and lightest type available. For the trans-radial amputee this would consist of a foam-filled glove, with wired fingers, fitted to a self-suspending socket. For higher levels of amputation where there is a need for a prosthetic elbow joint, an endoskeletal system may be supplied. This consists of the same type of hand attached to a foam-covered tube forearm and upper arm section with a hand-operated elbow joint. The upper section is attached to the socket. This prosthesis usually requires a simple figure-of-eight appendage for suspension; established amputees may manage a self-suspending socket. These prostheses give the best cosmetic replacement with minimal functional benefit, e.g. holding objects steady or carrying things over the forearm.

Individually sculpted silicon hands are also available, which are excellent cosmetically but expensive and not robust enough for any practical daily tasks.

Body powered

Body movement is harnessed to control the terminal device and elbow. This prosthesis is the simplest functional prosthesis. A set of appendages harness the body movement: biscapular protraction, shoulder flexion (and, for the transradial level of amputation, elbow extension) operates the terminal device. For the trans-humeral level of amputation, shoulder depression, internal rotation and abduction operate the elbow lock. This type of prosthesis is a working tool and is functional rather than attempting to be cosmetic.

Electric power

A battery-operated motor moves the hand/gripper, wrist or elbow by either myo-electric control, servo control or switch control. Rechargable batteries are usually mounted within the prosthesis and are issued to amputees complete with charger.

Myo-electric control. Electrodes pick up microvolts of electricity produced by contractions in the muscles of the residual limb – these are amplified and activate the motor. In operating the hand there may be two electrodes, one on the flexor and one on the extensor muscle groups, one opening and the other closing the hand (see Fig. 19.5). Alternatives include a single-site option of voluntary opening and automatic closing. Wrist operation may be myo-controlled using the two-site system. An electric elbow lock can be activated by a single site.

Servo control. The same movements required to operate the body powered prosthesis operates an electric hand but requires less shoulder girdle movement.

Switch control. This may take the form of a harness or touch pads, enabling control of the electric device to be achieved in different ways.

Electrically powered prostheses are not recommended for primary amputees because they are heavy, require a close fitting socket (especially myo-electric control) and are more complex

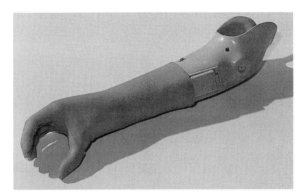

Figure 19.5   A myo-electric prosthesis for a trans-radial amputee. (Photograph by kind permission of Richmond, Twickenham and Roehampton Healthcare NHS Trust.)

to operate and care for. They could be considered at 6 months postamputation when oedema has completely resolved and the amputee has had some experience of a body-powered or cosmetic prosthesis. Careful assessment is essential (see page 261).

Terminal devices

The task of the hand is replaced by the terminal device that may be cosmetic and/or functional, passive or active. A variety of terminal devices are available for the body-powered prosthesis where the wrist unit is round allowing 360° of rotation and has a disconnect facility allowing the terminal devices to be changed.

The most commonly used active functional device is the split hook, which is designed purely for function and is the most useful tool comprising one static and one moving jaw; grip is provided by elasticated bands holding the two jaws together and the grip is increased by adding extra bands. The device is activated by a harness attached to the lever on the moving jaw (see Fig. 19.6). As the residual limb is moved the harness pulls the jaw open, giving good proprioceptive feedback.

If cosmesis is important, a cosmetic hand can be provided: the simplest is foam-filled with wire in the fingers, enabling them to be bent to an appropriate position. If cosmesis and function are required in the same device there must be

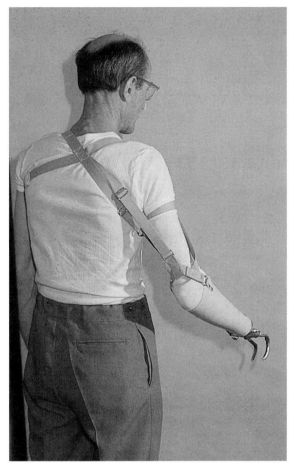

Figure 19.6   Split hook being activated by humeral flexion. (Photograph by kind permission of Richmond, Twickenham and Roehampton Healthcare NHS Trust.)

compromise: a mechanical hand, body power pulling the thumb and fingers apart. It is harder to operate than the split hook, has a poorer grip and is bulky, making precision difficult. It serves a purpose for amputees not demanding a high level of manipulative skill from the prosthesis.

There are terminal devices for specific tasks: *active*, e.g. pliers, tweezers, using the operating cord, and *passive*, e.g. hammer, fishing rod holder, tool holder. Thus the body powered prosthesis can be a tool to use with or without cosmetic replacement.

Some electrically powered prostheses have a

wrist disconnect allowing for change of terminal device, usually a powered hand to powered gripper.

Levels of amputation and prostheses

There are optimal levels of amputation in the upper limb as with the lower limb. For all active amputees these optimal levels should, as far as possible, be chosen. Preservation of length of residual limb is advantageous in order to act as a lever, but the residual limb should be short enough to allow the prosthetic components, such as wrist or elbow unit, to be fitted, thus enabling a functional and cosmetic artificial replacement to be supplied.

Partial hand amputation

This amputation is usually as a result of trauma. Cosmetic or functional replacement may be possible. However cosmetic replacement is likely to impede function. Functional devices will probably be activity specific.

Function should initially be assessed without hardware. Discussion is required between the amputee, occupational therapist, prosthetist and rehabilitation doctor about the amputee's needs and possible solutions; often the simplest solutions are best, e.g. a leather gauntlet with or without pockets.

Wrist disarticulation

This level of amputation is not ideal for prosthetic replacement due to the bulbous end created by the styloids. Some amputees have a split socket – one section at the elbow, the other at the distal end, the two sections joined by straps. This enables the amputee to utilise their own pronation and supination. A terminal device, e.g. split hook, can then be fitted directly to the socket. The whole of the lower section can be removed and replaced with a cosmetic hand. Alternatively, a whole forearm socket is made and a wrist unit fitted to allow pronation and supination. This makes the prosthesis 4 cm longer than the remaining limb.

A cosmetic prosthesis can sometimes be fitted using a silicone glove, the radial and ulnar styloids acting as suspension.

Trans-radial amputation

The optimum amputation level for fitting a trans-radial prosthesis is 8 cm above the ulnar styloid to allow room for the wrist unit and maintain the same length as the remaining arm.

The wrist unit, allowing rotation through 360° of any terminal device being worn, has a push-button mechanism to enable removal or locking of the device.

Active devices are operated by elbow extension and shoulder flexion and/or shoulder girdle protraction.

The socket can be of two types: (1) a cup socket, (2) a self-suspending/supracondylar socket.

Cup socket: held on by a harness that incorporates the operating cord, allowing the patient to activate the terminal device (Fig. 19.7). This socket is used for:

- amputees who require the prosthesis to carry heavy weights, as the appendages distribute the weight across both shoulders
- amputees with very short residual limbs, when a self-suspending socket may be very difficult to fit
- bilateral amputees.

The appendages should lie easily across the back; the cross-section should be just off centre. The operating cord should be just taut when the prosthesis is by the side. The buckle above the axilla strap should be below the clavicle and above the anterior axillary fold.

Self-suspending/supracondylar socket: (Fig. 19.8) in which the socket fits over the condyles and the olecranon. The operating cord is on a loop harness that activates the terminal device, which can be removed when the prosthesis is worn with a cosmetic hand or a passive terminal device.

The self-suspending type of socket is used for purely cosmetic prostheses; there is no operating cord, there is an oval wrist with no movement and a foam hand. It is also the type of socket used usually for the myoelectric prosthesis. There is

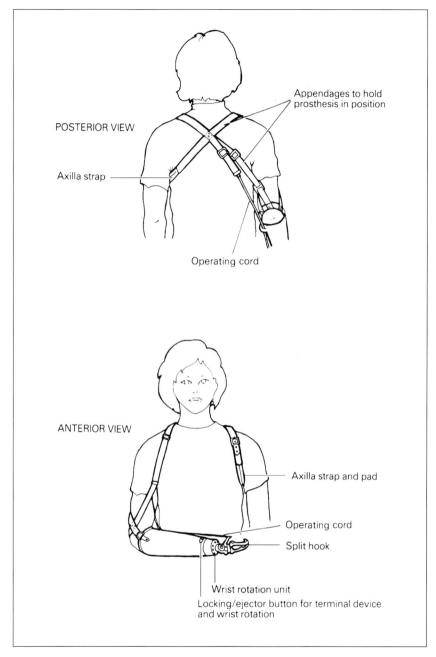

Figure 19.7   A body powered prosthesis with cup socket for a trans-radial amputee showing a full set of appendages.

no operating cord required. The electrodes are fitted in the most suitable position for the individual over the wrist flexor and extensor muscle bulks. There is a friction wrist or an electric wrist unit allowing 360° rotation. There may be a wrist disconnect facility.

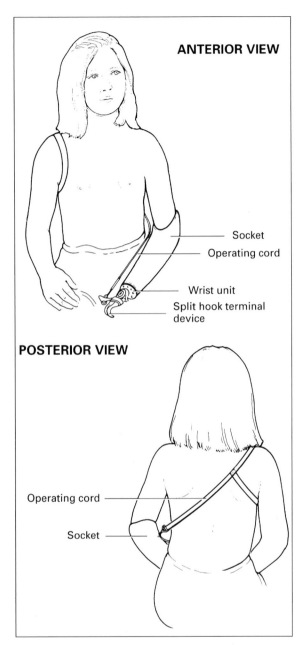

ANTERIOR VIEW

Socket

Operating cord

Wrist unit

Split hook terminal device

POSTERIOR VIEW

Operating cord

Socket

Figure 19.8 A body powered prosthesis with supracondylar self-suspending socket for a trans-radial amputee.

An alternative suspension is a silicone sleeve with a shuttle lock (Fig. 19.9), which fits into a hard outer socket. It can be used for cosmetic or body powered prostheses. The length of the residual limb is critical.

Elbow disarticulation

This level of amputation is not ideal for prosthetic replacement. It has the disadvantage that there is no space for the prosthetic elbow unit. This has to be fitted either under the socket making the upper arm 5 cm too long and the forearm too short. Alternatively the joint can be fitted externally with side steels up the socket and a simple joint on either side of the condyles. This makes the prosthesis very bulky and there can be no internal and external rotation. However, there may be situations where it is the optimum level for a particular patient, e.g. bilateral amputee or a non-prosthetic user.

Trans-humeral amputation

The optimum site for a trans-humeral amputation is 10 cm above the elbow joint, measured from the olecranon. This allows space for the elbow mechanism of the prosthesis to fit into the humeral section, and ensures that the prosthetic elbow joint is at the anatomical level. Additionally, it provides a good length of residual limb for leverage and prosthetic control. A residual limb shorter than 4 cm measured from the anterior axillary fold of the shoulder is considered prosthetically in the same way as a shoulder disarticulation.

A cosmetic trans-humeral prosthesis is usually endoskeletal, comprising of a socket that may be self-suspending or require minimal appendages. It has a simple hand operated elbow joint, manually moved and locked by the remaining hand, and a cosmetic hand with or without a friction wrist; usually the hand does not disconnect. A body powered prosthesis incorporates harnessing to hold the prosthesis in position and to allow the patient to activate it (Figs 19.10 and 19.11). The elbow joint is flexed by humeral flexion and shoulder girdle protraction, putting tension on the operating cord. To lock the elbow in the desired position the patient either pulls the locking strap with the remaining hand or uses the automatic locking mechanism. The latter is to be encouraged if it is possible, as it allows the remaining hand freedom. The mechanism is operated by a movement of the shoulder joint,

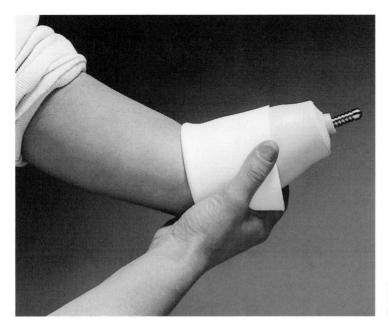

Figure 19.9   A silicone sleeve (with shuttle lock) for a trans-radial amputee. (Photograph by kind permission of Ossür UK).

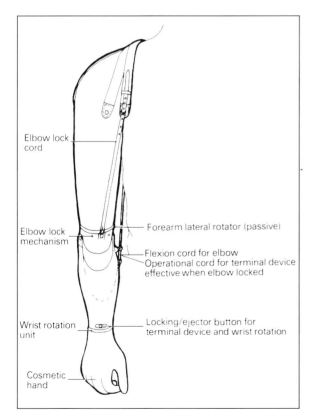

Elbow lock cord

Elbow lock mechanism

Forearm lateral rotator (passive)

Flexion cord for elbow
Operational cord for terminal device effective when elbow locked

Wrist rotation unit

Locking/ejector button for terminal device and wrist rotation

Cosmetic hand

Figure 19.10   A trans-humeral body powered prosthesis (anterior view).

which pulls on the lock cord: shoulder depression, extension, internal rotation and abduction, or 'nudging the ribs'. The same movement is required to unlock the elbow. An amputee with a very short residual limb or with brachial plexus damage will rarely achieve this movement and will operate the lock with the remaining hand. A hand operated elbow unit, i.e. a switch on the forearm, rather than a strap, may be considered. Once the elbow is locked, the movements and power used for elbow flexion are transmitted via the operating cord to the terminal device, which is then activated.

To compensate for loss of internal and external rotation at the shoulder, a friction joint is incorporated in the lower end of the humeral section above the elbow joint. It is passively rotated with the amputee's remaining hand in order to place the forearm in the desired position.

The appendages should lie easily across the back. The operating cord should travel from axilla to axilla allowing the greatest benefit from bilateral scapular protraction. The pulley section on the socket needs to be high enough not to wear on the sleeve hole of shirts. The buckle on the axilla loop should be below the clavicle and above the anterior axillary fold.

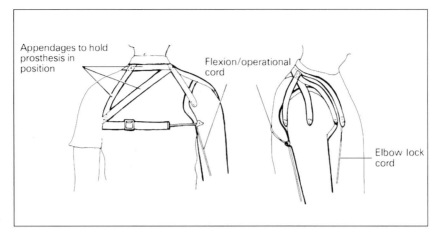

Figure 19.11 Suspension system for a body powered prosthesis (posterior and lateral views).

The servo controlled electric prosthesis fits the same way as the body-powered prosthesis, but requires less excursion to fully open the hand. The hand is heavier than the split hook so elbow flexion may be harder. A servo interlock should be fitted so that when the elbow is unlocked, power to the hand is off so shoulder girdle protraction flexes the elbow; when the elbow is locked, power to the hand is restored and protraction results in the hand opening.

Myo-electric power of the hand is possible but it is sometimes difficult for the amputee to isolate biceps and triceps muscle contractions. Myo-electric control can also be used for elbow flexion and extension, the elbow lock or wrist rotation. Electric power, myo and/or servo, can be used for all the functions of the prosthesis but careful assessment is needed. If electric power is used for hand, wrist and elbow operation, the prosthesis is heavy (as each function has a separate motor) and the operation complex; the prosthesis requires more maintenance and has greater possibility of breakdown.

Shoulder disarticulation

If it is possible, the head of the humerus should remain in situ to maintain the shape of the shoulder. If this is not possible, the clavicle and acromion process should be trimmed to have a rounded contour to prevent discomfort when wearing a prosthesis. The prosthesis is similar to that worn by trans-humeral amputees, but requires an extended shoulder cap. The elbow mechanism is locked and unlocked by the remaining hand. In the body powered prosthesis, the terminal device is activated by protraction of the shoulder girdle. The functional benefits of the prosthesis are limited and the prosthesis is used more as a steadying device for holding down objects whilst the amputee is writing, cutting, etc. Electric power may give extra benefits (see trans-humeral amputation section).

Forequarter amputation

This is usually performed for malignant disease. It involves the removal of the clavicle and scapula as well as the whole arm. Initially, the need is for replacement of body contour, and a light shoulder cap that will not cause pressure on the chest wall but allows clothing to be worn to give a normal outline, should be fitted post-operatively (Fig. 19.12). Early referral to the prosthetic service is essential to supply this shoulder cap, which is both for cosmetic replacement and protection. Many patients opt to wear this device permanently. A prosthesis may be supplied and it is made of light foam with a simple elbow and cosmetic hand. A functional prosthesis is usually

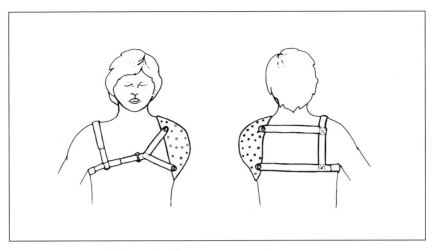

Figure 19.12   A shoulder cap for a forequarter amputation.

too heavy to be tolerated. However, patients who have a broad back may manage an electrically powered prosthesis where the heavy weight is tolerated because of the function.

PROSTHETIC REHABILITATION

Assessment

On the first visit to the prosthetic centre, the amputee will be assessed by the rehabilitation doctor, prosthetist and therapist. The therapist's assessment of the amputee will include all the general aspects of assessment, as detailed in Chapter 2. Particular attention is paid to the length of the residual limb, bony prominences, strength and range of movement of joints and muscles of both the residual limb and the remaining limb, and the amputee's overall mobility and posture. This physical assessment, along with information about their lifestyle, personality, psychological needs and employment is essential in the decision-making process regarding the most appropriate prosthetic prescription. If the amputee has poor posture, postural exercises and re-education are also necessary.

The amputee should have an opportunity to see the different prostheses and be fully informed about the advantages and disadvantages so that they can be actively involved in the prescription process.

Prosthetic training

Training with the prosthesis should commence on the day of delivery. This should be carried out by an occupational therapist in a centre with easy access to the prosthetist for adjustments that may be required during the period of training. It is important that the advantages of prosthetic rehabilitation are made known to the amputee early on; without this the amputee will not gain the full potential benefit of the prosthesis. If the amputee was not seen by the therapist on the first visit to the centre, it is essential that the full assessment is carried out prior to commencing training. The amputee may find the prosthesis uncomfortable initially, but should be encouraged gradually to build up their wearing tolerance. If there is pain or chafing, the prosthetist should check the fit of the socket and appendages.

The principles of training are the same, whatever type of prosthesis is supplied as detailed in Box 19.1.

Box 19.1   Principles of prosthetic training
1. Understanding the parts of the prosthesis 2. Donning and doffing the prosthesis 3. Checking the fit of the prosthesis 4. Prosthetic control 5. Functional tasks with the prosthesis 6. Care of the prosthesis 7. Care of the residual limb (see Ch. 11)

Prosthetic training with a cosmetic prosthesis

This is the simplest type of prosthesis and only minimal prosthetic training is usually required. However, psychological rehabilitation may take much longer.

Understanding the parts of the prosthesis. The trans-radial prosthesis is usually one piece with no moving parts; it may have a friction wrist. The foam hand has wired fingers that can be pushed into position by the remaining hand.

The type of cosmetic prosthesis for all higher levels has a simple elbow joint with locking knob in the forearm. This can sometimes be difficult to locate initially as it is under the cosmetic covering.

Donning the prosthesis. Some amputees choose to wear a stump sock – for the trans-humeral amputee this must be cut to come up over the shoulder. The trans-radial socket is donned and doffed with the elbow in flexion; some amputees find a twisting action assists them. The trans-humeral amputee may choose to wear a T-shirt under the appendages. Short trans-humeral amputees and those with higher levels of amputation will put the axilla loop onto the remaining limb first and lift the prosthesis round onto their residual limb. The longer trans-humeral amputees will fit the prosthesis onto their residual limb and then fit their appendages round their remaining limb. This can be difficult and requires practice.

Checking the fit of the prosthesis. This will be done by the prosthetist initially but it is important to check that problem areas do not appear during use. Particular areas of note for the trans-radial amputee are the olecranon and condyles, the socket rim (especially the anterior aspect) and the anterior aspect of the distal end of the residual limb. For all higher levels of amputation, areas of particular concern are the acromion and the clavicle.

Prosthetic control. Amputees using a cosmetic prosthesis require little training, but it is important that they know how to use the prosthesis appropriately. Care must be taken when bending fingers as too much movement may cause the wires to break.

The amputee with a prosthetic elbow requires practice locking and unlocking the joint. This involves pushing the locking knob while supporting the weight of the forearm.

Functional tasks with the prosthesis. The cosmetic prosthesis is not a functional tool, but it restores the body image better if it is incorporated into tasks, e.g. holding paper steady and carrying things over the forearm. The silicone prosthesis, which has excellent cosmetic appearance, cannot be used in this way as this would damage the surface. The therapist should ensure that the amputee is independent in daily living activities with special equipment or adapted techniques if necessary.

Care of the prosthesis. The cosmetic hand fitted with a PVC glove should be treated in the same way as the remaining hand, nail varnish and the remover can be used; it should be protected from heat, i.e. oven gloves should be used. However, it should not be immersed in water but be washed with a damp cloth as frequently as the remaining hand and as soon as possible after becoming dirty. If the cosmetic glove becomes damaged, a simple sticking plaster can be applied to prevent water from entering the foam hand. The glove can be changed if it becomes damaged or very stained. The socket should be wiped out regularly with a damp cloth, especially if the prosthesis is worn without a stump sock, to ensure the removal of perspiration.

Prosthetic training with a body powered prosthesis

This is the most functional type of prosthesis. Training amputees with higher levels of amputation will take longer than a trans-radial amputee. Skills learned need to be relevant to the amputee's daily life. Psychological support is part of the training and may need to be continued longer than the prosthetic training. Amputees with additional disabilities will require more training, e.g. damage to the remaining hand, blindness.

Understanding the parts of the prosthesis. Parts of the prosthesis are described earlier in this chapter (pp 252–256). It is important that the amputee has the opportunity to handle the prosthesis and find out how all the parts work. For the higher levels of amputation, this is best done after some initial training as the prosthesis has so many parts and concentrating on it too early can be overwhelming for the amputee.

Donning the prosthesis. Some amputees choose to wear a stump sock and some like to wear a T-shirt under the appendages. The self-suspending socket is donned in the same way as the cosmetic prosthesis and then the operating cord is put on the remaining limb. For the trans-radial amputee using a full set of appendages, the prosthesis should be laid across the amputee's lap with the appendages falling down to the side of the residual limb. The amputee should pick up the top strap, and place the residual limb through this and into the socket. The appendages are then passed round the back onto the remaining limb and up to both shoulders, like a shirt. The prosthetist will initially show the amputee how to don the prosthesis, but practice is required and the therapist should check that the appendages are positioned correctly.

The method used for the short trans-humeral or higher levels is the same as with the cosmetic prosthesis.

Those with a longer trans-humeral amputation will usually put the prosthesis on with the elbow locked and the terminal device supported on a table or chair. The residual limb is put into the socket first, then the appendages are passed round the back and the buckle of the axilla loop is fastened. This requires an agile spine and remaining limb. Many elderly trans-humeral amputees are unable to don the prosthesis without assistance. It is important however that they can doff the prosthesis independently: this involves undoing the axilla buckle and allowing the socket to come off with gravity. If an amputee is unable to manage the buckle, Velcro can be used instead.

Checking the fit of the prosthesis. During training, it is important to check that the socket is fitting comfortably; problem areas to note are as for the cosmetic prosthesis, i.e. the bony prominences and socket rim. The appendages must also be adjusted correctly without either tension or slackness, i.e. they should lie easily across the back and the operating cord should have minimal tension when the prosthesis is by the amputee's side.

The axilla loop can sometimes cause discomfort; personal hygiene in this area is very important. It is not advisable to increase padding here as this will exacerbate the problem. If the amputee is wearing a T-shirt, care should be taken that there are no seams or creases under the axilla loop that may cause discomfort. The skin will gradually become accustomed to the feel of the straps and will toughen up in time.

For the trans-humeral amputee, the neck section of the appendages should not cut in to the neck; if the amputee complains of headaches this section should be checked by the prosthetist. If the amputee complains of altered sensation in the residual limb when wearing the prosthesis, the position of the socket in the axilla should be checked; if they complain of altered sensation in the remaining limb, the tightness of the axilla loop should be checked.

Prosthetic control. Initially this should be using the split hook with the number of elasticated bands that can be easily operated, which at first may be only half a band. If the amputee feels unable to use it in their own environment it can still be used as a training tool in the therapy facility.

Learning control of the terminal device is carried out initially by unilateral exercise, at first by standing with the elbow at 45° of flexion. The movement required is protraction of the shoulder girdle and shoulder flexion; the trans-radial amputee will also use elbow extension. The movement should be as unobtrusive as possible. Examples of unilateral exercises and bilateral tasks for amputees are detailed in Boxes 19.2 and 19.3.

Box 19.2 Examples of unilateral exercises

- Removing pegs from a board, dropping them in a box: practising grasp and release
- Playing peg games, e.g. solitaire, draughts: practising grasp and positioning prior to release
- Moving objects of different shapes and sizes to different locations

---

Box 19.3 Examples of bilateral tasks

- Using scissors, holding the paper in the split hook and cutting with the remaining hand
- Using a stapler or hole punch, holding the paper in the split hook
- Using adhesive tape, holding the roll in the split hook
- Opening jars and bottles
- Undoing nuts and bolts
- Building construction models (see Fig. 19.13)

Box 19.4 Examples of functional tasks

- Rewiring an electrical plug
- Using a can opener
- Holding a knife in the terminal device and the fork in the remaining hand for eating
- Holding a fork in the terminal device and the kitchen knife in the remaining hand for food preparation
- Computer games and typing
- Other tasks related to the individual's leisure and work interests, e.g. gardening, carpentry, sewing, knitting, cooking and sports

---

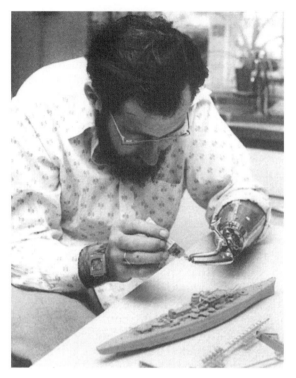

Figure 19.13 A trans-radial amputee using a split hook with a high degree of manipulative skill. (Reproduced by kind permission of Baillière Tindall, from Robertson E 1978 Rehabilitation of arm amputees and limb deficient children.)

Once the amputee has an understanding of how to control the terminal device, progression is from simple bilateral tasks and onto more complex tasks. The prosthesis becomes the non-dominant assistor to the remaining limb.

Functional tasks with the prosthesis. The use of the prosthesis should be incorporated into daily tasks. Examples of functional tasks that should be practised are listed in Box 19.4.

During the training period, the amputee should have the opportunity to see and try other terminal devices, e.g. spade grip for gardening and cricket and universal tool holder for mechanical work. Some amputees will want to use the more cosmetic mechanical hand at times. This is harder to operate than the split hook and it is necessary to return to simpler tasks when first trying the mechanical hand. The operating cord may not be the correct length for all terminal devices, therefore an extension piece must be fitted to the terminal device, e.g. if sometimes using a mechanical hand and sometimes a split hook, the split hook will need a 5 cm extension, which will then attach to the operating cord.

For those with a prosthetic elbow joint, control of this must be practised once the basic operation

of the split hook is achieved. For those with a high level of amputation or a brachial plexus lesion, automatic elbow operation is not possible and must be done with the remaining hand either pulling the elbow lock cord or a lever on the forearm.

Those able to operate the elbow lock automatically require practice and encouragement. The movement is depression, internal rotation, extension and abduction of the shoulder joint, like 'nudging someone in the ribs'. Careful adjustment of the lock strap is needed.

Initially with the elbow locked at 90°, the amputee practices unlocking the elbow. Watching another amputee do this is very helpful and doing the movement in front of a mirror gives visual feedback to the amputee. Once unlocking the elbow is achieved, locking it can be attempted. It is necessary for the elbow lock cord to return fully between each action. Once locking and unlocking are achieved, the skills should be incorporated into functional tasks.

Care of the prosthesis. The socket and outside of the prosthesis should be wiped with a damp cloth regularly. Appendages may require adjusting if they stretch. Split hook bands will need to be replaced regularly and the rubber covering on the inside of the split hook jaws may wear out, which will affect the grip. The prosthesis should not be dismantled by either the amputee or the therapist; this should only be done by the prosthetist.

Prosthetic training with the electrically powered prosthesis

These prostheses are not suitable for primary amputees as they are heavy and complex to operate. Myo-electric control requires a close fitting socket, oedema in the residual limb must have completely resolved.

Before an amputee is supplied with an electric prosthesis, it is important that they are reassessed. They should at this stage be fully rehabilitated physically, psychologically and prosthetically. They should have a high level of motivation as electric power necessitates extra visits to the prosthetic centre for fittings, training and maintenance. They should have realistic expectations of the powered limb. Those being fitted with a myo-electric control must have adequate myo signals to operate the device and be able to tolerate wearing the socket directly in contact with the skin. Electric power is not suitable for amputees requiring precise function or for use in heavy industry. The amputee should have a good understanding of its advantages and disadvantages (see Table 19.1) as it is not the answer to all prosthetic problems, but for some amputees it is an excellent prosthetic device.

Understanding the parts of the prosthesis. The method of operation should be explained in an appropriate manner for the individual (see p. 250). There is a friction wrist and maybe an on/off switch enabling power to the hand to be turned off. The adult sized hands have a thumb break enabling grip release, e.g. when the battery has run out. The battery, its removal and replacement in the battery case, should be explained, as well as the charging and care of the batteries.

Donning the prosthesis. This is done in the same way as the trans-radial self-suspending socket and, if trans-humeral, in the same way as the body powered prosthesis. A stump sock cannot be worn with a myo-electric prosthesis as there has to be direct contact between the skin and the electrodes.

Checking the fit of the prosthesis. Checking the socket, and appendages if used, will be the same as for the body powered prosthesis. With myo-electric power, marks showing where the electrodes are sited on the skin of the residual limb should be clear when the prosthesis has been worn for 10–15 min.

Prosthetic control. Training with the servo control will be similar to training with the body powered prosthesis; particular care must be given to the operating cord length, because the servo hand requires less movement to fully open.

Training with the myo-electric prosthesis may commence before delivery of the prosthesis. Practising the contractions required with electrodes

Table 19.1 Advantages and disadvantages of an electrically powered prosthesis

Advantages	Disadvantages
A hand that operates easily without body movement	Weight of the prosthesis is in the hand, at the end of the lever, making it appear even heavier than it is
Strong grip	Poor visibility of the gripping area
Myo can operate anywhere in space	Less cosmetic than cosmetic hand
Two-site myo may have variable grip force	No proprioceptive feedback from the operating cord
No harness required to operate myo	More daily care, i.e. charging batteries
	More maintenance required
	Hand operation is slow
	Cost

attached to the residual limb may operate a hand, or link to a computer to play computer games, or to an electric toy, e.g. a train set. Encouraging the amputee to move their phantom wrist, hand or fingers may help them understand the movements required to operate the electric device.

When the prosthesis is supplied, training commences with the same activities used for the body powered prosthetic training, starting with unilateral activities (Fig. 19.14), through to simple bilateral tasks and on to skills required for the amputee's daily living. If a two-site myo-electric control is used, one electrode opens the hand and one closes it; the settings of these two electrodes is critical. They will have been initially set by the prosthetist but may require adjustment. The lateral (outside) electrode opens the hand and the medial electrode closes it. If the amputee has difficulty opening the hand, the medial electrode setting can be turned down, i.e. making it more difficult to close the hand. The higher electrode settings require less muscle contraction to activate the motor, but may use more battery power, so lower settings should be used if possible. Operating the hand in space, e.g. for peg games,

can be tolerated for short periods, but this should be interspersed with work operating the hand while it is resting on a table, e.g. for clerical-type tasks. This is particularly important when the amputee finds the prosthesis heavy. Amputees who have previously worn a body powered prosthesis only have to learn how to operate the new device and how to take advantage of its benefits. Those who have previously used a cosmetic prosthesis need to be taught how to use a functional device actively using the grip rather than using it as a passive stabiliser.

Functional tasks with the prosthesis. Tasks similar to those used for training with the body-powered prosthesis can be used (Fig. 19.15). In addition, when training with the myoelectric control, the hand should be used with the arm in extension, e.g. for using a dustpan and brush or changing a light bulb, as well as in flexion, e.g. for doing up buttons.

Care of the prosthesis. The electric prosthesis is not robust and requires extra care. It must not be immersed in water; should this happen accidentally the cosmetic covering (glove) should be removed and the prosthesis put in a warm

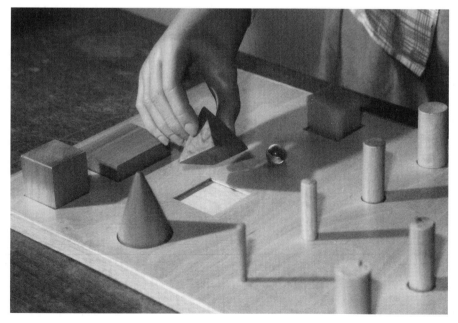

Figure 19.14 Unilateral exercise to train control of the myo-electric prosthesis. (Photograph by kind permission of Richmond, Twickenham and Roehampton Healthcare NHS Trust.)

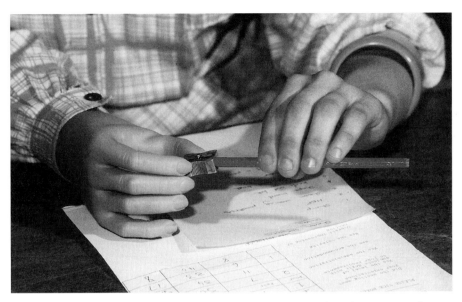

Figure 19.15 A trans-radial amputee using a myo-electric prosthesis to sharpen a pencil. (Photograph by kind permission of Richmond, Twickenham and Roehampton Healthcare·NHS Trust.)

dry place and returned for repair as soon as possible. If the glove is damaged, the hole should be covered immediately to prevent water or dust penetrating the motor and the glove should be cared for in the same way as the cosmetic prosthesis glove. No adjustment should be made to the electrode settings by the amputee unless it has been explained very clearly to them.

Electric power is very beneficial to some amputees – many find it a useful alternative to body power and become active users of both systems.

BILATERAL ARM AMPUTEES

Bilateral arm amputees are very small in number as their amputation is almost always acquired amputation; there are approximately two patients per year in the UK.

However, because of the severity of the disability, sensitive care must be given in the early stages of treatment. The pre-prosthetic programme should include all the objectives listed above for the unilateral arm amputee. From the very beginning, the problem-solving skills of therapist and amputee must be used to the full. The lead

of what to tackle first should come from the amputee and the therapist should give encouragement and set realistic goals. Use of the residual limbs together or with leather gauntlets or thermoplastic devices should be explored to achieve independence in feeding and some personal care. Use of feet, mouth and chin may also be useful in undressing and other skills. All possibilities should be tried. If the amputee is under 20 years of age, they may learn to use their feet; above this age it is likely that their lower limb joints are less flexible and will allow only minimal functional use of the feet (Fig. 19.16).

It is important to include family and other carers in discussions about independence skills so they can gain an understanding of what can be possible, rather than assuming that total assistance will be required. They will also need considerable support in adjusting to the new situation. When the bilateral amputee is ready (physically and psychologically) for prosthetic management, they should attend a specialised centre where there are expert therapists and specialised facilities for effective prosthetic rehabilitation. Most bilateral arm amputees, once they appreciate

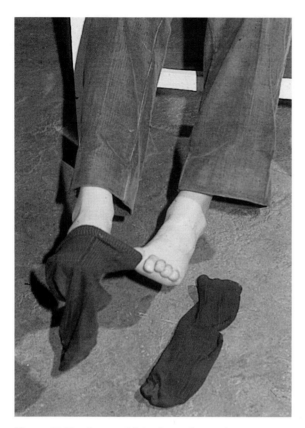

Figure 19.16 A young bilateral trans-humeral amputee demonstrating functional activity using his feet. (Photograph by kind permission of Richmond, Twickenham and Roehampton Healthcare NHS Trust.)

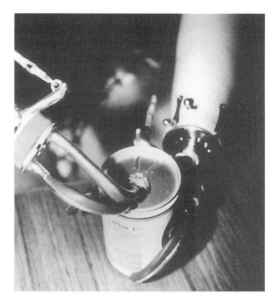

Figure 19.17 A bilateral trans-radial amputee using two split hooks to open a ring-pull can. (Photograph by kind permission of Richmond, Twickenham and Roehampton Healthcare NHS Trust.)

the functional possibilities that prostheses can offer them, are highly motivated towards success (see Fig. 19.17). They will find body powered prostheses the most functionally beneficial at this stage. The prostheses are usually attached to each other and the appendages lie across the back; moving the left residual limb operates the left terminal device, etc. Training will take a similar course to that for the unilateral amputee, but more practice will be required in functional tasks and independence training. Realistic goals for achievement are essential to build up confidence.

It may be helpful for the new amputee to meet an established bilateral arm amputee, who has adapted to life with two artificial arms and managed to assume a useful and acceptable lifestyle. This introduction must be carefully timed

and planned. The bilateral amputee may in the long term choose to use any type of prosthesis and in any combination depending on their needs. Some will choose to wear one or no prostheses. They may require advice and training to enable them to find the appropriate hardware or techniques for them at any one time; their needs will change as their social situation and physical health changes.

CONGENITAL LIMB DEFICIENCY

Parents occasionally know from the antenatal scan that their child will have have a limb deficiency. This enables them to gather information and meet relevant people, if they wish to, prior to the birth. It also enables them to separate the giving of 'good' and 'bad' news to relatives and friends. More commonly, however, the knowledge comes at the time of the birth and parents and medical personnel are equally shocked. The way this situation is handled is critical to the feelings of the family in the weeks and months to follow.

The family needs support, information and

advice. They should be referred to a prosthetic centre where children are regularly seen, ideally when their child is 4–6 weeks old. At this stage, the baby is assessed, but the visit is primarily for the parents. It is an opportunity to meet the rehabilitation consultant and therapist, to answer the parents' questions, to discuss the child's prosthetic management and to see some of the prosthetic options available. It may also be an opportunity to meet families in a similar situation.

Although all prosthetic services (in the UK) can deal with the simpler deficiencies, any child with complex deficiencies should be referred to a specialist centre. Families should be told of Reach, the Association for Children with Hand or Arm Deficiency (a parent self-help group), which is very supportive with regular newsletters, local groups and an information database.

Most children have a mid-forearm level of deficiency and they will normally be fitted with their first cosmetic prosthesis at 4–6 months. This is the time when a child is beginning to sit independently. The prosthesis enables the child to become used to having a full length arm, so hand/eye coordination is correctly formulated and the child becomes accustomed to wearing a prosthesis. Some parents find the concern and comments of the public hard to come to terms with; the presence of the cosmetic hand at the end of the sleeve makes the deficiency less obvious (Fig. 19.18).

The prosthesis can be used as a stabilising device, for hitting mobiles and towers, for holding large toys in a bimanual grasp. The prosthesis has to be replaced at regular intervals as the child grows. Some children find them helpful for crawling but others find the prosthesis a hindrance and reject it at this stage. Ideally, the prosthesis will be worn for part of each day but it is best that it does not become an area of conflict either between parent and child or between the two parents. If this is a possibility, the prosthesis should be kept in an accessible place, e.g. the toy box, so it is often seen by the child.

When treating a child with any form of deficiency, it is important that the therapist sees them in the context of the family since the parents are co-therapists, carrying out treatment regimes

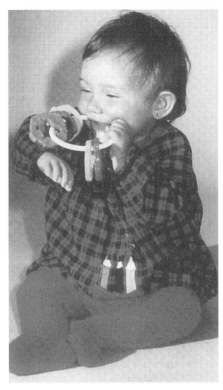

Figure 19.18   A cosmetic arm being used by a 9-month-old baby for bilateral play. (Photograph by kind permission of J.C. Lamparter and Richmond, Twickenham and Roehampton Healthcare NHS Trust.)

at home. Their ability to do this will depend on the advice and guidance given to them by the therapist. Siblings and grandparents may benefit from attending some training sessions.

When the child is walking securely and beginning to be interested in manipulative skills (at approximately the age of 18 months) their first functional limb is fitted, which has a self-suspending socket and an operating cord. This may be:

- an infant split hook (a small plastic-covered version of the adult hook). The hook can be removed and replaced with a cosmetic hand
- the Canadian Amputee Prosthetic Project (CAPP) device, with a larger top jaw and small lower jaw. It is not possible to remove this device so, if required, a second limb is provided for cosmesis

- a Scamp hand (Fig. 19.19), a small electric hand, initially with a pull switch operated by an operating cord but later can be changed to single site myo-electric control. This has a battery to power the motor
- other electric hands.

There are advantages and disadvantages to each of these functional limbs and the child needs to be assessed as an individual and the parents' views sought.

Training the child and parents begins when the first functional prosthesis is delivered and should consist of several short sessions as the child's concentration span at this age is limited. Play activities will be used and must be matched to the normal developmental milestones of the child. Initially, the child learns how to release objects, dropping small plastic toys into a bowl of water, then holding objects steady, e.g. con-

tainers in the sand pit, bilateral grasp holding larger toys, pushing a buggy or riding on toys. Activity choice will be determined by the maturity of the child. As the child grows, training will be required as new development milestones are reached or when the prosthetic prescription is changed. Training may take the form of unilateral activities, e.g. large knob puzzles, learning hand control, and bilateral activities of an appropriate level for the child, e.g. cutting, threading, playing with construction toys (Fig. 19.20).

During training, the fit of the socket should be checked and care of the prosthesis discussed with the parent. If the child is attending nursery, the staff should be contacted and given information about the prosthesis.

As the child approaches school age, the parents may need advice in how to introduce their child to the classroom situation. Most children with

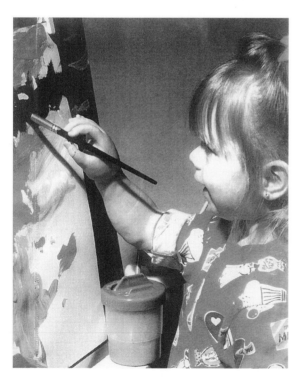

Figure 19.19 A 2-year-old child with mid-forearm deficiency experimenting with the use of a Scamp hand for painting. (Photograph by kind permission of P. Thomas and Hugh Steeper Ltd.)

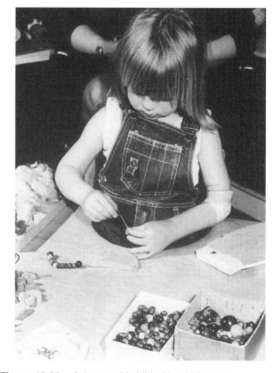

Figure 19.20 A 4-year-old child with mid-forearm deficiency using a myo-electric prosthesis to thread beads during a free-play activity session in the Arm Training Unit. Her mother is present as a co-therapist. (Photograph by kind permission of J.C. Lamparter and Richmond, Twickenham and Roehampton Healthcare NHS Trust.)

upper limb deficiencies attend normal school and it can be helpful, if the parents are in agreement, for the therapist to carry out a school visit and advise the teacher on how to accept and make the most of the child's potential.

Children's needs change dramatically as they grow. A constant dialogue must be maintained between the therapist and family to ascertain that these needs are being recognised and catered for, and if necessary further training may be arranged. This will increase the range of activities available to the child and will follow the type of bimanual approach used for adult amputees. The child should be given sufficient prosthetic information and training to make an informed choice of whether or not to wear the prosthesis, and if so, which system to choose. When the child is 8–9 years old, they should be very actively involved in discussions about prostheses. Some will choose no prosthesis and others will choose any of the options available. It is helpful for them to continue attending a prosthetic centre on a regular basis (3–4 monthly if they are an active prosthetic user, annually if not) so their socket fit can be monitored and their prosthetic, functional, social and educational needs can be addressed regularly. Children with higher levels of limb deficiency or with more than one limb affected will have a similar programme of rehabilitation, but each will be monitored individually. Problem-solving skills are essential for these children and their families (see Ch. 21). When these children reach adulthood, they should have acquired all the skills necessary to live a normal life with the means of choosing a career and lifestyle that will not be hampered by their limb deficiency.

PROSTHETIC INFORMATION

Detailed information regarding prostheses available in the UK can be obtained from manufacturers. The addresses are listed in Appendix 1.

BIBLIOGRAPHY FOR PREVIOUS EDITIONS

Angliss V 1981 Early referral to limb deficiency clinics. Prosthetics and Orthotics International 5:141–143

Bhala R P, Schultz C F 1982 Golf club holder for upper-extremity amputee golfers. Archives of Physical Medicine and Rehabilitation 63:339–341

Crosthwaite Eyre N 1979 Rehabilitation of the upper limb amputee. Physiotherapy 65(1):9–12

Curran B, Hambrey R 1991 The prosthetic treatment of upper limb deficiency. Prosthetics and Orthotics International 15:82–87

Enzinna A J 1975 Orientation and mobility for a totally blind bilateral hand amputee. New Outlook March:103–108

Hambrey R, Withinshaw G 1990 Electrically powered upper limb prostheses: their development and application. British Journal of Occupational Therapy 53(1):7–11

Hermansson L M 1991 Structured training of children fitted with myoelectric prostheses. Prosthetics and Orthotics International 15:88–92

Hughes S 1980 Abnormalities of the limbs. Nursing Mirror 16 October:17–20

Kulkarni J 1990 Partial hand prostheses: a clinical profile. British Journal of Occupational Therapy 53(5):200–201

Malone J M, Fleming L L, Roberson J, Whitesides T E, Leal J M, Poole J U, Sternstein Grodin R 1984 Immediate, early and late postsurgical management of upper-limb amputation. Journal of Rehabilitation Research and Development 21(1):33–41

Marquardt E G 1983 A holistic approach to rehabilitation for the limb-deficient child. Archives of Physical Medicine and Rehabilitation 64:237–242

Robertson E S 1971 How independent is the limb deficient child? Occupational Therapy Today-Tomorrow. Proceedings of the 5th International Congress of the World Federation of Occupational Therapy, Zurich, p 107–112

Sauter W F 1991 The use of electric elbows in the rehabilitation of children with upper limb deficiencies. Prosthetics and Orthotics International 15:93–95

Sorbye E 1977 Myoelectric controlled hand prostheses in children. International Journal of Rehabilitation Research 1:15–25

Trial of the Swedish Myoelectric Hand for young children. 1981 DHSS, London, Summarized in Physiotherapy 67(10):312

Trost F J 1983 A comparison of conventional and myoelectric below-elbow prosthetic use. Inter Clinic Information Bulletin 18(4):9–16

Van Lunteren A, Van Lunteren-Gerritsen G H M, Stassen H G, Zuithoff M J 1983 A field evaluation of arm prostheses for unilateral amputees. Prosthetics and Orthotics International 7:141–151

BIBLIOGRAPHY FOR THE THIRD EDITION

Atkins D J, Heard D C, Donovan W H 1996 Epidemiological overview of individuals with upper limb loss and their reported research priorities. Journal of Prosthetics and Orthotics 8(1):2–11

Carnegie F 1994 What treatment for the limb deficient child. British Journal of Hand Therapy 2(1):13–15

Day H J B 1991 ISO/ISPO classification of congenital limb deficiency. Prosthetics and Orthotics International 15(2):67–69

Doeringer J, Hogan N 1995 Performance of above elbow body powered prostheses in visually guided unconstrained motion tasks. IEEE Transactions on Biomedical Engineering 42(6):621–631

Eldestein J E, Berger N 1993 Performance comparison among children fitted with myoelectric and body powered hands. Archives of Physical Medicine and Rehabilitation 74(April):376–380

Esquenazi A, Meier R H III 1996 Rehabilitation in limb deficiency. 4. Limb amputation. Archives of Physical Medicine and Rehabilitation 77:S18–S28

Fixsen J A 1995 The upper limb. In: Harris N H, Birch R (eds) Other developmental abnormalities. Post graduate textbook of clinical orthopaedics, 3rd edn. Blackwell Science, Oxford, ch 8

Fraser C 1993 A survey of users of upper limb prostheses. British Journal of Occupational Therapy 56(5):166–168

Gavie W et al 1997 Upper limb traumatic amputees, review of prosthetic use. Journal of Hand Surgery 22B(1):73–76

Hal Silcox D et al 1993 Myo-electric prostheses, a long term follow up and study of use of alternative prostheses. Journal of Bone and Joint Surgery 75A(12):1781–1789

Jain S 1996 Rehabilitation in limb deficiency. 2. The pediatric amputee. Archives of Physical Medicine and Rehabilitation 77:S9–S13

Jones L, Davidson J H 1995 The long term outcome of upper limb amputees treated in a rehabilitation centre in Sydney Australia. Disability and Rehabilitation 17(8):437–442

Jones L, Davidson J H 1996 A review of the management of upper limb amputees. Critical Reviews in Physical and Rehabilitation Medicine 8(4):297–322

Kejlaa G 1993 Consumer concerns and functional value of prostheses to upper limb amputees. Prosthetics and Orthotics International 17:157–163

Kruger L, Fishman S 1993 Myoelectric and body-powered prostheses. Journal of Pediatric Orthopaedics 13(1):68–75

Kyberd P J, Beard D J, Morrison J D 1997 The population of users of upper limb prostheses attending the Oxford Limb Fitting Service. Prosthetics and Orthotics International 21(2):85–91

Levine E A, Warso M A, McCoy D M, Das Gupta T K, Vilendahl J, Keagy R 1994 Forequarter amputation for soft tissue tumour. The American Surgeon 60(5):367–370

Meredith J, Vilendahl J, Keagy R 1993 Successful voluntary grasp and release using the Cookie Crusher myoelectric hand in two year olds. The American Journal of Occupational Therapy 47(9):825–829

Pruit S et al 1996 Functional status of children with limb deficiency: development and initial validation of an outcome measure. Archives of Physical Medicine and Rehabilitation 77(12):1233–1238

Roeschlein R A, Domholdt E 1989 Factors related to successful upper extremity prosthetic use. Prosthetics and Orthotics International 13(1):14–18

Rout S N 1993 Lightweight prostheses for bilateral below elbow amputees. Prosthetics and Orthotics International 17:126–129

Verral T, Kulkarni J 1995 Driving appliances for upper limb amputees. Prosthetics and Orthotics International 19:124–127

Volpe C M et al 1997 Forequarter amputation with fasciocutaneous deltoid flap reconstruction for malignant tumour of the upper extremity. Annals of Surgery and Oncology 4(4):298–302

Weaver S, Large L L, Vogts V 1988 Comparison of myoelectric and conventional prostheses for adolescent amputees. The American Journal of Occupational Therapy 42(2):87–91

Wright T W, Hagen A D, Wood M B 1995 Prosthetic usage in major upper extremity amputation. The Journal of Hand Surgery 20A(4):612–622

20

Pain management

Maggie Uden
Benna Waites

Pain is a complex physiological phenomenon that is difficult to define in precise terms, but it has some clearly discernible characteristics. It is an unpleasant sensory and emotional experience commanding a response, which even when not expressed verbally, may be reflected in the individual's behaviour and often in other physical signs.

For the amputee, the presence of pain can have a significant effect on their lifestyle. Pain may be present prior to the amputation, in the early postamputation period and occasionally it can become a longstanding problem.

Assessment and management of pain for the amputee is best made with a multidisciplinary team approach, e.g. doctors, nurses, prosthetists, therapists and clinical psychologists. The underlying causes of any pain must be recognised and investigated thoroughly so that appropriate treatment can be initiated by the team member best able to do this.

TYPES OF PAIN

The amputee may report that pain is felt in the residual limb or in the phantom limb or both. It must be remembered that painless phantom sensation and phantom limb pain are two different feelings, perhaps best understood as two different ends of a continuum of phantom experience.

Phantom sensation

This can be described as 'a non-painful sensation or awareness of the presence of the amputated limb'. Three categories of sensation can occur. Kinaesthetic sensations, kinetic sensations and extroceptive sensations and may include itching, tingling, pressure, a telescoping limb, spontaneous movements, the presence of the amputated limb or part of it.

Phantom limb pain

This can be described as 'a painful feeling felt in the part of the extremity that has been amputated'. Phantom limb pain can include burning, stabbing, cramping, twisting, squeezing, an electrical shock like pain, or a crushing feeling. For many years, phantom pain was considered an emotional or psychiatric phenomenon representing an emotional response to the loss of a body part. However, more recently, Katz (1992) summarised current thinking on phantom limb pain and sensation, stating that it was a 'complex interaction of inputs from the periphery and widespread regions of the brain subserving sensory, cognitive and emotional processes'. Phantom pain is reasonably common, but often unpredictable in its predisposing factors, severity, frequency or duration. Nikolajsen et al (1997) state that clinical studies suggest that phantom pain is more likely to occur in patients who had pain in the limb before the amputation, e.g. diabetic foot ulcers or a critically ischaemic limb with gangrene, than those who were free of pain.

Residual limb pain

This can be described as 'pain arising in the residual limb often after a specific anatomical structure or pathological process has been identified'. Factors influencing residual limb pain will be discussed later in this chapter.

CAUSES OF PAIN
Pre-operative pain

The majority of patients who are waiting for an amputation whether as an acute emergency case, or following a longer term assessment, will present with pain in the affected limb, e.g.

pre-operative ischaemic pain. The degree of pain experienced may vary depending on the cause of the amputation and the overall patients condition. Effective pain control prior to surgery by use of analgesia and epidural may reduce the amount of postoperative pain experienced.

The ability of patients to talk freely about their feelings regarding the surgery to a team member may also diminish the fear of pain (see Ch. 2).

Early discomfort

All amputees experience discomfort in the early postoperative period and this may be caused by the following:

1. In the immediate postoperative phase, discomfort or pain is felt in the wound site and oedematous tissues. Excessive early pain may be caused by a haematoma; increasing pain 2–3 days after surgery may result from a developing infection.

2. Occasionally, the active exercise programme in the therapy facility may cause discomfort in the muscles and joints unaccustomed to movement and stretching.

3. During prosthetic rehabilitation, both when the early walking aid (EWA) is used and during the initial weeks of using the first prosthesis, the residual limb may become sensitive to the new pressures exerted on the tissues.

4. Phantom sensation may be experienced soon after the amputation, but will tend to fade gradually with time, as memory fades and the nervous impulses adapt to the new situation. Sensory re-education must be started from the first postoperative day, (see Ch. 4), with the amputee becoming accustomed to light pressure first, and as time progresses, to handling and resisted exercise.

Longer-term pain

In general, the majority of individuals will have adapted physically to life as an amputee by the time they have become mobile with their first prosthesis. This means that they will have learned to adjust to the appropriate pressure points and

> **Box 20.1**   Causes of longer-term pain
>
> *Pathological*
> - Scar contracture/adhesion
> - Unhealed wound
> - Oedema
> - Neuroma/nerve damage/hypersensitivity
> - Bony spur
> - Referred pain, e.g. from lumbar spine, sacroiliac joints or abdominal viscera
> - Ischaemic or claudication pain in the residual limb
> - Osteomyelitis
> - Arthritic conditions and joint pains
> - Neurological abnormalities, e.g. hemiplegia, spina bifida, diabetes mellitus
> - Fracture
> - Regrowth of tumour
> - Adverse neural tension
> - Sympathetic problems, e.g. reflex sympathetic dystrophy
> - Brachial plexus injury
>
> *Prosthetic*
> - Inappropriate prosthetic prescription
> - Prosthetic socket fitting problems
> - Low tolerance to pressure

prosthetic adjustments that may have been necessary at the early stage. However, a few amputees may experience either residual limb or phantom limb pain from the operation onwards. Other amputees who initially experienced no problems, may in time present with longer-term pain. The causes of longer-term pain are listed in Box 20.1.

TREATMENT OF PAIN

Although the knowledge of treatment of pain in general has improved in the last few years, it still has a long way to go. Recent literature on one aspect of pain, i.e. phantom pain is highly contradictory as studies are limited by short-term follow-up and small groups of patients. Different causes of pain require different approaches to treatment. However, it is not always easy to diagnose the exact cause. A wide range of treatments are available, but most of the commonly used treatments for phantom limb pain do not appear to have good long-term success rates, particularly when they are not related to the underlying causes. For example, burning, tingling phantom limb pain is often caused by decreased blood flow in the residual limb, whereas a cramping, squeezing pain may be caused by spasms in the residual limb.

A multidisciplinary approach, a supportive attitude and an intelligent understanding of the causes of pain, as well as the use of the various methods of treatment available, will in most cases help amputees to overcome the unpleasant experience of their pain. Three areas of treatment will be outlined:

1. Physical therapy
2. Medical treatment, e.g. pharmacological and surgical
3. Psychological management of chronic pain.

PHYSICAL THERAPY

The therapist is frequently one of the first team members approached with a problem of pain and must consider every aspect of the pain while assessing the amputee. This assessment may be carried out with the use of pain charts, e.g. visual analogue scales, pain questionnaires, a diary in which patients can record their own pain pattern, or by careful questioning.

It must be realised that assessment in these cases often requires a number of sessions to investigate a possible cause for the pain or to formulate an accurate impression of the problem. Observation of the amputee over a period of time enables an accurate picture to emerge. At some hospitals, the assessment is carried out by outpatient visits, and at others, the amputee is admitted for a period of time.

Assessment

Subjective examination

The therapist must record all relevant history of the present condition as well as past medical history. The nature and behaviour of the pain must also be known and recorded. Considering the amputee's answers to the following questions can help to determine the extent to which the amputee is feeling pain:

1. How does the amputee describe their pain, e.g. is it nagging, burning, dull or sharp?
2. Is the pain intermittent or constant?

3. How long has the amputee had the pain?
4. What is the intensity of the pain (0–10)?
5. Where is the exact site of pain?
6. Is the pain originating from the phantom limb, the residual limb or both?
7. What aggravates or relieves the pain?
8. Is there any radiation of pain?
9. Is there any paraesthesia?
10. At what time of day is the pain felt?
11. What is the daily pattern of pain, e.g. throughout a 24-hour period, including night-time and disturbance of sleep?
12. What is the lifestyle of the amputee?
13. Is the pain related to prosthetic use and activity?

The following are also relevant pieces of information:

- types of medication taken currently (prescribed or non-prescribed) and the frequency with which it is taken
- amount of alcohol and tobacco consumed or other addictive substances
- impact on social interaction
- impact on occupational function.

Objective examination

A physical assessment of the residual limb must be carried out and may be compared with the non-affected limb. This may include:

- range of movement of all joints of the residual limb, in particular, assessing to see if there are any flexion contractures, unstable, painful and non-functional joints
- muscle strength
- sensation
- pulses
- temperature
- skin condition
- observation and palpation of the tissues of the residual limb.

The cervical, thoracic and lumbar spine may be examined, as pain can be referred distally.

If the amputee is a prosthetic user, the fit and alignment of the prosthesis during all activities is examined, including a gait assessment.

The general state of hygiene and physical fitness of the amputee is assessed.

The possible underlying cause of the amputee's pain can be assessed by the physiotherapist, both from this formal assessment and from an informal observation of the amputee during activities of daily living over a period of time. Following assessment, the therapist should formulate a problem list and attempt to set achievable and realistic goals with the amputee.

A medical opinion should be sought for a diagnosis to be made following further investigation. Sometimes it may take weeks or months for a diagnosis to be confirmed, and only after a period of trial and error with various treatments.

Physical treatment modalities

The therapist should undertake treatment for phantom limb pain or residual limb pain where there is evidence that underlying physical mechanisms which may be influenced by physical treatments are responsible for the pain. If after careful evaluation the whole team considers it to be appropriate, it may be necessary to use physical therapy in combination with other treatments (e.g. pharmacological, psychological or psychiatric treatments). It is the therapist's responsibility to check the fit of the prosthesis, its state of repair and the type of socks used, and refer the amputee back to their prosthetic service if the pain experienced relates to a problem with the prosthesis.

There are many treatment modalities that can be effective, but whichever is selected must be given a reasonable trial before stopping, modifying or changing to another modality. Clear records must be kept of each treatment used, the individual technique employed and the amputee's response to the treatment.

The following treatments are merely suggestions – individual techniques and preferences vary. The accepted contraindications for these modalities apply to the amputee as for all patients.

Desensitising techniques

Sensory re-education must be started from the first postoperative day following the amputation (see Ch. 4). It is important that the amputee becomes accustomed to light pressure on their residual limb in order to settle the sensitive nerve endings. Residual limb handling and gentle massage should be encouraged as part of a daily programme throughout the amputee's life.

Exercise programme

A graded exercise programme for the muscles and joints of the residual limb and remaining limbs should be given to maintain or increase joint mobility and muscle strength. Muscle tone and circulation will also be promoted. If an amputee complains of pain in their affected limb, they may hold their limb in a tensed position and be reluctant to move their joints. Muscle weakness and atrophy can develop as a result of this situation. More often than not, it is essential that the amputee continues with an exercise programme to prevent further complications of joint contractures developing and the possibility of fitting problems with their prosthesis. (see 'Graded exercise' section under 'Psychological Management of Chronic Pain' later in this chapter for more detail).

Oedema control techniques and tissue support

Where the residual limb pain is seen to be caused by oedema, a variety of methods of treatment are available (see Ch. 4). Occasionally, merely a sensation of contained tissue support is required, e.g. a Juzo sock.

Percussion

A small rubber hammer, an electrical vibrator or manual techniques can be used. Percussion is best employed while the amputee is experiencing pain. It should not be used during the periods of freedom from pain.

Thermal modalities

The use of hot and cold therapy can have a dramatic effect on increasing the circulation to the affected area and thereby decreasing pain, oedema and reducing muscle spasm.

Heat therapy can be applied in a variety of forms to the residual limb, e.g. a heat pad or towels can be used. Cold therapy can include ice packs, towels, ice-cube massage or even contrast techniques.

In clinical practice, there are circumstances where one of these modalities is preferable to the other. Careful assessment and accurate clinical judgement by the therapist is essential in order to decide if thermal treatment is appropriate for the amputee. It must be remembered that an assessment of the amputee's sensation is carried out prior to any use of hot or cold therapy. Diabetic amputees and those with peripheral vascular disease must be carefully assessed due to probable altered sensation, and another approach to their treatment may be preferable.

Electrical modalities

Various forms of electrotherapy can be used, predominantly to provide pain relief. Ultrasound can have a beneficial effect if soft tissue structures are found to be the cause of pain. Adherent scars on the residual limb can be mobilised with ultrasound. If the residual limb has particularly bony prominences, care must be taken when using ultrasound. Recent studies have also shown that ultrasound may have some effect in relieving pain from a neuroma in the residual limb.

Megapulse, interferential therapy and laser treatment can also be used at the discretion of the physiotherapist.

Spinal treatment

Where there is residual or phantom limb pain that is reproducible on spinal movements, an accurate spinal assessment must be carried out and appropriate treatment can then be given. This may include techniques such as mobilisation or manipulation, traction and exercises. Adverse neural tension can be relieved by mobilising the neural tissue. It may be necessary to refer the amputee for specialist spinal physiotherapy.

Peripheral joints

Where joint range limitations exist, appropriate mobilising modalities should be carried out. This may include an exercise programme, stretches and proprioceptive neuromuscular facilitation (PNF) techniques such as hold–relax.

Transcutaneous electrical nerve stimulation

Transcutaneous electrical nerve stimulation (TENS) has become increasingly used in treating phantom and residual limb pain over recent years, with varying results. TENS works by inhibiting pain through the gate control theory. Stimulation of large diameter myelinated nerve fibres closes the gate to pain at a cordal level, thereby over-riding pain input from non-myelinated small diameter nerve fibres (see Fig. 20.1).

TENS is a useful adjunct to therapy as it can be used in a treatment facility or at home.

If TENS is chosen as the optimum form of treatment for the amputee, accurate assessment, careful instruction and monitoring are needed in terms of placement of electrodes, frequency of current and duration of treatment. Various TENS machines are available on the market and therefore it is essential that the therapist and amputee follow the guidelines for use and precautions set by each manufacturer.

Contraindications to treatment must also be considered. Too often, TENS is abandoned as a form of treatment due to an inadequate length of treatment time, poor electrode position or inappropriate patient selection.

Some controversy lies over the positioning of electrodes for treating phantom and residual limb pain. Wells et al (1991) state:

The guidelines to follow for electrode placement are that the pads should be placed:

- over the affected nerve where it is most superficial
- over the affected dermatome or the adjacent dermatome
- over the nerve trunk
- above or below the painful area
- not over anaesthetic areas
- over areas which will still allow functional use of the limb or part.

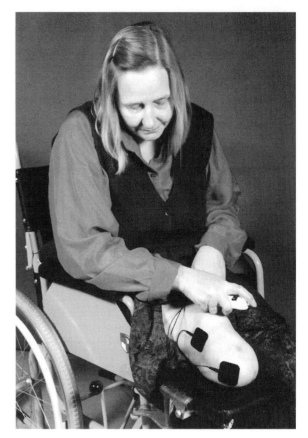

Figure 20.1 A trans-tibial amputee controlling her pain using a transcutaneous electrical nerve stimulation machine (TENS). (Photograph by kind permission of Richmond, Twickenham and Roehampton Healthcare NHS Trust.)

One or more of the above principles may be applied. If the treatment is at first unsuccessful, the amputee should be encouraged to try different electrode positions before the treatment is abandoned. Electrode placement on the contralateral limb can also be tried.

If the amputee is to use TENS for a home trial, pain charts or a diary should be kept to record pain site and severity, electrode placement and frequency of use, time and duration of treatment and the effect produced. Re-assessment by the therapist is important. If TENS is to be considered for treatment, it is essential to have the amputee's full understanding and compliance with treatment sessions.

Hydrotherapy

Hydrotherapy can be used as a treatment modality for the amputee. The effect of residual limb exercises in warm water can be beneficial in pain relief as well as mobilising the joints. Before commencing hydrotherapy, care should be taken in assessing the amputee to ensure there are no open wounds on the residual limb. The standard assessment checks for this modality must be made and recorded.

Acupuncture

Acupuncture or electro-acupuncture have been used to help relieve phantom limb pain. Acupuncture should always be performed by a suitably trained therapist.

Prosthetic rehabilitation

Increased prosthetic use and mobility can have the effect of decreasing phantom limb pain. A good fitting socket that encases and supports the residual limb is essential.

Other treatments

Relaxation techniques and Biofeedback are also available as a form of treatment and have been used with varying results. (See 'Relaxation' section under 'Psychological Management of Chronic Pain' later in this chapter).

Education

The therapist's role is also extended to offering education and advice. This may include a re-evaluation of the amputee's gait pattern and the use of appropriate walking aids. Advice may also be needed in terms of hygiene of the residual limb and the prosthesis, footwear and encouraging a home exercise programme. (see Ch. 11). Therapy may often only provide temporary pain relief and therefore pain management techniques may be appropriate in the absence of a cure. Referral to other specialists may be appropriate in promoting the multidisciplinary approach to pain management for the amputee.

MEDICAL TREATMENT

If the cause of residual or phantom limb pain is diagnosed, a variety of pharmacological treatments and surgical procedures may be indicated.

Pharmacological

Treatment of limb pain by pharmacological methods might include:

- non-opiate analgesia
- anti-inflammatory agents
- vasodilators
- muscle relaxants
- anti-depressants
- injections (these may be in the form of a sensory nerve block, a sympathetic block or anti-inflammatory injections).

Surgical

Surgical procedures may include:

- excision of neuroma
- revision of scar
- release of nerve entrapment
- revision of bone end
- refashioning of residual limb
- revascularisation
- excision of inflamed bursa
- insertion of spinal cord stimulator
- re-amputation at a higher level.

PSYCHOLOGICAL MANAGEMENT OF CHRONIC PAIN

Chronic pain is defined as 'pain which lasts longer than 6 months despite appropriate treatment'.

During the 1980s, psychologists and others developed a series of techniques, based largely on a cognitive-behavioural approach (see Ch. 3) designed to help people living with chronic pain learn to live with the pain as best they could and reduce its impact on quality of life. The approach is likely to be most effective when patients perceive themselves to be at 'the end of the road' as far as conventional medical interventions are concerned, and when the medical team are no longer pursuing any active treatment or investigations. Psychologists often lead pain management programmes, though therapists are also often closely involved. In some cases, psychiatrists, anaesthetists and nurses also take part. There are specialist centres that offer intensive programmes, sometimes on an inpatient basis and often using group as well as individual work. However, with an appropriately trained multi-disciplinary team (training is often provided by specialist centres in the form of conferences, workshops and visits), there is no reason why the approaches described as follows cannot be introduced outside of specialist centres. What follows should be taken only as a summary of pain management techniques and not as a 'how to do it' guide.

Assessment

In addition to the suggestions in the therapy section earlier in this chapter, and as well as a full psychological assessment of the amputee, particular attention should be paid to the following:

- factors that make the pain better or worse
- the amputee's beliefs about the pain and its consequences
- the impact of the pain on the amputee's life
- the responses of the family and friends to the pain.

Pain diaries and visual analogue scales can be used and where a more detailed, formalised and standardised assessment is required, various questionnaires are available (see Turk and Melzack 1992). All of these methods are important for evaluating intervention outcomes.

Education about chronic pain management

Education about chronic pain is an essential start to using a pain management approach as it engages patients with the model and clarifies some basic assumptions and attitudes on which the approach rests. This education should include:

- the basic assumption that the amputee's pain is real and is not 'all in the mind', even

though there may not be a clearly diagnosable pathology. Amputees may often be feeling that their pain is not fully believed, and clarifying from the start that their experience of pain is not in question can be a relief and reduce defensiveness.
- the emphasis that pain management is aimed towards living with pain more effectively rather than curing it. Some programmes have shown reductions in overall levels of pain, but it is more common for people to experience changes in mood, activity levels, coping strategies and quality of life.
- the difference between acute and chronic pain, including the statement that while acute pain often acts as a warning signal to the body and a sign of underlying disease or injury, chronic pain is not generally a warning signalling new damage.
- some explanation of the poorly understood phenomenon of chronic pain, referring to possible changes in the nervous system leading to pain signals being sent out even when no new damage has occurred.
- an illustration of some of the vicious circles that commonly compound the difficulties of people living with chronic pain (such as the way in which depression and pain make each other worse).

Graded exercise

Because acute pain is often a signal to our bodies to rest, amputees with chronic pain have often been relatively inactive for long periods of time. This can lead to a dramatic loss of fitness and muscle weakening and stiffening. Sometimes the symptoms of this secondary deterioration in physical state can become confused with the pain problem itself and a vicious circle is set up whereby the aching and fatigue experienced on performing a physical activity is taken as evidence confirming the problem, so less activity is attempted and fitness worsens further still. It is essential to start from a manageable baseline from which exercise can be gradually increased, and this can be aided by using pulse rates to determine appropriate limits.

Goal setting

Goal setting is used to help build activities back into an amputee's life in a planned and achievable way in order to try to combat the avoidance that often occurs in chronic pain. Avoidance can appear to work well in the short-term, but over time it can set up vicious circles (where an individual starts to do less, causing reductions to their fitness and/or confidence and leading them to feel less inclined to do things, and so on). Goal setting may involve re-establishing old activities or developing new ones but an essential ingredient in its success is making goals achievable. This may require breaking goals down into a series of smaller steps, which can then be gradually worked towards.

Pacing

Pacing is a key technique in any pain management approach and to some extent underlies the success of the approach as a whole (particularly in the use of graded exercise and goal setting). It combats the amputee's tendency to 'overdo it' on a good day, which leads to periods of increased pain and enforced rest and thus causing highly inconsistent activity patterns over time. This is known as 'activity cycling'. Pacing encourages the deliberate restriction of activities to a manageable level: taking regular rests, doing little but often to enable a gradual, steady and planned increase of activity over time. Amputees are warned to not to fall into the '5 minutes more syndrome' in order to finish tasks as this often leads to unhelpful overactivity. The essence of pacing is that activity levels are based on a pre-determined plan (of graded exercise and goals) rather than how the patient feels on any particular day.

Relaxation

Muscular tension is a natural response to pain and often occurs without our awareness. This tension can increase pain as well as having an effect on psychological well being. Teaching progressive muscular relaxation can help amputees to detect muscular tension more rapidly and diffuse it before it becomes a problem.

Cognitive therapy

Cognitive techniques in pain management involve identifying and challenging unhelpful beliefs and thoughts and replacing them with more helpful and reality-based alternatives. Beliefs can have a powerfull effect on people's moods and activity levels. Relevant beliefs to target may include specific beliefs about pain such as: 'pain is always a sign of illness' or 'being in pain stops me from enjoying anything'. More general beliefs can also be targeted, such as: 'I'm no good at anything anymore' or 'my friends won't want to see me'. It is essential that this process of challenging beliefs occurs within a collaborative relationship where the amputee is encouraged to evaluate their thinking style and consider alternatives. A confrontational approach is rarely beneficial.

Distraction techniques can be used as both stress and pain management techniques, and are probably most helpful for short periods. Visual imagery can also be used, whereby the amputee imagines an image that is calming and associates the image with the pain.

Changing pain behaviour

'Pain behaviour' refers to the often habitual responses people develop to their pain, which are generally visible to those around them. This behaviour can contribute to the amputee's own self-evaluation, but can also have a powerful effect on how others react to the individual. In some cases, others' reactions can serve to reinforce and maintain the problem. For example, a wife who becomes used to responding to her husband's wincing at the end of a day's activity by chiding him that he should not take on things that make his pain worse, may be unwittingly reinforcing his 'sick role'. Amputees are encouraged to weigh up the pros and cons of changing behaviours that lead to people responding to them as if they were sick. This may also involve people developing better communication and assertiveness skills as pain behaviour can sometimes be an unhelpful substitute for this.

Medication reduction

Amputees often use medication (both prescribed and non-prescribed) to try to reduce their pain, and are often too scared to stop for fear of making pain worse. However, many medications, particularly when used over the longer term can cause unwanted side-effects and the negative effects may outweigh any benefit to the amputee. Medication can also provide diminishing returns as continuing use may reduce its effectiveness over time. The first step to reducing medication is often to medicate on a time-based rather than a pain-based schedule, as research has found that regular medicating has a more powerful effect on pain levels than sporadic medicating. Having established a routine, a planned reduction then becomes more manageable. It is clearly important, however, that any reduction be carried out in a planned and gradual way with medical support.

Stress management

This is a useful adjunct to any pain management programme as pain always seems worse at times of stress and better management of stress can lead to an improved quality of life.

Value of pain management techniques

Pain management programmes generally run over several weeks if not months and have long follow-up periods to ensure maintenance of gains and management of setbacks. While this requires considerable investment of staff resources, the gains in terms of improvements in amputee quality of life and reductions in consultations to other parts of the medical system, as well as any savings made on medication costs, may well be thought to be worthwhile.

CONCLUSION

The management of pain is not easy. It will require precise evaluation by many different professions and intricate combinations of treatment over a period of time. However, it is advisable that one team member has overall responsibility for an amputee so that continuity and coordination is maintained.

Whatever the cause, it must be remembered that the pain is real to the amputee and can totally disrupt both their life and that of family and friends. However, both residual and phantom limb pain can be cyclic in nature with spontaneous remission and relapses. With good assessment and investigation, appropriate treatments can often be found. There are cases in which amputees have residual and phantom limb pain that cannot be relieved. This situation is very difficult for amputees and for their carers. No individual should be labelled as having psychological problems and dismissed without help or support, whatever the real cause may be. Whichever drug or treatment method helps most should be used and the amputee should not 'shop around' by attending hospital after hospital for a 'magic cure' (see Fig. 20.2). Amputees should be encouraged to adjust to living with the pain, though the frustration and difficulty of this task should not be underestimated. Once the process of medical investigation and intervention has come to an end and if the amputee is still significantly debilitated by their pain, referral to a psychologist or specialist pain management unit should be considered.

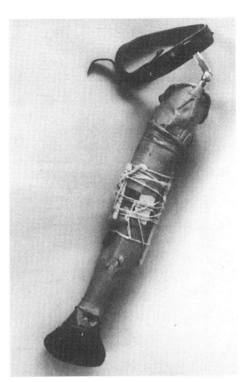
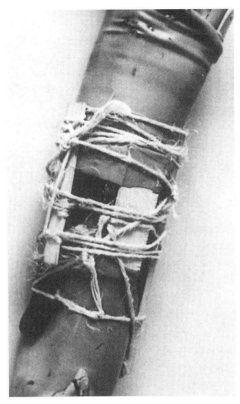

Figure 20.2 One individual's attempted cure for phantom pain. This amputee had phantom pain and was convinced that there were 'little devils' in the artificial limb causing the pain. His solution was to beat the limb and stick nails into it. He then had to splint the knee so that he was still able to walk.

BIBLIOGRAPHY FOR PREVIOUS EDITIONS

Berger S M 1980 Conservative management of phantom limb and amputation-stump pain. Annals of the Royal College of Surgeons 62:103–105

Connolly J 1979 Phantom and stump pain following operation. Physiotherapy 65(1):13–14

Doliber C M 1984 Role of the physical therapist at pain treatment centres. Physical Therapy 64(6):905–909

Feldman R S 1983 Phantom limb pain. Blesmag Spring: 19–21

Frampton V M 1982 Pain control with the aid of transcutaneous nerve stimulation. Physiotherapy 68(3):77–81

Hittenberger D A 1982 Use of electric stimulation in prosthetics for the control of pain. Orthotics and Prosthetics 36(2):35–41

Kristen H, Lukeschitsch G, Plattner F, Sigmund R, Resch P 1984 Thermography as a means for quantitative assessment of stump and phantom pains. Prosthetics and Orthotics International 8(2):76–81

Lewith G T 1981 Acupuncture. World of Medicine Update 509–520

Melzack R 1975 The McGill pain questionnaire: major properties and scoring methods. Pain 1:277–299

Melzack R, Wall P D 1965 Pain mechanisms: a new theory. Science 150(3699):971–979

Monga T N, Jaksic T 1981 Acupuncture in phantom limb pain. Archives of Physical Medicine and Rehabilitation 62:229–231

Mouratoglou V M 1986 Amputees and phantom limb pain: a literature review. Physiotherapy Practice 2(4): 177–185

Ottoson D, Lundeberg S 1985 Conservative management of painful stumps in the upper limb amputee. Newsletter of the British Association of Hand Therapists (January)

Parkes C M 1973 Factors determining the persistence of phantom pain in the amputee. Journal of Psychosomatic Research 17:97–108

Reading A E 1980 A comparison of pain rating scales. Journal of Psychosomatic Research 24:119–124

Sacks O 1986 Phantoms. In: The man who mistook his wife for a hat. Picador, London, ch 6

Sedgwick E M 1991 Phantom limbs. Step Forward Issue 25 (Winter)

Steinbach T V, Nadvorna H, Arazi D 1982 A five year follow-up study of phantom limb pain in post traumatic amputees. Scandinavian Journal of Rehabilitation Medicine 14:203–207

Swerdlow M 1980 The treatment of shooting pain. Postgraduate Medical Journal 56:159–161

Wall P D 1980 The gate control theory of pain mechanisms – a re-examination and restatement. Brain 101:1–18

Wall P D, Devor S 1981 The effect of peripheral nerve injury on dorsal root potentials and on transmission of afferent signals into the spinal cord. Brain Research 209:95–111

Withrington R H, Wynn Parry C B 1984 The management of painful peripheral nerve disorders. Journal of Hand Surgery 9B(1):24–28

Wyke B D 1981 Neurological aspects of pain therapy: a review of some current concepts. In: Swerdlow M (ed.) The therapy of pain. MTP Press, Lancaster

Wynn Parry C B 1981 The 1981 Philip Nichols Memorial Lecture. International Rehabilitation Medicine 4:59–65

Wynn Parry C B 1984 The management of painful peripheral nerve disorders. In: Wall P D, Melzack R (eds) Textbook of pain. Churchill Livingstone, Edinburgh, p 395–401

BIBLIOGRAPHY FOR THE THIRD EDITING

Esquenazi A, Meier R H III 1996 Rehabilitation in limb deficiency. 4. Limb amputation. Archives of Physical Medicine and Rehabilitation 77:S18–S28

Flor H, Fydrich T, Turk D C 1992 Efficacy of multidisciplinary pain treatment centres: a meta analytic review. Pain 49:221–230

Gifford L 1998 Pain, the tissues and the nervous system. A conceptual model. Physiotherapy 84(1):27–36

Hettiaratchy S P, Stiles P J 1996 Rehabilitation of lower limb traumatic amputees: the Sandy Gall Afghanistan Appeal's experience. Injury 27(7):499–501

Hill A, Niven C A, Knussen C 1995 The role of coping in adjustment to phantom limb pain. Pain 62:79–86

Houghton A D, Nicholls G, Houghton A L, Saadah E, McColl I 1994 Phantom pain: natural history and association with rehabilitation. Annals of the Royal College of Surgeons England 76:22–25

Katz J, France C, Melzack R 1989 An association between phantom pain limb sensations and stump skin conductance during transcutaneous nerve stimulation (TENS) applied to the contralateral leg: a case study. Pain 36:367–377

Katz J, Melzack R 1990 Pain 'memories' in phantom limbs: review and clinical observations. Pain 43:319–336

Katz J 1992 Psychophysiological contributions to phantom limbs. Canadian Journal of Psychiatry 37:811–821

Katz J 1997 Prevention of phantom limb pain by regional anaesthesia. The Lancet 349(22):519–520

Kerns R D, Turk D C, Hollzman A D, Rudy T E 1986 Comparison of cognitive-behavioural approaches to the outpatient treatment of chronic pain. Clinical Journal of Pain 1:195–203

Krane E J, Heller L B 1995 The prevalence of phantom sensation and pain in paediatric amputees. Journal of Pain and Symptom Management. Jan 10(1):21–29

Larbig W, Montoya P, Flor H, Bilow H, Weller S, Birbaumer N 1996 Evidence for a change in neural processing in phantom limb pain patients. Pain 67:275–283

Lyth 1995 Invisible problem: amputation, phantom limb. Nursing Times May 10(91):19

Meilman P W, Skultety F M, Guck T P, Sullivan K 1985 Benign chronic pain: eighteen months to ten year follow up of a multidisciplinary pain unit treatment programme.

The Clinical Journal of Pain 1:131–137

Moore J E, Chaney E F 1985 Outpatient group treatment of chronic pain. Effects of spouse involvement. Journal of Consulting and Clinical Psychology 53:326–344

Nikolajsen L, Ilkjaer S, Kroner K, Christenson J H, Jensen T S 1997 The influence of preamputation pain on post amputation stump and phantom pain. Pain 72:393–405

Pavey T J G, Doyle D L 1996 Prevention of phantom pain by infusion of local anaesthesia into the sciatic nerve. Anaesthesia and Intensive Care 24(5) October

Quinlivan D 1995 Use of ANT stretches and techniques for treating phantom limb pain in amputees. British Association of Chartered Physiotherapists in Amputee Rehabilitation Journal. Autumn Edition 10

Snow B R, Gusmorino P, Pinter I, Jimenez A, Rosenblum A 1988 Multidisciplinary treatment of physical and psychosocial disabilities in chronic pain patients: a follow up report. Bulletin of the Hospital for Joint Diseases Orthopaedic Institute 48:52–61

Spires M C, Leonard J 1996 Prosthetic pearls: solutions to thorny problems. Physical Medicine and Rehabilitation Clinics in North America 7(3):509–526

Turner J A, Calsyn O A, Fordyce W E, Ready L B 1982 Drug utilisation patterns in chronic pain patients. Pain 12:357–363

Uygur F, Sener G 1995 Application of ultrasound in neuromas. Experience with seven below-knee stumps. Physiotherapy 81:12

Van Dongen V C P C, Liem A L 1995 Phantom limb and stump pain and its treatment with spinal cord stimulation. Journal of Rehabilitation Sciences 8(4):110–114

Warton S W, Hamann W, Wedley J R, McColl I 1997 Phantom pain and sensation among British Veteran amputees. British Journal of Anaesthesia 78:652–659

Weinstein S 1994 Phantom pain. Oncology 8(3): 65–70

Weiss S A, Lindell B 1996 Phantom limb pain and etiology of amputation in unilateral lower extremity amputees. Journal of Pain and Symptom Management 11(1):3–17

Wells P, Frampton V, Bowsher D 1991 In: Pain management and control in physiotherapy, 2nd edn. Butterworth Heinemann, London, ch 10, p 89–112

Williams A M, Deaton S B 1997 Phantom limb pain; elusive yet real. Rehabilitation Nursing Mar–April 22(2):73–77

21

Multipathology and complex cases

People who have undergone an amputation may well have other medical problems. These may be apparent before the amputation or may appear years afterwards. In the case of those with dysvascular conditions, there are obvious associated problems that have already been discussed (see Chs 2 & 4).

Younger persons with amputations due to trauma and congenital deficiencies may experience other medical problems as they grow older – they may have other musculo-skeletal or neurological pathologies, which cause problems in subsequent years while wearing prostheses. The therapist must be aware of potential issues and assess and treat the individual symptomatically.

Some of these complex cases are described in this chapter with some ideas on problem solution; which forms a summary of the authors' experience in treatment of these varied conditions over the years.

CHILDREN

Congenital lower limb deficiency

Children's problems are very complex. In the case of congenital limb deficiency, the local prosthetic centre should be informed by the obstetric team/paediatrician as soon as possible after the birth of the affected child. The first appointment should be when the child is 6–8 weeks old, in order to ensure that the family feels less isolated, gains confidence and learns about the rehabilitation programme. At this stage, they should be put in touch with self-help groups (e.g. Reach and STEPS in the UK; addresses can be found in Appendix 1). These organisations provide support and information for parents, especially in the first few years of their child's life.

The child's development must be monitored, and intervention, either prosthetically or surgically, should be made at the right time. It is essential that this is carried out in a specialist centre, where all the disciplines involved have a highly developed knowledge of rehabilitation in these complex cases. This can mean fitting a child's first lower limb prosthesis between 6 and 8 months of age, to coincide with the child's first attempts to pull up into a standing position. For

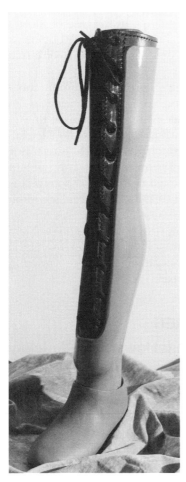

Figure 21.1 An extension prosthesis for a congenital lower limb deficiency. (Photograph by kind permission of Vessa Ltd.)

children with severe lower limb abnormalities it may be necessary either to supply an extension prosthesis during the early stages of their development (see Fig. 21.1) or to amputate severely deformed limbs. This surgical decision should not be taken lightly and should only be carried out after full consultation with the rehabilitation team, including the prosthetist, the family and the child (if old enough to understand the situation). It must be remembered that the same reaction to ablative surgery will be felt by these children as by normally developed people who undergo an amputation.

Children with a unilateral lower limb prosthesis will have little difficulty learning to walk, however their parents will need considerable support. The parents must be aware of the fit and function of the prosthesis and have an understanding of a good gait pattern. They should

Case study 1: Complex limb deficiency

K is the oldest of three children in her family. She has congenital deficiency, bilateral terminal transverse at mid-humeral level and longitudinal deficiency of her right leg (femur partial, fibula total, rays 4 and 5 total). Her left leg has an unstable knee and ankle. In the early years she required supportive cushions to enable her to sit; she used her feet to explore her environment, play, and later to feed herself and write. She learned to bottom shuffle and had a buggy that she rode in for longer journeys.

At 4 years of age she was fitted with a right extension prosthesis and a left KAFO (knee/ankle/foot orthosis), standing initially and then learning to walk holding 'hands' and then progressing to using a rollator with arm sockets attached. She progressed to walking independently at 7 years of age.

Her function is limited when she is wearing her prosthesis and orthosis. She has tried arm prostheses, but they have been bulky and complex to use. She now has arm sockets into which tools are fitted, e.g. a typing peg. She walks daily for exercise and enjoyment, but she has greater ability using her feet and no prostheses for all functional tasks. She continues to bottom shuffle and also uses an electric wheelchair operated by her arm. At 7 years of age, she can undress, put on some of her clothes, transfer on and off chairs, bed and toilet, and can feed herself. She will require regular therapy assessment until she reaches adulthood and thereafter will need support when changes in her life occur, e.g. employment, childrearing and ageing. (See Fig. 21.2)

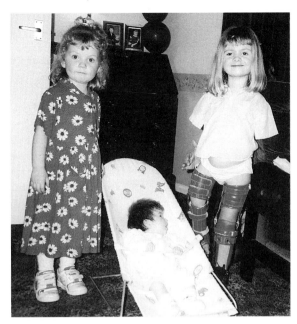

Figure 21.2 K with her siblings, wearing her right extension prosthesis and left KAFO. (Photograph by kind permission of Mrs O'Halloran.)

always attend the prosthetic service with their child. The child will require regular appointments to maintain the correct prosthetic prescription and fit. Gait training will not be required on a regular basis, but at times of change of prosthetic prescription or developmental milestones, it is important to check that the correct progress is being made. It may be helpful for the therapist to visit the child's school to talk to the teachers about realistic walking distances, and sports and activities that the child may undertake.

Acquired lower limb amputation

The rehabilitation of the child with acquired lower limb amputation will depend on their age, the cause of amputation, their personality and developmental maturity at the time of amputation. Children should be fitted with a prosthesis as soon as possible and, if very young, when they start to pull up into a standing position. Younger children will have little difficulty learning to walk, but their parents require considerable support. The child's progress will be similar to that of the congenitally limb-deficient child. Those

becoming amputees in their adolescence may have considerable psychological difficulties and they and their parents may require a great deal of help adjusting with the support of the services of clinical psychologists, nurses or counsellors experienced in the needs of adolescents. They will need similar prosthetic training as an adult amputee, with particular attention given to their leisure and sports interests (see Fig. 21.3). They will benefit from meeting other children and young people who have had amputations and who have been successfully rehabilitated.

Those suffering from conditions such as spina bifida or arthrogryphosis, or who have experienced severe burns or trauma in childhood, may after expert consultation and assessment decide on amputation to improve function and cosmesis.

How children cope with disability and a prosthesis will largely depend on the parental attitude and the child's peer group. Children from a stable home who remain in the same locality

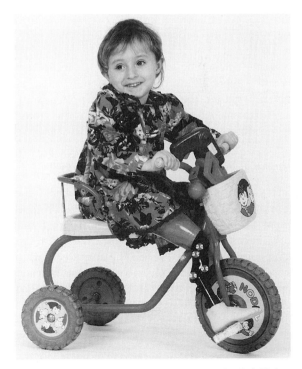

Figure 21.3 A child with a trans-femoral prosthesis (with four bar linkage knee component) riding on a tricycle. (Photograph by kind permission of C.A. Blatchford and Sons Ltd.)

generally do well as they are encouraged from an early age to socialise with others familiar to them at playgroups, nursery schools, etc. The potential crisis points are when young amputees are starting school, moving to the upper school (which is often at the time of puberty) and leaving school for employment or higher education. These difficult periods can be anticipated and provided for by way of meetings between the rehabilitation doctor, therapist, teacher, social worker, child psychologist, potential employer, the child and parents. Adolescents of both sexes become much more conscious of the appearance both of themselves and of their prosthesis at puberty.

NEUROLOGICAL CONDITIONS

Stroke

Amputation with stroke resulting in hemiplegia is a common combination of problems. Mobility will depend on the severity and time of onset of the stroke, the level of amputation and most importantly, whether the stroke and amputation affect opposite sides. Careful evaluation at pre-operative and postoperative stages with an early walking aid (EWA) will help the assessment of whether prosthetic rehabilitation is indicated. Positive rehabilitation in a wheelchair must be given whether the amputee is supplied with a prosthesis or not (see Ch. 6) and the home environment should be reassessed.

Stroke and amputation on the same side

Successful rehabilitation may be possible if the amputation is at the trans-femoral level. Trans-tibial amputations are unsuccessful prosthetically because of insufficient muscle control at the knee joint and altered tone. The amputee with a knee disarticulation and stroke, who has marked increase in flexor tone at the hip has similar problems, as flexion cannot be accommodated in the long socket (see Ch. 14).

Stroke and amputation on opposite sides

Prosthetic rehabilitation is sometimes successful with the lower levels of amputation, i.e. Symes or trans-tibial, but this applies only if there is an uncomplicated postoperative course and a prosthesis is supplied as soon as possible.

Bilateral amputation followed by stroke

Hemiplegic amputees require a simple light-weight prosthesis with easy fastenings using Velcro attachments. For those who were active prosthetic users prior to the stroke, prosthetic re-education should be recommenced. Walking aids are chosen according to their suitability for each individual; learning again to don and doff the prosthesis may be necessary using a different method and a carer may have to help. For those who have the amputation above the knee joint on the stroke side, it may be possible to continue using prostheses with a prosthetic knee component that can be locked to provide stability on the weaker side. However, overall management should be very carefully considered and the energy cost of ambulation taken into account. Wheelchair independence and home assessments must be completed before prostheses are considered.

The established amputee suffering a stroke

Amputation and stroke may occur within a short space of time, particularly for those with dysvascular conditions. However, there is a small number of amputees who experience stroke many years after amputation. The same indications for the success of prosthetic rehabilitation regarding side of amputation and side of stroke apply here as described previously, although these amputees usually walk extremely well after recovery from the initial neurological disturbance. Sometimes the prosthesis may require alteration to provide greater stability.

Spina bifida

Teenagers or young adults who are able to walk with suitable orthoses may find that as they mature, their hyposensitive feet or chronic ulceration are unacceptable. The orthoses may appear to be heavy and ungainly. Trans-tibial amputation may be considered in these cases to increase mobility and improve cosmesis. However, it is essential that this decision is taken only after careful consideration by both the orthopaedic surgeon and the rehabilitation consultant, and after the patient has had the opportunity to visit the prosthetic service to look at prostheses.

Careful assessment and recording of muscle power and skin sensation is important to evaluate whether knee function will be adequate to use a prosthesis. People with spina bifida need careful gait re-education and this should be carried out where there is immediate prosthetic help. In many cases, although muscle power is reasonable there may be unequal muscle pull, which creates some torsion and friction at the residual limb/socket interface. As skin sensation may be imperfect, the therapist must check the skin constantly and teach the amputee to do this. If there is any rubbing or soreness, the socket must be adjusted immediately by the prosthetist and the skin must return to normal before gait re-education recommences.

Walking aids will again be chosen for each individual. There is usually little problem in using the prostheses as these people are already familiar with orthoses and are extremely capable.

Hygiene and care of the residual limb and prosthesis should be explained in detail (see Ch. 11) as many have problems with sweating and incontinence.

Paraplegia

Occasionally, a person with paraplegia may require an amputation. Gross ischaemia, fractures which are impossible to stabilise and extensive infection may be life endangering, and after many months of treatment, amputation of the affected part may be the only treatment left.

These people rarely use prostheses. It is sometimes difficult for them to appreciate this, particularly if long-leg orthoses had been used prior to the amputation. Both the doctor and the therapist must explain that skin tolerance and pressure sensitivity is vital for the use of any prosthesis. It may be necessary to retrain sitting balance, transfers and general wheelchair independence.

Progressive neurological conditions

Amputees with neurological conditions such as multiple sclerosis (MS), Parkinson's disease, motor neurone disease (MND), etc. have complicated rehabilitation needs. During the early stages of these progressive conditions, the therapist may feel it is necessary to alter the type of walking aid. A frame may give more stability if spasticity or balance problems are present, whereas people with Parkinson's disease may do better with walking sticks for balance. All the issues regarding rehabilitation of people with these conditions are more difficult when there is also a prosthesis. Each case must be treated individually, but some may have to stop using the prosthesis because it becomes too difficult.

Wheelchair independence and functional capabilities in the activities of daily living should be reassessed in the home. Both the rehabilitation centre and the community therapy team must be aware of the potential difficulties that may arise for these amputees and provide ongoing help and advice.

SENSORY DISORDERS
People with visual impairment

Diabetes mellitus is a common cause of visual impairment among amputees. Successful prosthetic rehabilitation will depend on whether the visual impairment is long-standing and whether the person has adjusted their mobility well. These people are usually extremely capable of coping with their situation and, once the prosthesis is understood, gait rehabilitation must be aimed at full weightbearing. This is because the amputee will need a hand free to use a white stick or long cane to locate obstacles, or to hold a guide dog's harness. Two walking sticks would therefore be impractical and cumbersome, unless there was a full-time carer involved.

The less fortunate people with visual impairment and amputation are those whose sight is gradually diminishing at the same time as the limb is becoming ischaemic and the amputation is needed. Here progress will be slow as so many aspects of the person's life will need to be re-taught as they adapt to gradually changing circumstances.

For all people with visual impairment, the fit of the prosthesis and the sensations transmitted from it must be carefully explained and in the early stages of gait re-education, the therapist must take responsibility for checking the weight-bearing areas for redness, rubbing, etc. unless there is a full-time carer who can do this for the amputee. This is particularly necessary if there is hyposensitivity in the residual limb. The prosthesis must be designed for simplicity of donning and doffing. Once a correct fit of the prosthesis has been achieved and initial mobility outside of the parallel bars mastered, it is more relevant to continue gait re-education and activities of daily living in the amputee's own home environment.

People with hearing impairment and vestibular disorders

Balance problems should be assessed prior to prosthetic use and intensive rehabilitation given where necessary.

Carers of profoundly deaf people may have to attend the therapy sessions during prosthetic re-education if communication is difficult.

People with hearing aids should ensure that their batteries are working well and it may be helpful to keep spares in the therapy facility. Some may benefit from a reassessment in the ear, nose and throat department of the hospital, where minor problems, such as excessive wax, can be dealt with quickly.

ORTHOPAEDIC CONDITIONS
Arthrodesed lower limb joints

Arthrodesed lower limb joints can cause problems for the amputee during gait training. The mechanics of walking with a fixed knee or hip joint, either on the remaining leg or the residual limb can be extremely complicated, tiring and uncomfortable.

There are certain points to consider when carrying out an assessment pre-operatively. If the hip joint is arthrodesed on the side of the proposed amputation, the amount of flexion in the hip and the flexibility of the lumbar spine should be noted. It is not easy for an amputee to sit down or stand up wearing a prosthesis if the hip joint is fixed. Additionally, the therapist must check there is sufficient trunk flexion to reach down to the residual limb to don the prosthesis, or that a carer is available to do this. If the knee joint is arthrodesed on the side of the proposed amputation, there is no benefit in carrying out a trans-tibial amputation.

When an amputee with an arthrodesed joint learns to walk with a prosthesis, standing up and sitting down need close attention; chair, toilet and bed heights may require modification.

Fractures and joint replacements

Those amputees with fractures in the lower limb generally have to wait until full weightbearing is permitted before using their prosthesis again. It is therefore essential that an exercise programme is performed daily to strengthen muscles and preserve joint mobility. If the fracture is on the amputated side, the residual limb will become oedematous; this oedema must be controlled where possible (see Ch. 4) and must have subsided considerably before a prosthetic fitting.

If the orthopaedic surgeon permits, an EWA can be used at the partial weightbearing stage (see Ch. 6). Amputees must not attempt to re-mobilise in their existing prosthesis after fracture before the alignment and fit have been checked by the prosthetist, or a different design of prosthesis has been supplied with more proximal weightbearing areas.

Amputees with hip arthroplasty are limited in the range of movement permitted in the affected hip. The type of prosthesis supplied and the method of donning will need careful consideration to avoid dislocation of the joint prosthesis.

Limb lengthening procedures

An amputee's function with a prosthesis depends on the length of the residual limb. A stable suspension of the socket and the effective lever arm for its motion both relate to length. The residual muscle mass is less in a shorter residual limb. Preservation of the knee and elbow joints results in a better outcome in terms of function and cosmesis for the amputee, but in some challenging surgical situations, only a short residual limb can be fashioned.

Various techniques have been used to lengthen the residual limb: lengthening osteotomies, callous distraction (the Ilizarov method) and a custom tissue expander with custom elongation prosthesis.

It must be remembered that most of these amputees will have already been through long surgical and rehabilitative procedures before the assessment for this further procedure; it is important that all prosthetic avenues have been explored to the full and that the amputee is fully aware of the time these procedures will take before a decision to proceed is taken.

Limb lengthening procedures have also been used in cases of congenital lower limb deficiency, particularly when there is a partial or complete absence of the fibula. In this situation, the management of severe shortening by amputation of the foot is controversial. Lengthening using the Ilizarov method preserves the foot and can provide simultaneous correction of leg length discrepancy and foot and ankle deformities. The major consideration for the amputee, their family and the surgeons is that amputation is a single procedure whereas with limb lengthening, multiple and unpredictable operations are needed along with long periods of rehabilitation. Furthermore, some of these procedures fail to achieve the results anticipated and result in amputation in the end.

Multiple amputations

Young people who have experienced gross trauma or who have extreme Buerger's disease, resulting in multiple loss of limbs, will need to attend a specialist prosthetic centre.

Those with bilateral lower limb amputations, or a single upper and lower limb combination, have the lower limb prosthesis fitted first and independence in walking is gained before arm training begins.

Case study 2: Traumatic multiple amputations

A 19-year-old scaffolder was admitted to a specialist rehabilitation unit following an accident at work, which resulted in multiple limb amputations (bilateral trans-radial and bilateral trans-tibial). A complex assessment and treatment regime involving all members of the multidisciplinary team was necessary to achieve a successful functional outcome. He and his family required psychological support throughout the rehabilitation process.

A daily programme was co-ordinated to ensure physical fitness pre-prosthetically. He was fitted with thermoplastic gauntlets enabling him to hold cutlery, a hair brush, toothbrush, etc., to encourage independence in activities of daily living. He was encouraged to use a problem-solving approach to all tasks and to devise his own solutions where possible. He used the forwards/backwards method for bed and toilet transfers.

Prosthetic rehabilitation started with his upper limbs due to delayed healing and further surgery to his left trans-tibial residual limb. Arm training progressed quickly with his upper limb body-powered prostheses with split hooks. He was well motivated and the new prostheses increased his independence considerably.

Initially, lower limb gait training commenced using a patellar tendon bearing (PTB) prosthesis on his right leg and a Ppam aid on the left. He needed the support of two therapists to help with his walking as he was unable to hold onto the parallel bars or use adapted crutches. Within 2 months post-amputation, and as soon as the left transtibial residual limb had healed sufficiently, he was cast for his left prosthesis and gait rehabilitation continued with two PTB prostheses. There was an intense daily programme of walking and he soon became independent in donning and doffing his lower limb prostheses (see Fig. 21.4). The therapists worked closely with the prosthetists who were on site at this specialist centre.

During prosthetic training, the amputee and the team discussed his future more thoroughly. This led to more thought and practise with recreational activities and referral to other specialists as appropriate, e.g. for a driving assessment.

He was discharged from hospital 7 months after his amputations when he was walking independently with his prostheses and had excellent functional use with his upper limb prostheses. Over the next few months, he successfully completed a driving tour of the UK and felt he had achieved the goals he had set for himself.

He continues to be an active upper limb prosthetic user 8 years postdischarge, but no longer wears his lower limb prostheses. As he is financially secure, he no longer needs employment and has opted to use an electric wheelchair for mobility due to an increase in his weight and the high energy expenditure used in walking.

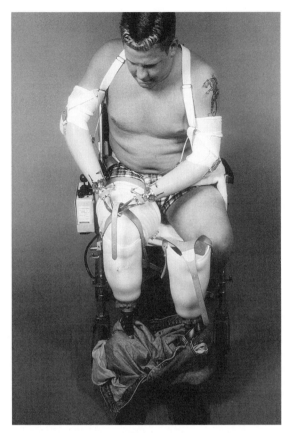

Figure 21.4 A young bilateral trans-radial and bilateral trans-tibial amputee donning his lower limb prostheses using body-powered prostheses with split hook terminal devices. Note that a powered wheelchair is used. (Photograph by kind permission of Richmond, Twickenham and Roehampton Healthcare NHS Trust.)

Those with bilateral upper limb amputations remain in a wheelchair and concentrate first on arm training with prostheses.

For multiple amputees, independence in the activities of daily living is of primary importance and how this is achieved may or may not be with the assistance of prostheses. Careful assessment involving the whole rehabilitation team, along with the amputee and their carers, is essential.

BURNED/GRAFTED SKIN

The skin of amputees with burns or grafts on the residual limb or under suspension straps or appendages must be carefully examined when using prostheses. Any tissue abnormality that gives rise to altered sensation, adhesions, lack of viability or frank breakdown is potentially dangerous. The amputee must be meticulous in checking pressure areas of the socket and suspension.

Care is needed with the timing of the first trial of the EWA and the fitting of the prosthesis, so that skin tolerance to pressure is gradually built up. It is often advisable to allow the skin time to mature, i.e. for up to 3 months, otherwise the amputee can become demoralised because of constant skin breakdown during prosthetic training. If minor skin breakdown occurs initially, it is advisable to wait a little longer, possibly for 2 weeks, before carrying out another trial.

The first prosthesis supplied to those with burns or grafts may be very basic; progression to more sophisticated prostheses is possible if the skin toughens adequately, but this can often take more than 1 year. These amputees must not become disheartened and may require frequent attendances to the prosthetic service for psychological support and prosthetic adjustment (see Ch. 3).

INFECTIONS

Leprosy (Hansen's disease)

Leprosy is a chronic infectious disease, essentially of the peripheral nerves, but also affecting the skin and sometimes other tissues such as the eye, the mucosa of the upper respiratory tract, muscle, bone and testes. It takes two principle forms: tuberculoid and lepromatous and between these forms, the disease covers a broad immunological spectrum.

One feature of leprosy bacilli is that they grow in the cooler parts of the body, particularly exposed skin. Furthermore, early parasitisation of nerves occurs and this results in early acute nerve damage in tuberculoid leprosy; this condition may be reversible if treatment is started soon after the neural deficit occurs. In lepromatous leprosy the neural deficit may not be clinically obvious for many years. All forms of leprosy may develop abnormalities of sensory perception, even to total loss of feeling and pain. Hence patients are likely to neglect trauma and this may result in infections and tissue loss. Motor nerve involvement causes paresis and paralysis, which results in abnormal pressures on anaesthetic limbs and increases the risk of trauma and deformity.

The main thrust of rehabilitation is to provide education on care of the insensate limb and the healing of neuropathic ulcers, in very much the same way as for those with diabetes mellitus, and to correct any deformities present by reconstructive surgery. Active splints are not used as they may cause more pressure and trauma as they grip tightly or rub insensate skin.

The need for amputation should only arise in patients with delayed diagnosis or those who have been mismanaged with poor medical treatment and no education in self-care. It is usually possible to save at least part of a damaged foot; a short weightbearing foot is preferable to an amputated leg, as the skin of the residual limb is also often anaesthetic, creating problems for the prosthetist with suitable socket construction. Should major amputations be needed because of an accident (such as burns) or malignancy, the major considerations are care of the insensate residual limb and a highly skilled understanding of prosthetic intervention, using total contact socket design (as for spina bifida and familial neuropathies).

Indeed, much of the modern understanding of the management of insensate limbs comes from the vast experience with leprosy over the years. The treatment of neuropathic ulcers by total contact casting was pioneered by Dr Paul Brand for leprosy patients in the 1950s and it is used in diabetic ulceration today. Furthermore, the reconstruction of neuropathic feet by arthrodesis and osteotomies to correct marked deformity that is compatible with ulcer-free walking was shown to be practical by the operations on the feet of leprosy patients in the 1960s and 1970s.

Meningococcal septicaemia

This is a systemic illness that can result in skin and extremity necrosis leading to single or multiple amputations. Patients become extremely ill and develop a haemorrhagic rash due to bleeding into the skin. Damage to the tissues, skin necrosis and disseminated intravascular coagulation (DIC) causing gangrene can result in amputation of the toes, fingers and limbs (see Fig. 21.5A and B).

Rehabilitation for the multiple amputee is a challenging and lengthy process. Independence in the activities of daily living is of primary importance and how this is achieved may or may not be with the assistance of prostheses. Careful assessment of the amputee by all members of the multidisciplinary team with the setting of realistic goals is essential.

PROSTHETIC SUSPENSION

Osseointegration

Osseointegration is defined as 'a method of anchoring a prosthesis directly to bone tissue via a fixture of titanium (see Fig. 21.6). This technique has been developed by Professor Brånemark and his team at the Osseointegration Centre, Göteborg, Sweden. It was first introduced as a method for prosthetic tooth replacement 25 years ago. More recently, finger and thumb replacements have been perfected. A multidisciplinary team of experts from Queen Mary's University Hospital, Roehampton and the Bioengineering Department of the University of Surrey in the UK, are currently working with the Brånemark team to study the technique and assess amputees using external prostheses fitted directly to the residual skeleton for both upper and lower limbs. This technique is at present in the early stages of development with approximately 20 lower limb amputees having been successfully treated by the end of 1997.

The osseointegration procedure takes place in two stages. Stage one is when the titanium fixture is inserted into the medullary cavity of the femur. The amputee then mobilises either on crutches or with their prosthesis for 6 months to ensure secure fixation of the inplant. At stage two an abutment is attached to the fixture to allow it to protrude through the end of the residual limb and for fixation of the prosthesis.

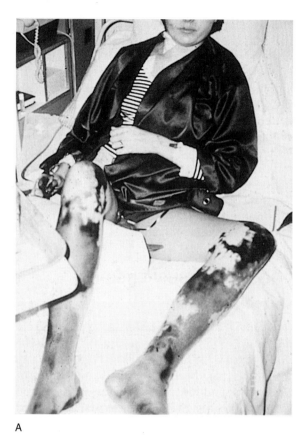

A

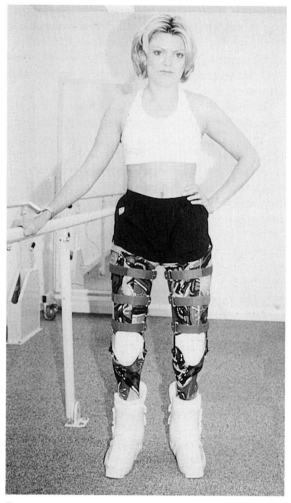

B

Figure 21.5 A patient with meningococcal septicaemia. (A) pre-operatively; (B) following bilateral trans-tibial amputations and rehabilitation. She is wearing adapted thigh corset prostheses designed for snow skiing. (Photographs by kind permission of Richmond, Twickenham and Roehampton Healthcare NHS Trust.)

The rest of the rehabilitation process consists of a programme of exercises first with a short training prosthesis and then progressing to the full-length prosthesis. The rehabilitation programme is very intensive and needs strict supervision by a therapist; it can last from a minimum of 18 months to 2 years.

Colostomy

When a person with a colostomy needs an amputation, it is important that particular attention is given to the design of auxiliary suspension encompassing the waist or pelvis (should it be required) prior to prescription of the prosthesis.

Similar consideration should be given to the prosthetic design for amputees with inguinal hernias wearing a support.

Those patients who have experienced gross trauma requiring an amputation and a colostomy are often able to use prostheses and the authors know of amputees with hindquarter amputation who have managed this well. Expert help is required from the prosthetist during gait re-education and it is advisable that these amputees attend the therapy facility in the prosthetic centre.

Occasionally an established amputee will need a colostomy. It is advisable that the surgeon observes the patient wearing their prosthesis and

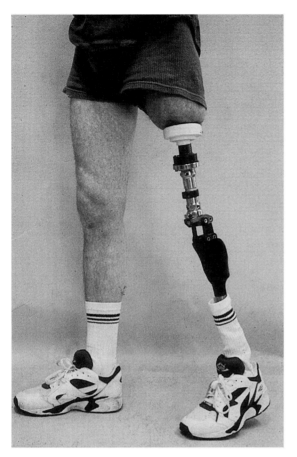

Figure 21.6 A trans-femoral amputee with a prosthesis suspended by intra-medullary osseointegration. (Photograph by kind permission of Professor Brånemark, Institute for Applied Biotechnology, Göteborg.)

notes the position of any auxiliary suspension used so the stoma can be created in a suitable position that will make the colostomy bag easier to manage. Alternatively, the surgeon can contact the rehabilitation consultant at the prosthetic centre should the suspension need to be altered. The local stoma therapist may also need to give added support and advice to the amputee during the recovery and rehabilitation stages.

MENTAL HEALTH
Residual limb abuse (stump abuse)

This condition, the deliberate and normally secretive damaging of the residual limb by the amputee exists but is uncommon. It can occur in the context of a history of self-harming/self-neglecting behaviour or may arise as a specific adjustment reaction to amputation. It is important to have as full an understanding as possible of the medical situation before considering abuse. It should not be used to explain unresolved medical problems where there is no other evidence that residual limb abuse is occurring. In centres where there are no staff with suitable qualifications in this field, it is recommended that suspected cases are referred on to the local psychology department or liaison psychiatrist for a full assessment.

Other mental health issues

Some amputees may have a history of mental health problems such as depression, schizophrenia, anxiety disorders (e.g. agoraphobia), or obsessive compulsive disorder. They will often be under the care of a psychiatrist who may operate within a community mental health team. It can be helpful to establish links with this service in order to gain some understanding of the individual's condition and any particular requirements for support they may have during their rehabilitation. A life event such as an amputation can trigger off a recurrence of a previous mental health problem and in such cases contact with psychiatric services should be re-established where appropriate. This can normally be done through the amputee's general practitioner (GP).

Occasionally the issue of mental health is particularly acute in cases where the amputation is caused by the result of a failed suicide attempt (e.g. throwing self in front of a train or cutting wrists). Such cases require particularly sensitive handling and liaison with psychiatric services is essential. It will be their role to assess the individual's risk of further suicide attempts and to provide follow-up support. Some patients may feel very embarrassed about the circumstances of their amputation and may opt to share this with very few people (e.g. the psychologist/counsellor only). Their desire for confidentiality should be respected where possible.

WOMEN'S HEALTH

Issues associated with menstruation and pregnancy

Some females suffer from a 'pre-menstrual syndrome', one facet of which is a feeling of fluid retention. In some amputees this can affect the size of the residual limb and the fit of the socket for a few days each month. This is more noticeable with intimately fitting sockets and may be so severe as to prevent the amputee from wearing the prosthesis for those few days.

It is often the therapist or prosthetist who is first made aware of this problem. Referral to a gynaecologist for symptomatic treatment (such as diuretics) may be required if simple methods of socket adjustment are unsuccessful. Amputees with diabetes should seek the help of their physician, who will need to monitor any treatment given.

The pregnant amputee will generally be advised by the obstetrician to remain as mobile as possible for as long as it is comfortable. This may mean frequent visits to the prosthetic centre for alteration to socket size and auxiliary suspension. The centre of mass in the pregnant female alters after 20–24 weeks of pregnancy and even non-amputees can experience balance problems. Therefore balance may be even harder to maintain for amputees either when wearing the prosthesis or using crutches. In higher levels of amputation, when prosthetic wear is no longer possible in late pregnancy, crutch hopping can continue without any damage to the mother or baby. Swimming is an excellent activity to maintain general fitness during pregnancy.

BIBLIOGRAPHY FOR PREVIOUS EDITIONS

Altner P C, Rusin J J, DeBoer A 1980 Rehabilitation of blind patients with lower extremity amputations. Archives of Physical Medicine and Rehabilitation 61:82–84

Bernd L, Blasius K, Lukoschek M, Lucke R 1991 The autologous stump plasty. Treatment for bony overgrowth in juvenile amputees. Journal of Bone and Joint Surgery 73B(2):203–206

Bowker J H, Rills B M, Ledbetter C A, Hunter G A, Holliday P 1981 Fractures in lower limbs with prior amputation. Journal of Bone and Joint Surgery 63A (6):915–920

Clark G S, Naso F, Ditunno J F 1980 Marked bone spur formation in a burn amputee patient. Archives of Physical Medicine and Rehabilitation 61:189–192

Grundy D J, Silver J R 1983 Amputation for peripheral vascular disease in the paraplegic and tetraplegic patient. Paraplegia 21:305–311

Grundy D J, Silver J R 1984 Major amputation in paraplegic and tetraplegic patients. International Rehabilitation Medicine 6:162–165

LaBorde T C, Meier R H 1978 Amputations resulting from electrical injury: a review of 22 cases. Archives of Physical Medicine and Rehabilitation 59:134–137

Malin A S et al 1991 Leprosy in reaction: a medical emergency. British Medical Journal 302:1324–1326

Milling A W F 1984 Multiple traumatic limb amputations. Injury 16(6):6

Pfeil J et al 1991 The stump capping procedure to prevent or treat terminal osseous overgrowth. Prosthetics and Orthotics International 15:96–99

Stavrakas P A, Sanders G T 1983 Sling support during pregnancy after hemipelvectomy: case report. Archives of Physical Medicine and Rehabilitation 64:331–333

Stillwell A, Menelaus M B 1983 Walking ability in mature patients with spina bifida. Journal of Pediatric Orthopedics 3:184–190

Varghese G, Hinterbuchner C, Mondall P, Sakuma J 1978 Rehabilitation outcome of patients with dual disability of hemiplegia and amputation. Archives of Physical Medicine and Rehabilitation 59:121–123

Wood M R, Hunter G A, Millstein S G 1987 The value of stump split skin grafting following amputation for trauma in adult upper and lower limb amputees. Prosthetics and Orthotics International 11:71–74

BIBLIOGRAPHY FOR THE THIRD EDITION

Alman B A, Krajbich J I, Hubbard S 1995 Proximal femoral focal deficiency: results of rotationplasty and Syme amputation. The Journal of Bone and Joint Surgery 77A(12):1876–1882

Chalmers I M, Arneja A S 1994 Rheumatoid nodules on amputation stumps: report of three cases. Archives of Physical Medicine and Rehabilitation 75(10):1151–1153

Coleman S S 1995 The lower limb: congenital pseudarthrosis of the tibia. In: Hanis N H, Birch R (eds) Post Graduate Textbook of Clinical Orthopaedics, 3rd edn. Blackwell Science, Oxford

Cotter D G, Neumann V, Geddes J M, Waxman R 1997 The influence of stroke on prosthetic rehabilitation in lower limb amputees. Proceedings of ISPO UK NMS:34

Diamant D S 1996 Lower extremity amputation secondary to heparin-associated thrombocytopenia with thrombosis.

Archives of Physical Medicine and Rehabilitation 77(10):1090–1092

Dunne G, Fuerst K 1995 Breastfeeding by a mother who is a triple amputee: a case report. Journal of Human Lactation 11(3):217–218

Eriksson E, Brånemark P I 1994 Osseointegration from the perspective of the plastic surgeon. Plastic and Reconstructive Surgery 93(3):626–637

Ethans K D, Kirby R L, Adderson J A 1997 Trans-tibial prosthesis for a patient with Kaposi's sarcoma lesions on the residual limb. Archives of Physical Medicine and Rehabilitation 78(1):106–108

Evans D G R, Thakker Y, Donnai D 1991 Heredity and dysmorphic syndromes in congenital limb deficiencies. Prosthetics and Orthotics International 15(2):70

Fernandez-Palazzi F, De Gutierrez D P, Paladino R 1991 The care of the limb deficient child in Venezuela. Prosthetics and Orthotics International 15(2):156–157

Garrison S J, Merritt B S 1997 Functional outcome of quadruple amputees with end-stage renal disease. American Journal of Physical Medicine and Rehabilitation 76(3):226–230

Genoff M C, Hoffer M, Archauer B et al 1992 Extremity amputations in meningococcal induced Purpura Fulminans. Plastic and Reconstructive Surgery 89(5):471–472

Grogan D P, Holt G R, Ogden J A 1994 Talocalcaneal coalition in patients who have fibular hemimelia or proximal femoral focal deficiency. The Journal of Bone and Joint Surgery 76A(9):1363–1370

Harris N J, Gosh M 1994 Skin and extremity loss in meningococcal septicaemia treated in a burn unit. Burns 20(5):471–472

Herbert L M, Engsberg J R, Tedford K G, Grimston S K 1994 A comparison of oxygen consumption during walking between children with and without below-knee amputations. Physical Therapy 74(10):943–950

Herman T, David Y, Ohry A 1995 Prosthetic fitting and ambulation in a paraplegic patient with an above-knee amputation. Archives of Physical Medicine and Rehabilitation 76:290–293

Hirons R R, Williams K B, Amor R F, Day H J B 1991 The prosthetic treatment of lower limb deficiency. Prosthetics and Orthotics International 15(2):112–117

Jain S 1996 Rehabilitation in limb deficiency. 2. The pediatric amputee. Archives of Physical Medicine and Rehabilitation 77:S9–S13

Jones L E, Lipson A 1991 The care of the limb deficient child in Australia. Prosthetics and Orthotics International 15(2):140–142

Kakurai S, Kida M 1991 The care of the limb deficient child in Japan. Prosthetics and Orthotics International 15(2):146–151

King R, Powell D F 1995 The lower limb: congenital shortening. In: Hanis N H, Birch R (eds) Post Graduate Textbook of Clinical Orthopaedics, 3rd edn. Blackwell Science, Oxford

Kour A K, Seo J S, Pho R W H 1995 Combined free flap, Ilizarov lengthening and prosthetic fitting in the reconstruction of a proximal forearm amputation – a case report. Annals of the Academy of Medicine 24(4):135–137

Lachmann S M 1993 The mobility outcome for amputees with rheumatoid arthritis is poor. British Journal of Rheumatology 32(12):1083–1088

Landham T L, Datta D, Nirula H C 1991 Amputation for gangrene of the limbs following severe meningococcal infection. Journal of the Royal College of Surgeons 36:11–12

Letts M, Vincent N 1993 Congenital longitudinal deficiency of the fibula (fibular hemimelia). Parental refusal of amputation. Clinical Orthopaedics and Related Research 287:160–166

Loro A, Franceschi F, Dal Largo A 1994 The reasons for amputations in children (0–18 years) in a developing country. Tropical Doctor 24:99–102

Naudie D, Hamdy R C, Fassier F, Morin B, Duhaime M 1997 Management of fibular hemimelia. The Journal of Bone and Joint Surgery 79B(1):58–65

Oppenheim W L 1991 Fibular deficiency and indications for Syme's amputation. Prosthetics and Orthotics International 15(2):131–136

Persson B M, Broomé A 1994 Lengthening a short femoral amputation stump. A case of tissue expander and endoprosthesis. Acta Orthopaedica Scandinavica 65(1):99–100

Sharma V P 1991 The care of the limb deficient child in India. Prosthetics and Orthotics International 15(2):143–145

Shatilov O E, Rozkov A V, Cheminova T V 1991 Reconstructive surgery for fibular deficiency. Prosthetics and Orthotics International 15(2):137–139

Sliman N, Mrabet A, Daghfous S, Douik M 1991 The care of the limb deficient child in North Africa. Prosthetics and Orthotics International 15(2):152–155

Smith W D F, Clark P F, MacArthur D, Allatt R D, Hayes K C, Cunningham D A 1997 Oxygen costs using a reciprocating gait orthosis in a paraplegic (T9) patient with a bilateral below-knee amputation: case report. Spinal Cord 35(2):121–123

Stricker S J 1994 Ilizarov lengthening of a posttraumatic below elbow amputation stump. Clinical Orthopaedics and Related Research 306:124–127

Torode I P, Gillespie R 1991 The classification and treatment of proximal femoral deficiencies. Prosthetics and Orthotics International 15(2):117–126

Viscardi P J, Polk Jr H C 1995 Outcome of amputations in patients with major burns. Burns 21(7):526–529

22

A different perspective: the importance of user involvement

Ann Stead

Users? Patients? Clients? Customers? Whatever the term, this is simply a shorthand description of 'a person with needs', in this case the needs relate to limb loss. Dealing with *people* is, by definition, the day-to-day work of any healthcare professional. Therefore, most would say that they are constantly taking account of their 'patients' views, in their daily work. If this is so, why does the issue of user involvement need special mention in a book of this type? The answer is complex and lies in recognising where the *expertise* lies. It also needs a clear understanding about what the term *'disability'* really means. Only when these issues are clear, can *what users want* from the service be met in full. Before considering this in detail it might be helpful to reflect on how services for disabled people have developed to date.

BACKGROUND

Western society's perceptions of disability are at last moving from 'welfarism' to 'empowerment' and the services supporting disabled people are beginning to change in line with these more enlightened attitudes. However, affecting attitudinal change in society has always been a slow process. Over the last century, the foundations of most disability services stemmed from efforts to support the war wounded and victims of industrial accidents. Prior to this, charities were the only hope for many disabled people. However, large numbers of newly disabled people, like the war wounded, can have a marked effect on attitudes; the freedom of expression in the 1960s coincided with America's involvement in the Vietnam war. In the USA, huge numbers of young, angry and articulate war veterans with other disabled people forced through new anti-discrimination legislation and gave birth to the Independent Living Movement, the effects of which are still being felt throughout the rest of the world. It has taken 20 years for similar anti-discrimination legislation to reach the UK. Therefore, the concept of active user involvement in shaping the way services are delivered to disabled people is not new. The methods, however, can and do vary.

EXPERTS

Following the surgical removal of a limb, patients will ideally be referred for rehabilitation where the processes involved relate to sharing information so that 'patients' can learn new behaviours. In this postoperative, rehabilitative phase, information and knowledge is given to the patient in order to train them in the use of their first prosthesis. As knowledge is power, the healthcare professional is unquestionably the most powerful of the two parties involved at this stage. At this point, the term 'patient' is an entirely appropriate description of an amputee. However, in time the 'patient' will eventually return to a new state of both psychological and physical health. In this new and altered state of normality the term 'patient' may no longer apply. However, the system will continue to use this terminology. A person with a physical impairment or disability is a person first and foremost with the same needs and wishes as the rest of the population; their new-found motor impairment may give them some additional needs. From the amputee's point of view, learning to walk (or manipulate objects) again will be the initial priority. However, concerns of a more social nature, i.e. will they still be attractive to the opposite sex, have children, have bills paid, and return to work, etc. are also likely to dominate their thoughts. These feelings will persist long after the initial recovery stage and this progression from health to social needs also corresponds

with the transfer back to the individual of responsibility for their own healthcare.

Patients   RESPONSIBILITY   Customers
Medical ◄━━━━━━━━━━━━━━━━━━━► Individuals

This shift in responsibility does not always sit comfortably with western healthcare systems as services often fail to recognise the importance of the distinction between a 'patient' and a 'person with disabilities'. Equally, the purpose of rehabilitation is not just to return people to independent mobility, it is also to enable people to regain conrol and exercise choices in their lives. If prosthetic services are too prescriptive and do not encourage this need for control, they can be seen to be oppressive.

Another important factor is that not all people who are referred to as 'amputees' have in fact gone through the experience of amputation surgery as they may have been born with partially formed or absent limbs. To them, 'disability' is a normal state and by the time they reach adulthood they are likely to know far more about living with a disability than any health or social care professional. This kind of experience of living with the day-to-day problems that artificial limbs can bring is an invaluable adjunct to the support of newly disabled people and is often an underused resource.

All of this means that whilst healthcare professionals are undoubtedly expert in the process of rehabilitation, the only experts in disability are those that experience it for themselves. Many disabled people therefore feel it is unreasonable that those who design services for them come from the healthcare professions alone and they are demanding that their voices should also be heard.

UNDERSTANDING DISABILITY

It is now well recognised that disability and illness are not synonymous and that medical control over disability is inappropriate. However, most healthcare professionals receive very little education about disability. The most commonly recognised definitions are the World Health Organisation's International Classification of Impairments, Disabilities and Handicaps (ICIDH). Whilst this model does acknowledge a socio-logical dimension of handicaps, it focuses on physical impairments as the causes of disability and handicaps. Many groups of disabled people reject the causal link between these groups, e.g. someone with a facial disfigurement might be severely handicapped (unable to gain employ-ment or make friends) but not have a disability. They believe that disability and handicap are caused by physical and attitudinal barriers within society, which could be removed if there was the political will to do so. The ICIDH model also defines disability as 'abnormality', inevitably leaving disabled people excluded and isolated from the mainstream of life. Therefore, the model leaves little room for disabled people to be embraced as equal and integral participants in society, despite having all the personal attributes and sense of good citizenship to do so. Disabled people's organisations, therefore, are insisting on approaches based not on restoring normality but on a socially inclusive model of disability which, rather than tolerating difference and diversity, rejoices in it.

In 1998 The World Health Organisation published new terms and vocabulary, in draft, in the ICIDH-2, replacing the word 'disability' with 'activity limitation' and introducing the terms 'participation' and 'participation restriction'. These changes are an attempt to respond to the negative and welfarist connotations associated with the language used at the time of writing. The importance of language in the development of values and beliefs is well recognised; however, attitudinal change cannot come from language alone. Understanding the intent behind the words being used is just as important as using the correct terminology, indeed political correctness taken to extremes can itself be a barrier to progress.

The politics of disablement are complex and the western world has adopted a very medical approach to disability, which has led to conflicts about professional dominance but this is not the same everywhere. As disability is beginning to be recognised as a social issue it follows that different cultures and social groups will interpret it differently. Amputees will therefore find very different reactions to their situation in different parts of the world.

WHAT DO USERS WANT?

It is impossible to list everything that users want from a quality service as every individual will have different needs. There are, however, three essential ingredients:

- a *flexible service* that will change in harmony with them
- highly *skilled professionals* for giving the right advice and making the prosthesis
- a feeling that they have the *best product* available to them.

Flexible service

A prosthetic service will see people of all ages with differing causes of limb loss at various times in their lives. Not all of those who are referred will become prosthetic users but if they do, it is essential that they feel comfortable in visiting the service as they may be totally dependent upon it throughout their lifetime. The ideal is that people should be able to 'shop around' to find a service that suits them, but the reality is that there are often very few options and people do not always have the resources to travel long distances to access alternatives. This places an enormous responsibility on services to continu-ously ensure that they are being sensitive to the needs of their clientele. If people are fearful of attending the clinic, the prosthesis may not be reviewed as regularly as it should be or they may be wearing uncomfortable sockets unnecessarily.

Whether it is an adult who has lost a limb through illness or accident or a child born with congenital limb deficiencies, the whole family will require tremendous emotional support from every member of staff in the service from the onset. They are likely to have many miscon-ceptions about the level of present day prosthetic technology and unrealistic expectations about how long it will take to learn to use an artificial limb for the first time. But as time moves on and people become competent limb wearers, the service must accommodate the changing needs of the individual. This is not to imply that artificial limb wearers always instantly accept what has happened to them; the emotional scars of limb loss can reappear at any time in a person's life and services should be flexible enough to recognise this and support people as necessary. Life events such as adolescence, marriage, redundancy, getting older, etc. can all re-awaken anxieties about coping, which may or may not be related to the original loss but the artificial limb can become an easy target to be blamed in times of difficulty. The general ambience of the service therefore needs to be warm, welcoming, sensitive and courteous at all times. Having somewhere to enjoy refreshments and comfortable seating in a pleasant waiting area and being kept informed about delays in carrying out repairs, etc. all help to make a visit less stressful than it might be. Making it clear who to ask if there are concerns or even who to complain to if things seem to be going wrong are all very important features in making users feel valued and supported.

Skilled professionals

There is an assumption within the general public that all professionals automatically have up-to-date knowledge and qualifications in their field of work. This assumption might be misplaced and users should have the right to expect all those involved in their care to be highly competent in their work. Additionally, the importance of the relationship any amputee has with those involved in their prosthetic provision cannot be underestimated. Trust and respect for one another are fundamental prerequisites for successful outcomes for all concerned. Staff therefore must be approachable and good communicators as well as being skilled practitioners. In state-run systems, users may also be reliant on these professionals to provide independent, accurate and up-to-date information on prosthetic advances. Seeing the same prosthetist or therapist at each visit also ensures continuity of care, which is vital as it allows time for the development of a good rapport between prosthetic users and professionals.

The best products

To begin with, new amputees will trust the professionals to decide which prosthesis is the most appropriate for them. As they become competent limb wearers they may become more adventurous and decide to try new activities in the form of work, play, sport, etc. Initially, they may expect the prosthetist to ask the right questions and may not be aware that some of their new ambitions require a change in limb design. As people become more experienced and have tried a range of products, they are likely to know when to ask for help or when they need a new device. However, the frail elderly amputee may not be so confident and the service should be able to recognise those who need continuous guidance and support.

However, the real dilemma for users is: how do they know that they are getting the best deal? How can they tell if they are attending a good centre or if it is the right artificial limb for them? How do they know that the prosthesis is as comfortable, controllable and functional as it possibly can be or that there is not something more aesthetically pleasing elsewhere? The Internet is opening up new opportunities for information but this currently relates to the products. Any standards that have been developed in prosthetic services have been of a clinical nature providing little information about the long-term use of artificial limbs. The majority of amputees, therefore, have little option but to place their trust in service providers and hope that the care they receive is of a high standard. An important source of information also comes from other amputees via support groups, newsletters or informal discussions in centres, etc.

PATIENTS, CLIENTS OR CUSTOMERS – WHAT IS THE DIFFERENCE?

Patients are by definition people who are ill or have had accidents – they may therefore be very frightened. People who have recently undergone amputation surgery are undoubtedly in this category and they may enter the prosthetic service in a very vulnerable state. At this time they are usually more than happy that the healthcare professionals take control and guide them through what happens next. At this point, a prescriptive model is entirely appropriate but as time goes on and people recover their health and mobility, responsibility for their care is handed back to the individuals themselves – this is the whole purpose of rehabilitation. But having been 'given' this responsibility, are users free to demand what they want from the service? Are they really customers?

In many countries, people purchase their artificial limbs themselves and are customers in every sense of the word – they choose the provider, the prosthetist and the type of limb they want. Health insurance may be available but this varies enormously and some policies provide cover for ongoing equipment but others exclude it or provide for very basic products. The high costs involved mean that it is not unusual for some people to have to take out second mortgages to cope with the expense.

In countries that operate national health schemes such as in the UK, the state covers the costs of any equipment needed throughout a person's lifetime through National Insurance contributions. This may mean providing a prosthesis free at the point of delivery or partial funding.

Where the state provides an all-inclusive service, the 'customer' is a composite of three elements:

1. those with the money, i.e. the local health authority, which is responsible for commissioning the service
2. those with the authority: this could be a medical consultant or someone else of similar standing who prescribes the prosthesis
3. those with the need: the amputee.

For this model to work, all of those involved must understand the amputee's needs. Whilst many people are content with this type of decision making, there are those (usually experienced users), who feel frustrated by it. They argue that they feel more than competent to make their own judgements about what type of prosthesis they need and would prefer to go to a supplier of their own choice. Some countries have listened to these wishes and have provided vouchers so that people can add to the value of these to increase the range or specification of a new prosthesis.

METHODS OF SECURING USER INVOLVEMENT

It is notoriously difficult to achieve accurate feedback about services. Meetings can be problematic in identifying broad representation. It is critical that the views of the majority are heard, e.g. those with limited mobility are unlikely to be able to get to meetings. Most centres will have clients who would say 'don't trouble them, they're busy' or 'oh, don't say anything, they're doing their best'. These are probably the silent majority and a great deal of creative thought needs to be given to canvassing their views. Minority groups also need to be considered, e.g. parents of disabled children and people from varying ethnic backgrounds who are likely to have particular needs that should be brought to the attention of management. Important concerns about clinic appointments clashing with school times or issues about cosmetic developments that to date have largely concentrated on Eurasian complexions should all be given an opportunity for discussion in this way. Other important groups that are often missed are the families of amputees and carers.

Quality standards

The development of quality standards and clinical effectiveness measures have become key priorities in all healthcare systems in an attempt to determine value for money. Quality circles, audit groups and recording compliments and complaints are all very laudable in the clinical world but to date these have made no real changes to what really matters to an amputee. Service standards nearly all relate to administrative procedures or clinical care, whereas a successful outcome to an amputee could well be that they are able to ride a bicycle again or to go shopping. Because of the medical bias, services standards have tended to focus on the rehabilitative phase, which is an important but comparatively minor component of an amputee's life. Technical mobility grades, which are useful to physiotherapists and doctors, make no impression when what users want is a comfortable socket or an acceptable cosmetic cover. It is recognised that measuring subjective information is difficult but it is not impossible and services must react to this challenge. Where amputees do not have the buying power of real customers, there is an urgent need for services to work in active partnership to develop standards that are meaningful to the users as well as professionals. They must relate to lifestyles and ideally should be adopted nationally for comparison. It is only by doing this that real choices about issues that are fundamental to the quality of people's lives can be made.

Canvassing opinion

Satisfaction questionnaires are a useful tool but they need to be constructed professionally to be made fully objective. Services that design their own questionnaires invariably use leading questions which are biased in favour of the organisation. They are useful if views are needed about specific issues, e.g. a move to new premises, but they tend to limit subjective views. Structured interviews are better for this but are time-consuming – again professional guidance should be sought before embarking. Commissioning an independent audit ensures questions are completely neutral as there is no vested interest in the outcome.

Advocacy

One-to-one communication with someone who can empathise is one of the most useful methods of hearing the truth and supporting people. Users often feel overwhelmed by what is happening to them and feel unable to speak out. New amputees are particularly at risk of not being heard as they may not have the confidence to share their concerns no matter how welcoming the service. Keeping a register of those willing to talk to other amputees and matching together people in similar circumstances, such as two families with a disabled child, can bring enormous relief as people realise they are not alone. Some prosthetic services use volunteers or employ advocates specifically for this purpose.

User groups

User consultative groups can be very informative and have been formed in the majority of NHS prosthetics services in the UK. In 1994, The Limbless Association of the UK published model Terms of Reference to help centres set up user consultative committees. Many groups have outgrown this form, although these may be useful as a starting point.

The major problem with working in groups like this is that people can use meetings to fulfil their own agenda. They may fail to speak for a constituency or use meetings to focus attention on themselves. This not only risks the subject matter going off at a tangent, it can also use up a disproportionate amount of time. If these issues are not managed well, groups can become destructive. It is therefore vital for success that they are well chaired, have a broad membership and have clear aims and objectives. It can be equally damaging for management to pay lip service to the concept of consultation and hand pick a passive membership, deliberately avoiding any possible conflict and ensuring compliance with management's wishes. It is only by being open to the concept of consultation that meaningful dialogue can occur.

National support groups

National support groups offer a variety of support including: information, one-to-one befriending, financial help, respite holidays and political lobbying, etc. Not all have a political dimension but it is the groups that include lobbying that have effected the greatest change in recent years. Like many situations where minority groups are struggling to be heard, frustration can lead to extremist views that can be off-putting to some members. Furthermore, this can lead to confrontational behaviour. However, inevitably some middle ground has to be found before progress can be made. Whilst the disability rights movement is embryonic in many parts of the world, countries that have been leading the way have now progressed to a point of serious dialogue with governments effecting much needed progress.

FUTURE

Information technology and increased media attention to hi-tech innovation is leading to raised expectation, and services that operate on limited budgets are struggling to cope with current demands. Advances in cosmetic finishes are also giving those concerned about appearance and body image, hope of progress in this much needed area, but each new development tends to mean higher costs. Services are beginning to see the effects of the present consumer culture, which is empowering users to express their dissatisfaction. This kind of pressure will inevitably bring change but as healthcare systems across the world are coping with diminishing resources, this may not all be positive. Options might be to change funding priorities to identify the necessary resources or to find alternative methods of funding including self-finance or insurance. Whilst this may introduce some choice into the system it may not suit everyone. What could happen is that those who have been able to benefit from a 'free' system will now have to pay for what has been theirs by right. For those living on state benefits, and many disabled people fall into this category, this is likely to feel like a retrograde move.

SUMMARY

Recent years have seen massive progress in attitudes towards disability and the type of support available to disabled people in general. In addition, there have been major advances in new technology that have improved the style and capability of specialised equipment such as artificial limbs. There can be no doubt that all of this has contributed to major improvements in the quality of life of thousands of amputees. As the millennium approaches, the new challenge is for services to keep pace with advancing technology at a time of diminishing public sector resources. It is, therefore, critical that professionals begin to work in partnership with disabled people so that services can face these problems together, ensuring that the real experts in disability are involved in service developments. In the commercial world, no new product or service would be considered without first carrying out market research to test the idea. This would then be followed by continuous customer feedback to inform any advancement. As people who use artificial limbs are not always seen as consumers, this critical aspect of service provision has not always been given the attention it deserves. This chapter started out by asking why user involvement was necessary. Perhaps the question should have been: 'how could services develop effectively without it?'

BIBLIOGRAPHY FOR THE THIRD EDITION

Department of Health 1996 User involvement: community service users as consultants and trainers. NHS Executive Community Care Branch

Editorial 1995 Rights for disabled people now: civil rights or a discriminating law. Rights Now

Lee T, Rodda M 1994 Modification of attitudes toward people with disabilities. Canadian Journal of Rehabilitation 7(4):229–238

Nicholas J J, Robinson L R, Schulz R, Blair C, Aliota R, Hairston G 1993 Problems experienced and perceived by prosthetic patients. Journal of Prosthetics and Orthotics 5(1):16–19

Oliver M 1996 Defining disability and impairment: issues at stake. In: Barnes C, Mercer G (eds) Exploring the divide: illness and disability. The Disability Press, Leeds

Prince of Wales Advisory Group on Disability and The

King's Fund 1992 Planning services for people with severe physical and sensory difficulties. Living Options in Practice Project Paper No. 3

Prince of Wales Advisory Group on Disability and The King's Fund 1995 The power to change: commissioning health and social services with disabled people. Living Options Partnership

Shakespeare T 1994 Cultural representation of disabled people: dustbins for disavowal? Disability and Society 9(3):283–299

Vasey S 1992 Disability culture: it's a way of life. In: Rieser R, Mason M (eds) Disability equality in the classroom: a human rights issue. Disability Equality in Education

Wood P 1980 International classification of impairments, disabilities and handicaps. World Health Organisation, Geneva

23

Therapy service quality

The purpose of this chapter is to create a general awareness of quality issues in healthcare and specifically indicate which organisations set standards relevant to the rehabilitation of amputees. Most of the chapter is based on the UK: undoubtedly parallel activity will be happening in other countries, and there is a continuous process of development in all the issues raised. All therapists will wish to know that the service they are providing to amputees is of a proven (or known) effectiveness, and is of an acceptable standard. It is appreciated that few therapists work full-time in the rehabilitation of amputees, as frequently this work only forms a small part of a more general rehabilitation service: therefore therapists should be able to network and gather the information needed for their particular facility. However, there is a lack of standardisation in terminology, which can be very confusing to the clinical therapist. The reader must first identify what they want to know and the bias any publication may have, e.g. professional association, government directive, etc.

The Chartered Society of Physiotherapy (CSP) in the UK defines a quality assurance programme as 'one which provides a systematic method of evaluating the quality of services and facilitates continuous improvement'. In the field of amputee rehabilitation, once the unidisciplinary approach to quality is appreciated, multidisciplinary standards should be set, which should bring together all the professions involved and include patient groups. This is to ensure there is an holistic approach with agreed aims between all involved in patient treatment.

Quality in healthcare was originally defined in terms of service dimensions by Maxwell as follows:

1. Access
2. Equity
3. Responsiveness
4. Relevance to need
5. Efficiency
6. Effectiveness (encompassing both the organisational and human aspects of quality).

All these are relevant to the quality of rehabilitation services to amputees.

According to Donabedian (1980), measuring quality is possible at three stages:

1. Inputs: the resources and personnel available and how they are organised
2. Process: how the patient experiences the service or care
3. Outcome: the results of care.

BACKGROUND

In the developed and the developing world, there is now a much greater emphasis on quality issues. Quality initiatives have been driven by the economic climate in healthcare, the political climate and demographic factors, increased expectations of patients and clinicians and improved technology. These factors influence the demand for clinical interventions to be based on sound evidence of effectiveness and value for money. Therefore government agencies and professional organisations have all been involved in promoting standard setting, clinical audit, measurement, evaluation of outcomes, setting up care plans/guidelines/pathways, evidence-based practice, etc. In the UK, the health service reforms from the late 1980s resulted in the development of clinical audit, technological assessment and outcome measurement. These policies have evolved into one promoting clinical effectiveness. All purchasers and providers within the public healthcare system have been involved. Annual reports are published to which the public have access, which in turn have developed public awareness. In private healthcare provision, the

need for effective treatment at a reasonable cost has meant an equal interest in this subject.

Quality assurance is demanded in all aspects of healthcare provision. Therapists must not only be concerned with actual clinical treatments and their documentation, but also with the safety of the equipment and the environment in which they work and treat their patients, the management of identified risks, and communication standards with the patient and other healthcare professionals in the team.

A variety of groups have been formed in the UK to help take this work forward. One group was set up by the Disablement Services Authority (see Ch. 1), which covered prosthetic and wheelchair services. This enabled a facilitator to work nationally with all specialist centres on clinical audit, patient satisfaction and making improvements where indicated. This national work ceased in 1994, but now each service carries out its own local initiatives. Even though the services are now fragmented in the UK, communication between teams and individuals working in the same profession in different services is essential in order to learn from others' experiences. Commercial competition between centres in the past has hampered this communication, but now the climate is one of collaboration, which has enabled these organisations to work together in a more meaningful way, e.g. with benchmarking (see p. 308).

EVIDENCE-BASED PRACTICE

Muir Gray (1997) states that 'evidence-based clinical practice is an approach to decision making in which the clinician uses the best evidence available, in consultation with the patient, to decide upon the option that suits the patient best'. Evidence should be used to formulate criteria in standard setting (see Figs 23.1 and 23.2).

Therapists must therefore keep up to date by reading relevant literature and networking with professional colleagues and the national clinical interest group of their professional organisation in order to be aware of the best available evidence. Those who have good library and on-line

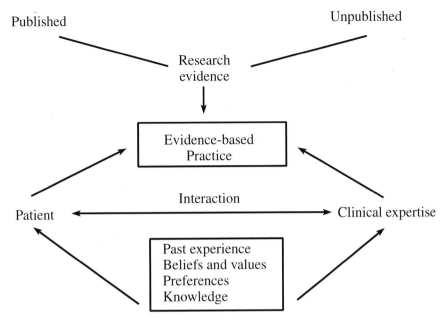

Figure 23.1   Evidence-based practice. (Illustration by kind permission of The Chartered Society of Physiotherapy, UK.)

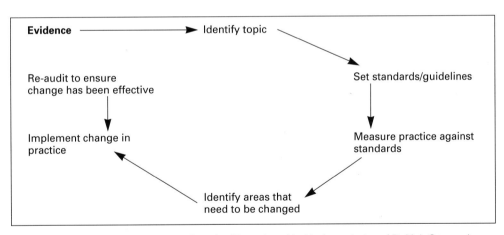

Figure 23.2   The evidence-driven audit cycle. (Reproduced by kind permission of Dr Muir Gray and Churchill Livingstone.)

search facilities obviously can do this easier than those in remote locations without computer links.

Dunning (1995) states that 'clinical effectiveness is the application of interventions, which have been shown to be efficacious to appropriate patients, in a timely fashion to enhance patient outcomes and value for the use of resources. Professional staff therefore need up-to-date knowledge and skills, as well as the appropriate attitude which embraces clinical effectiveness and the need for change'. The therapy professions must demonstrate that they produce health benefits in order to remain at the forefront of rehabilitation and as Muir Grey (1997) states:

Evidence-based healthcare plus quality management equals maximum benefit at lowest risk and cost.

STANDARDS

There are many different definitions of what a standard is; Øvretveit (1992) defines it as 'a specific expectation of staff, described in terms of an activity or outcome against which their actions can be measured. The expectation is specified in terms of a level of performance to be achieved on a defined measure or indicator'. They are created first by formulating criteria: these are the mechanisms that have to be in place in order to achieve the standard and they should be specific, measurable, achievable, realistic and have timescales for implementation. From these criteria the standard is developed, which states an expected level of performance, e.g. a standard in the field of amputee rehabilitation may state that 'all lower limb amputees are provided with a temporary wheelchair on the first post operative day'.

The quality of a service is the degree to which it conforms to pre-set standards of care whether national or local, e.g. bearing in mind most dysvascular, unilateral, trans-tibial amputees' life expectancy is short, if the outcome of rehabilitation is that it takes 1 year to reach an objective of care (i.e. walking independently 50 meters), then this cannot be considered to be an acceptable standard. Literature indicates that if the input of the team and the process through rehabilitation is well defined, this outcome should be achieved by 85% in 3–4 months.

Taking Donabedian's view of standards:

- An example of an *input standard* is in the following statement: 'there is a programme which maximises the patient's functional independence' (The Chartered Society of Physiotherapy's *Standards of practice for people with amputations*, Standard 7).
- An example of a *process standard* is ISO 10328, which is a process testing standard for the manufacture of lower limb prostheses.
- 3. An example of an *outcome standard* is the mobility of an amputee following rehabilitation, expressed on the Harold Wood/Stanmore mobility scale (Hanspal 1991).

Who sets standards?

The national government, through the local health authority, sets standards of performance for the healthcare provision for local populations. A provider unit (i.e. where therapy is delivered) is interested in both these performance standards for the whole population it serves and also for clinical standards delivered to individual patients. The therapist must be aware of standards required by purchasers, which are normally stated in contracts for service provision, and any national targets, such as the Patient's Charter in the UK. They must then be aware of those set by their professional body, both for general working practice (e.g. documentation, health and safety) and specifically for the client group (e.g. people with amputations). Discussion between team members will identify a range of standards set by the medical, nursing, prosthetic, therapy and psychologist/counsellor professions and from these national standards (which are considered to be the minimum acceptable level, below which no service should fall without urgent remedial action being taken) local standards should be set by the team, bearing in mind the views of the users.

Audit

The definition of clinical audit given by the Department of Health in the UK in 1989 was: 'the systematic, critical analysis of the quality of clinical care, including the procedures used for diagnosis and treatment, the use of resources and the resulting outcome and quality of life for the patient'.

Audit is a quality assessment mechanism, which has a continuous and developing programme through re-audit, the major objective being improved services to consumers. Standard setting encourages thoughtful planning that leads to valid information collection and subsequently to informed decision making. Audit must cover all aspects of service provision and an example of an audit of patient satisfaction is Smith C et al (1995).

While there remains a need for individual

professions to maintain and develop their own standards of care and to audit these, the focus of clinical audit in recent years has been on the performance of the whole clinical team. This is particularly relevant to amputee rehabilitation and can be used to compare one amputee rehabilitation team's performance with another's, where broadly the same service is provided to the same type of population (e.g. in the UK), and to compare outcomes from the regional specialist prosthetic rehabilitation centres.

Measurement

Measurement is the way in which the change in a patient's status over time as a result of an intervention is evaluated. Measurements should be distinguished from clinical impressions or clinical opinions, which are beliefs or opinions that therapists may hold about their patients.

Measurements may be quantitative, i.e. the assignment of numbers to measure a performance or characteristic, or qualitative, i.e. the assignment of categorical names as a measurement (e.g. improved, no change, worse).

Therapists are advised to use validated standard tests or measuring instruments wherever possible to show that the instrument intended for use yields results that can be reproduced. However, it is appreciated that there are few such scales that are sufficiently sensitive to the changes/achievements attained in therapy. A variety of different scales are being used and there is ongoing work by various organisations, e.g. the Scottish Physiotherapy Amputee Research Group (SPARG) that are seeking better methods of measuring the results of rehabilitation.

Audit and research

A note must be made of the relationship between research and audit. Research advances our knowledge about the most effective form of treatment that can be extended to the general population. Audit looks at local practice against expectation: it compares local care to a general standard (formulated from research evidence), i.e. what *should* be done. Audit results demand

an action plan locally and a re-audit will check whether improvement has been made or whether new standards should be set.

QUALITY IMPROVEMENT TOOLS

In the UK, extensive work is being carried out looking at various methods to improve the overall quality of care. All of the following are tools that can be used for amputee management.

Multidisciplinary care pathways (MCPs) or integrated care pathways (ICPs)

These terms are defined as a multidisciplinary process of patient-focused care that specifies key events, tests and assessments, occurring in a timely fashion, to produce the best prescribed outcomes, within the resources and activities available for an appropriate episode of care. One of these processes is illustrated by Schaldach (1997). These processes are a risk management tool and aim to improve the documentation and communication of patient care and the process and quality of healthcare delivery.

Designing a pathway is a local facility activity and is good for team building and sharing of evidence and standards. The integrated care management approach involves debate and agreement by the team, who establish consistent and realistic goals. They provide the agreed guidelines and a working collaborative document of patient care, but they are no substitute for professional judgement and individualised patient care – they are there to assist the process.

MCPs cannot be imported from one healthcare setting to another as local ownership and commitment are needed and local resources differ.

A variance from the pathway is a deviation from the plan of care, e.g. the plan may indicate that a trans-tibial amputee at 5 days postoperatively should start to use an early walking aid (EWA): if the wound is insufficiently healed for this to be possible, there will be a variance from this plan.

Enquiry into the number of variences indicates enquiry into clinical practice and identifies remedial factors to improve practice, e.g. as in the example above, the method of suturing or post-operative dressing may be causing the problem.

This enquiry into the appropriateness of the plan can also be viewed as clinical audit.

Patient-focused care

This is a concept of care delivery management that involves relying on a small team of multi-skilled practitioners to meet all the clinical needs of the patients close to the bedside. It is supposed to increase patient satisfaction by reducing the number of staff in direct contact with them and reducing hospital costs.

Clinical guidelines

According to Field (1992); clinical guidelines are: 'Systematically developed statements to assist practitioner and patient decisions about appropriate healthcare for specific clinical circumstances'. Guidelines are the scientific evidence in accessible form and are advisory in nature (not compulsory). They are one element in the wheel to promote improvements in clinical practice.

Care protocols

A care protocol indicates the method of care to be employed for an identifiable group of patients (e.g. trans-tibial amputees or those with total hip replacement): it guides the team step-by-step through the care process, from diagnosis, to treatment, to evaluation of outcome.

Care plan

A care plan is a team protocol that also involves the patient and carer, is applied to the individual and adapted and tailored to their needs. Information from patients is a component of the evidence base in clinical effectiveness (see Fig. 23.1).

Benchmarking

Benchmarking is the means of comparing data by which outcome of performance can be measured

and ultimately ensures that best practice is constantly improved. It involves seeking, finding, implementing and sustaining good practice, which is a continuous process. Healthcare organisations have to be able to demonstrate to both patients and purchasers that they are highly productive, effective, efficient and innovative.

Once local benchmarks have been identified by audit, the service can decide to join with a similar service elsewhere and search together for best practice in common areas of concern, and share information, experience and initiatives in clinical practice. It is essential to benchmark like with like and all parties involved must use the same definitions for the data they collect.

Managed care

Hale (1995) defines managed care as: '... an organisational process which identifies specific case types and spells out the sequence of care and treatment that is to be given by professionals in order to achieve previously determined patient outcomes'.

Within a managed care system, standard care is delivered to groups of patients who have certain common conditions for which it is possible to define a core set of interventions and services, e.g. care of people with diabetes mellitus. It is a way of controlling costs and improving quality. The issue with the system is that there are some individual patients with specific problems who may not fit into the system, e.g. elderly dysvascular patients requiring amputation may be the specific case type/group. However, if a young patient has an amputation as a result of meningococcal septicaemia (see Ch. 21), the clinicians must agree on a different sequence of care and treatment to be given. It can also be seen as a form of rationing healthcare.

Continuous professional development

The input standard of an individual professional in a clinical team is dependent on their knowledge and experience. CSP (1997) state that: 'Continuous professional development (CPD) is the educational process by which professional people maintain, enhance and broaden their professional competence. It is a systematic process that is undertaken throughout the career to develop and enhance the individual's work. It is an ongoing process which is professionally owned and underpinned by day-to-day evaluation and reflection of practice'.

For therapists concerned with amputee rehabilitation in the UK, the following organisations will be able to provide information on learning opportunities in this field:

- The Chartered Society of Physiotherapy (CSP) and clinical interest group, the British Association of Chartered Physiotherapists in Amputee Rehabilitation (BACPAR)
- The College of Occupational Therapy (COT) and clinical interest group, the Clinical

Interest Group in Orthotics, Prosthetics and Wheelchairs (CIGOPW)
- The British Association of Prosthetists and Orthotists (BAPO)
- The International Society for Prosthetics and Orthotics (ISPO)

Addresses for these organisations can be found in Appendix 1.

Therapists must explore every avenue available to them to improve the quality of service given to amputee rehabilitation. Many of the quality standards briefly described in this chapter will be further developed and expanded in future years and it is the responsibility of the individual therapist to keep their knowledge up to date, and to understand and work with initiatives in their own country.

BIBLIOGRAPHY FOR THE THIRD EDITION

Amputee Medical Rehabilitation Society 1992 Amputee rehabilitation: recommended standards and guidelines. Royal College of Physicians, London
Amputee Medical Rehabilitation Society 1997 Congenital limb deficiency: recommended standards of care. Royal College of Physicians, London
Baker R 1997 What is the role of evidence-based guidelines. Health Care Risk Report February:15–17,24
Bardsley M, Cole J 1991 Measured steps to outcomes. Health Service Journal 101(S274):18–20
Bardsley M J, Coles J M 1992 Practical experiences in auditing patient outcomes. Quality in Health Care 1:124–130
Bury T 1996 Evidence-based practice: survival of the fittest. Physiotherapy 82(2):75–76
Buttenshaw P, Dolman J 1992 The Roehampton approach to rehabilitation: a retrospective survey of prosthetic use in patients with primary unilateral lower-limb amputation. Topics in Geriatric Rehabilitation 8(1):72–78
Chesson R, Macleod M, Massie S 1996 Outcome measures used in therapy departments in Scotland. Physiotherapy 82(12):673–679
Condie E, Jones D, Treweek S, Scott H 1996 A one-year national survey of patients having a lower limb amputation. Physiotherapy 82(1):14–20
Cotter D H G, Hanspal R S, Lachmann S M, Morrison J D 1992 Amputee rehabilitation – recommended standards and guidelines. Report by the Working Party of The Amputee Medical Rehabilitation Society
Datta D, Ariyaratnam R, Hilton S 1996 Timed walking test – an all-embracing outcome measure for lower-limb amputees. Clinical Rehabilitation 10(3):227–232
De Clive Lowe S 1996 Outcome measurement, cost effectiveness and clinical audit: the importance of standardised assessment to occupational therapists in

meeting these new demands. British Journal of Occupational Therapy 59(8):357–362
De Fretes A, Boonstra A M, Vos L D V 1994 Functional outcome of rehabilitated bilateral lower limb amputees. Prosthetics and Orthotics International 18:18–24
Deutsch A, Braun S, Granger C 1996 The functional independence measures (FIMsm Instrument) and the functional independence measure for children (WEEFIM Instrument): ten years of development. Critical Reviews in Physical and Rehabilitation Medicine 8(4):267–281
Donabedian A 1980 The definition of quality: a conceptual exploration. In: Exploration in Quality Assessment and Monitoring, Vol 1 The definition of quality and approaches to its assessment. Health Administration Press, Ann Arbour
Dunning M 1995 Promoting action on clinical effectiveness (correspondence). The King's Fund, London
Esquenazi A, Meier III R H 1996 Rehabilitation in limb deficiency. 4. Limb amputation. Archives of Physical Medicine and Rehabilitation 77:S18–S28
Field M J, Lohr K N 1992 Institute of medicine. Guideline for clinical practice: from development to use. National Academy Press, Washington DC
Fricke J et al 1993 Reliability of the functional independence measure with occupational therapists. Australian Journal of Occupational Therapy 40(1):7–15
Hale C 1995 Key terms in managed care. Nursing Times 91(29):29
Hanspal R S, Chakrabarty B K, Fisher K, Morton M, Roberts A 1991 Mobility grades in amputee rehabilitation. Clinical Rehabilitation 5:344
Heafey M L, Golden-Baker S B, Mahoney D W 1994 Using nursing diagnoses and interventions in an inpatient amputee program. Rehabilitation Nursing 19(3):163–168

Heasell S 1995 Economics of clinical guidelines – risks and resources. Health Care Risk Report October:23–25

Hendry J A 1995 The utilization of physiotherapy services after lower-limb amputation in an academic hospital in South Africa. Proceedings of 12th International Conference of the World Confederation for Physical Therapy, Washington

Hubbard W A, McElroy G K 1994 Benchmark data for elderly, vascular trans-tibial amputees after rehabilitation. Prosthetics and Orthotics International 18(3):142–149

Humphries D, Littlejohns P 1995 The development of multiprofessional audit and clinical guidelines – their contribution to quality assurance and effectiveness in the NHS. Journal of InterProfessional Care 9(3):207–225

Humphries D, Littlejohns P 1996 Implementing clinical guidelines: preparation and opportunism. Journal of Clinical Effectiveness 1(1):5–8

Johnson V J, Kondziela S, Gottschalk F 1995 Pre and post-amputation mobility of trans-tibial amputees: correlation to medical problems, age and mortality. Prosthetics and Orthotics International 19(3):159–164

Jutai J, Ladak N, Schuller R, Naumann S, Wright V 1996 Outcomes measurement of assistive technologies: an institutional case study. Assistive Technology 8(2):110–120

Kane R L 1994 Looking for physical therapy outcomes. Physical Therapy 74(5):425–429

Keith R A, Granger C V, Hamilton B B, Sherwins F S 1987 The functional independence measure. Advances in Clinical Rehabilitation 1:6–18

Kitchener D 1995 Multidisciplinary pathways of care series – analysis of variance in patients. Health Care Risk Report September:16–17

Klein D, Campbell A 1995 The CQI pathway ... to decrease the length of stay for amputee patients. Rehabilitation Management 8(4):89–90,92,94–95

Law M et al 1990 The Canadian occupational performance measure for occupational therapy. Canadian Journal of Occupational Therapy 57(2):82–87

Leung E C-C, Rush P J, Devlin M 1996 Predicting prosthetic rehabilitation outcome in lower limb amputee patients with the functional independence measure. Archives of Physical Medicine and Rehabilitation 77(6):605–608

Mann T 1996 Clinical guidelines: using clinical guidelines to improve patient care within the NHS. Department of Health, Wetherby, Yorkshire

Mawson S J, McCreadie M J 1993 TELER: the way forward in clinical audit. Physiotherapy 79(11):758–761

Maxwell R J 1984 Quality assessment in health. British Medical Journal 288:1470–1472

McCulloch D 1991 Can we measure output: quality adjusted life years, health indices and occupational therapy. British Journal of Occupational Therapy 54(6):219–221

Muir Gray J A 1997 Evidence based healthcare: how to make health policy and management decisions. Churchill Livingstone, Edinburgh

Newdick C 1996 The status of guidelines. Health Care Risk Report October:14–15

National Health Service Management Executive 1996 Promoting clinical effectiveness: a framework for action in and through the NHS. NHSME, London

Nicholson J 1997 Care pathways – a tool for improving quality and managing risk. Health Care Risk Report March:16–17,24

Øvretveit J 1992 Health service quality. An introduction to quality methods for health services. Blackwell Scientific Publications, Oxford, p 100

Pratt D J 1995 British Standard (BS) 5750 – quality assurance. Prosthetics and Orthotics International 19(1):31–36

Pruitt S D, Varni J W, Setoguchi Y 1996 Functional status in children with limb deficiency: development and initial validation of an outcome measure. Archives of Physical Medicine and Rehabilitation 77:1233–1238

Pruitt S D, Varni J W, Seid M, Setoguchi Y 1997 Prosthesis satisfaction outcome measurement in pediatric limb deficiency. Archives of Physical Medicine and Rehabilitation 78:750–754

Reynolds J P 1995 Prosthetics under management care. Magazine of Physical Therapy November 3(11):58–62

Rommers G M, Vos L D W, Groothoff J W, Eisma W H 1996 Clinical rehabilitation of the amputee: a retrospective study. Prosthetics and Orthotics International 20:72–78

Sackett D L, Rosenburg W M C, Gray J A M et al 1996 Evidence based medicine: what it is and what it isn't. British Medical Journal 312:71–72

Sapp L, Little C E 1995 Functional outcomes in a lower limb amputee population. Prosthetics and Orthotics International 19(2):92–96

Schaldach D E 1997 Measuring quality and cost of care: evaluation of an amputation clinical pathway. Journal of Vascular Nursing 15(1):13–20

Scottish Physiotherapy Amputee Research Group 1997 The further development of a national system of clinical audit for lower limb amputees (CA95/01 Final report). National Centre for Training and Education in Prosthetics and Orthotics, Strathclyde

Sener S, Yakut Y, Uygar F, Karaduman A 1995 Living with disability: Quality of life in rehabilitated lower limb amputees. Physiotherapy 81(8):455

Shaw C D 1994 Quality and audit in rehabilitation services. Clinical Rehabilitation 8:183–187

Simpson J M, Harrington R, Marsh N 1998 Guidelines for managing falls among elderly people. Physiotherapy 84(4):173–177

Smith C, McCreadie M, Unsworth J, Wickings H I, Harrison A 1995 Patient satisfaction: an indication of quality in disablement services centres. Quality in Health Care 4(1):31–36

Stead L, Arthur C, Cleary A 1995 Multidisciplinary pathways of care series – do multidisciplinary pathways of care affect patient satisfaction? Health Care Risk Report November:13–15

Subbarao K V, Bajoria S 1995 The effect of stump length on the rehabilitation outcome in unilateral below-knee amputees for vascular disease. Clinical Rehabilitation 9:327–330

Sumsion T 1997 Client centered implications of evidence-based practice. Physiotherapy 83(7):373–374

UK Clearing House 1993 Outcomes briefing, introductory issue 1. Nuffield Institute for Health, Leeds

Wilson J 1995 Multidisciplinary pathways of care series introduction. Health Care Risk Report June:21–22

Wood P 1980 The International classification of impairments, disabilities and handicaps: a manual of classification relating to the consequence of disease. World Health Organisation, Geneva

Woodman R 1995 Quality systems: going for ISO 9000. Health Care Risk Report April:19–20

Zander K 1992 Focusing on patient outcomes: case management in the 90's. Dimensions of Critical Care Nursing 11(3):127–129

The Chartered Society of Physiotherapy

1992 Standards of physiotherapy practice for the management of patients with amputations. The Chartered Society of Physiotherapy, London

1993 Standards of physiotherapy practice, 2nd edition. The Chartered Society of Physiotherapy, London

1994 Quality assurance: co-ordinating a consumer satisfaction survey, information paper PA 15. The Chartered Society of Physiotherapy, London

1996 Standards for administering tests and taking measurements. The Chartered Society of Physiotherapy, London

1996 How to … set standards. Information paper PA 16. The Chartered Society of Physiotherapy, London

1996 Clinical guidelines reference list, information paper PA 36. The Chartered Society of Physiotherapy, London

1997 Standards for continuing professional development (CPD). The Chartered Society of Physiotherapy, London

1997 Current awareness bulletin: Amputee Rehabilitation. The Chartered Society of Physiotherapy, London

1997 Clinical effectiveness strategy. The Chartered Society of Physiotherapy, London

The College of Occupational Therapists

1991 Standards, policies and proceedings: standards of practice for audit, SPP 180. The College of Occupational Therapists, London

1991 Standards, policies and proceedings: standards of practice for setting up a quality assurance programme, SPP 175. The College of Occupational Therapists, London

1991 Standards, policies and proceedings: standards of practice for occupational therapy services for consumers with physical disabilities, SPP 105A. The College of Occupational Therapists, London

Clinical Interest Group in Orthotics Prosthetics and Wheelchairs 1997 Occupational therapy in the treatment of lower limb amputees: standards and guidelines. The College of Occupational Therapists, London

CONTENTS

Appendix 1: General information and some helpful addresses

PATIENT AND CARERS ORGANISATIONS

The Limbless Association

Roehampton Rehabilitation Centre
Roehampton Lane
London SW15 5PR

The Association offers an advisory service for amputees and their families and publishes *Step Forward*.

British Limbless Ex-Servicemen's Association (BLESMA)

Frankland Moore House
185 High Road
Chadwell Heath
Essex RM6 6NA

BLESMA offers help and advice for war pensioners with amputations, and publishes Blesmag and Driving After an Amputation.

STEPS

15 Stratham Close
Lymm
Cheshire WA13 9NN

STEPS is the national association for families of children with congenital abnormalities of the lower limb; they publish a Newsletter.

Reach

12 Wilson Way
Earls Barton
Northamptonshire NN6 0NZ

Reach is the association for children with hand or arm deficiency; they publish Within Reach.

The Carers National Association

20–25 Glass House Yard
London EC1A 4JS

Pain Concern

PO Box 318
Canterbury
Kent CT2 0DG

Lady Hoare Trust for Physically Disabled Children

4th Floor, Mitre House
44–46, Fleet Street
London EC4Y 1BN

SPORTS AND LEISURE ASSOCIATIONS

British Sports Association for the Disabled (BSAD)

Mary Glen Haig Suite
Solecast House
13–27 Brunswick Place
London N1 6DX

British Amputee and Les Autres Sports Association (BALASA)

35a Clarence Road
Moseley
Birmingham B13 9FY

The British Ski Club for the Disabled

Spring Mount
Berwick St John
Shaftsbury
Dorset SP7 0HQ

The British Disabled Water Ski Association

The Tony Edge National Centre
Heron Lake
Hythe End
Wraysbury
Middlesex TW19 6HW

British Wheelchair Sports Foundation (BWSF)

Guttman Sports Centre
Harvey Road
Stoke Mandeville
Buckinghamshire HP21 9PP

Jubilee Sailing Trust Ltd

Jubilee Yard
Merlin Key
Hazel Road
Wooton
Southampton SO19 7GB

Handicapped Anglers Trust (HAT) and Boating for the Disabled

Hazelhope
Stalisfield
Faversham
Kent ME13 0HY

Riding for the Disabled Association

Avenue R
National Agricultural Centre
Kenilworth
Warwickshire CV8 2LY

Gardening for the Disabled Trust

Hayes Farmhouse
Hayes Lane
Peasmarsh
East Sussex TN1 6XR

Camping for the Disabled

20 Burton Close
Dawley
Telford
Shropshire

TRAVEL ASSOCIATIONS AND INFORMATION

Disabled Drivers Association

Ashwell Thorpe
Norwich NR6 1EX

Disabled Motorists Federation

National Mobility Centre
Unit 2a, Atcham Estate
Shrewsbury SY4 4UG

Banstead Mobility Centre

Damson Way
Fountain Drive
Queen Mary's Avenue
Carshalton
Surrey SM5 4NR

The Automobile Association (AA)

Fanum House
Basingstoke RG21 2FA
The AA publishes the *Guide for the Disabled Traveller*

Motability

Gate House
West Gate
The High
Harlow
Essex CM20 1HR

HOLIDAYS AND INFORMATION
Calvet Trust

Little Crosthwaite
Keswick
Cumbria CA12 4QD

John Grooms Association for Disabled People

50 Scrutton Street
London EC2A 4PH

Holiday Care Service

2 Old Bank Chambers
Station Road
Horley Surrey RH6 9HW

The Winged Fellowship Trust

Holidays for Disabled People
Angel House
Pentonville Road
London N1 9XD

OTHER INFORMATION SERVICES FOR AMPUTEES
Local Social Services Departments

These addresses can be located in local telephone books and will supply and give information covering housing, aids and adaptations, education, benefits, employment, etc.

The Association of Community Health Councils for England and Wales (CHCs)

30 Drayton Park
London N5 1PB

The Royal Association for Disability and Rehabilitation (RADAR)

12 City Forum
250 City Road
London EC1V 8AF

A registered charity producing monthly publications with much useful information on access, mobility and travel, sports and leisure, etc.

The Disabled Living Foundation (DLF)

380–384 Harrow Road
London W9 2HU

One of many centres throughout the UK.

The Disability Alliance

1st Floor East
Universal House
88–94 Wentworth Street
London E1 7SA

This organisation publishes the annual *Disability Rights Handbook*, a comprehensive guide to benefits and services.

Disability Information Trust

Mary Marlborough Centre
Nuffield Orthopaedic Centre
Headington
Oxford OX3 7LD

They publish *Equipment for the Disabled* (see Bibliography).

Disability Scotland

Princes House
5 Shandwick Place
Edinburgh EH2 4RG

Disability Wales

Llys Ifir
Crescent Road
Caerfilly CF83 1XL

Citizens Advice Bureaux

(Addresses can be found in local telephone books.)

Sexual and Personal Relationships for Disabled People (SPOD)

286 Camden Road
London N7 0BJ

National Council of Voluntary Organisations (NCVO)

Regent's Wharf
8 All Saints' Street
London N1 9RL

INFORMATION SOURCES FOR THERAPISTS

International Society for Prosthetics and Orthotics (ISPO)

UK National Member Society Secretary
Mrs R. Ham
Camden and Islington Wheelchair Service
Peckwater Centre
6 Peckwater Street
London NW5 2TX

The international centre is:
ISPO
Borgervaenget 5
2100 Kobenhaven Ø
Denmark

ISPO International publishes *Prosthetics and Orthotics International*, a quarterly journal.

National Centre for Training and Education in Prosthetics and Orthotics

Curran Buildings
131 St James' Road
Glasgow G4 0LS

RECAL, a current awareness list, is available from this centre.

The Chartered Society of Physiotherapy

14 Bedford Row
London WC1R 4ED

The British Association of Chartered Physiotherapists in Amputee Rehabilitation (BACPAR) is contactable here and they publish a regular newsletter.

The College of Occupational Therapy

106–114, Borough High Street
London SE1 1LB

The Clinical Interest Group in Orthotics, Prosthetics and Wheelchairs (CIGOPW) can be contacted here.

British Association for Counselling

1 Regent Place
Rugby
Warwickshire CV21 2PJ

British Association of Prosthetists and Orthotists (BAPO)

Secretariat: Sir James Clark Building
Abbey Mill Business Centre
Paisley
Renfrewshire PA1 1TJ

BAPO publish *BAPOMAG*.

British Dietetic Association

7th Floor, 22 Suffolk Street
Queensway
Birmingham B1 1LS

British Psychological Society

St Andrews House
48 Princes Road East
Leicester LE1 7DR

The Forum for Clinical Psychologists in Physical Disability is contactable here.

Society of Chiropodists and Podiatrists

53 Welbeck Street
London W1M 7HE

The Appropriate Health Resources and Technologies Action Group Ltd (AHRTAG)

Farringdon Point, 2nd floor
29–35 Farringdon Road
London EC1M 3JB

AHRTAG's objective is to promote successful techniques in support of primary healthcare in developing countries.

REMAP

Hazeldene
Ightham
Sevenoaks
Kent TN15 9AD

This group of individuals produce one-off technical equipment for disabled people: there is usually a local panel.

The National Centre for Clinical Audit (NCCA)

BMA House
Tavistock Square
London WC1H 9JP

MANUFACTURERS, DESIGNERS AND DISTRIBUTORS OF PROSTHETIC COMPONENTS

C. A. Blatchford and Sons Ltd

Lister Road
Basingstoke
Hampshire RG22 4AH

Dorset Orthopaedic Company Ltd

Headlands Business Park
Salisbury Road
Ringwood
Hampshire BH24 3PB

North Sea Plastics

Lillyburn Works
Milton of Camsie
Glasgow G65 8EE

OrthoEurope Ltd

Napier Court
Abingdon Science Park
Barton Lane
Abingdon
Oxfordshire OX14 3YT

Ossür UK

Synergy House
Manchester Science Park

Guildhall Close
Manchester M15 6SY

Otto Bock UK

32 Parsonage Road
Englefield Green
Egham
Surrey TW20 0JW

PI Medical (suppliers of the LIC Femurett)

Box 67
Sylveniusgatan 8A
S-751 03 Upssala
Sweden

Rehabilitation Services Ltd

Riverside Orthopaedic Centre
51 Riverside
Medway City Estate
Rochester
Kent ME2 4DP

Hugh Steeper Ltd

Roehampton Rehabilitation Centre
Roehampton Lane
London SW15 5PN

Vessa Ltd

Mill Lane
Alton
Hampshire GU34 2PK

THE INTERNET

The vast amount of information on the Internet can open up new horizons for many. Factual information on a wide range of diagnoses and disabilities, and user and news groups, allow people with common interests to share experiences and knowledge. Both amputees and therapists can find further information via this medium; the skill will be in interpreting this information correctly for the individual circumstances.

CONTENTS

Appendix 2: Wheelchairs

Wheelchair Education and Training Group

CHECKLIST FOR ASSESSMENT, PRESCRIPTION, PROVISION AND REVIEW

1. Establish the reason for referral and the client's/parents'/carers' wishes.

2. Observe the current prescription of wheelchair/seating and the way that the client is using these.

3. Assess, measure and/or record the client's posture and function in current equipment.

4. With client out of equipment, examine the components and their condition.

5. Assess the client in positions of lying, sitting and standing in order to determine his abilities in each of these positions. **Do not use prescribed equipment for this process**.

6. Measure and note presence of deformity, particularly of the spine and hips, taking care to check for any asymmetric deformities. Determine whether deformity is fixed or postural and the degree of correction achievable.

7. Define pressure distribution needs.

8. Determine the treatment/management programmes related to the client's postural support needs.

9. Determine environmental and social constraints on the prescriptions.

10. Use the collected data to determine the posture (upright or alternatives) and the support required by the client. Simulate this support with the aim of drafting the prescription, bearing in mind the following:

10a. **For tissue trauma considerations**: determine the appropriate pressure distributing or pressure re-distributing cushion either commercially available or purpose made.

10b. **For postural considerations**, whenever possible:
   a. Aim for symmetry and distribution of loadbearing through both ischial tuberosities and the whole of the thighs and buttocks.
   b. Avoid pelvic tilt, i.e. pelvis to be neutral.
   c. Avoid asymmetry, e.g. windswept hips scoliosis, etc.
   d. Provide appropriate support to stabilise the pelvis and lower limbs in all the postures being considered.
   e. Once the lower part of the body has been stabilised, determine the postural support required at the trunk level without diminishing functional ability.

11. Use support surfaces that provide bio-mechanically correct application of forces (references 1, 2, 3, 6).

12. If the foregoing is not readily achievable, referral to a specialist centre is required.

13. Choose, or design and manufacture (an iterative process), the most appropriate support system to provide the biomechanically correct postural stability to achieve the above objectives. The equipment should preferably be adjustable to meet the changing needs of the client.

14. Determine the type of wheeled mobility into which this postural support system will fit and which will also be compatible with the client's lifestyle, the family's/carer's lifestyles, physical abilities and mental abilities. Consider the following:

    a. Self-propelled, attendant propelled or powered mobility
    b. Indoor or outdoor or both
    c. Size – open and folded (for seating system, access to buildings, transportation, space, convenience)
    d. Need for various components to be removable
    e. Weight with or without removable components
    f. Ease of use including manoeuvrability and removable components

    g. Footrest position with reference to sitting posture
    h. Castor position with reference to desired foot position
    i. Stability of chair with occupant
    j. The wheelchair or other wheeled mobility devices should permit the full range of adjustment of the postural support equipment.

15. Determine whether or not provision is through NHS or by private purchase using published lists of wheelchairs and other vehicles.

16. The prescribed wheelchair must be tested for static stability with client in place. If unstable, determine modifications required or new prescription and retest on completion.

17. Instruct the client and/or carers in the particular features and functions of the seating system and wheelchair(s) and other vehicle(s), including maintenance and responsibilities for correct use.

18. Identify intervals for review and set dates.

Reproduced courtesy of Roy Nelham, Carolyn Nichols and Pauline Pope (1989).

CONTENTS

Further reading

Amputee rehabilitation

American Academy of Orthopaedic Surgeons 1965 Joint
    motion: method of measuring and recording. Churchill
    Livingstone, Edinburgh
Atkins D J, Meier R H 1989 Comprehensive management of
    the upper limb amputee. Springer-Verlag, New York
Banerjee S N 1982 Rehabilitation management of amputees,
    Williams and Wilkins, Baltimore
Barsby P, Ham R, Lumley C, Roberts C 1995 Amputee
    management: a handbook. King's College School of
    Medicine and Dentistry. London
Beck A T 1973 The diagnosis and management of
    depression. University of Pennsylvania Press,
    Philadelphia
Coates H, King A 1982 Patient assessment: handbook for
    therapists. Churchill Livingstone, London
Croucher N 1981 Outdoor pursuits for disabled people.
    Woodhead Faulkner, Cambridge
Galley P M, Forster A L 1982 Human movement: an
    introductory text for physiotherapy students. Churchill
    Livingstone, Edinburgh
Ham R, Cotton L 1991 Limb amputation from aetiology to
    rehabilitation. Champman and Hall, London
Humm W 1977 Rehabilitation of the lower limb amputee,
    3rd edn. Baillière Tindall, London
Kolb L C 1954 The painful phantom: psychology, physiology
    and treatment. C C Thomas, Springfield, IL
Kostuik J P 1981 Amputation surgery and rehabilitation: the
    Toronto experience. Churchill Livingstone, Edinburgh
Kottke F J, Stillwell G K, Lehmann J F 1982 Krusen's
    handbook of physical medicine and rehabilitation, 3rd
    edn. W B Saunders, Philadelphia
Krueger D W 1984 Rehabilitation psychology: a
    comprehensive textbook. Aspen Systems, Maryland
Kubler-Ross E 1970 On death and dying. Routledge, London
Lamb D, Law H 1988 Upper limb deficiencies in children.
    Prosthetic, orthotic and surgical management. Little
    Brown, Boston
Lewin A 1996 Life and limb. Plasma Print, Princes
    Risborough
Macdonald E M (ed) 1976 Occupational therapy in
    rehabilitation, 4th edn. Baillière Tindall, London
Mensch G 1987 Physical therapy management of lower
    extremity amputation. Heinemann Medical, London

Pendleton D, Hasler J 1983 Doctor and patient communication. Academic Press, London

Robertson E 1978 Rehabilitation of arm amputees and limb deficient children. Baillière Tindall, London

Rusk H 1977 Rehabilitation medicine, 4th edn. C V Mosby, St Louis

Saunders G T 1986 Lower limb amputations: a guide to rehabilitation. F A Davis, Philadelphia

Setoguchi Y, Rosenfelder R 1982 The limb deficient child. C C Thomas, Springfield

Troup I M, Wood M A 1982 Total care of the lower limb amputee. Pitman, London

Willard H S, Spackman C S 1971 Occupational therapy, 4th edn. JB Lippincott, Philadelphia

Biomechanics and gait

Basmajian J V 1978 Muscles alive, 4th edn. Williams and Wilkins, Baltimore

Carlsoo S 1972 How man moves. Heinemann, London

Gage J R 1991 Gait analysis in cerebral palsy. MacKeith Press, London

Hughes J 1976 Human locomotion. In: Murdoch G (ed) The advance in orthotics. Edward Arnold, London, p 57–73

Hughes J, Paul J P, Kenedi R M 1970 Control and movement of the lower limb. In: Simpson D C (ed) Modern trends in biomechanics 1. Butterworth, London, P 147–179

Le Veau B 1977 Williams and Lissner – Biomechanics of human motion, 2nd edn. W B Saunders, Philadelphia

MacConaill M A, Basmajian J V 1969 Muscles and movement: a basic for human kinesiology. Williams and Wilkins, Baltimore

Perry J 1992 Gait analysis: normal and pathological function. Slack Incorporated. Thorofare, N J

Rose G K, Butler P, Stallard J 1982 Gait: principles, biomechanics, and assessment. Orlau Publishing, Oswestry

Rose J, Gamble J G 1994 Human walking, 2nd edn. Williams & Wilkins, Baltimore

Sutherland D H, Olshen R A, Biden E N, Wyatt M P 1988 The developments of mature walking. Mac Keith Press, London

Whittle M 1996 Gait analysis: an introduction, 2nd edn. Butterworth Heinemann, London

Winter D A 1991 The biomechanics and motor control of human gait, 2nd edn. University of Waterloo Press, Ontario

Videotape

Normal walking. Gillette Children's Hospital, 200 East University Avenue, St Paul MN 55101, USA. Tel: +1 612 291 2848

Quality

Adler J, Tofts A 1995 Health service manager. Croner publications Ltd, Surrey

Bowling A 1997 Measuring health: a review of quality of life measurement scales, 2nd edn. Open University Press, Buckingham

Bury T, Mead J 1998 Evidence based healthcare: a practical guide for therapists. Butterworth Heinemann, London

Cole B, Finch E, Gowland C, Mayo N 1995 Physical rehabilitation outcome measures. Williams and Wilkins, Balitmore

Crombie I K, Davies H T O, Abraham S C S, Forey CduV 1993 The audit handbook. John Wiley and Sons, London

Muir Gray J A 1997 Evidence based healthcare: how to make health policy and management decisions. Churchill Livingstone, Edinburgh

McIver S 1991 Introduction to obtaining the views of users of health services. Kings Fund Bookshop, London

Øvretveit J 1992 Health service quality: an introduction to quality methods for health services. Blackwell Scientific Publications, Oxford

Sackett D L, Scott Richardson W, Rosenberg W, Haynes R B 1997 Evidence based medicine: how to practice and teach EBM. Churchill Livingstone, Edinburgh

Spath P L 1989 Innovations in healthcare quality measurement. American Hospital Publishing Inc, Chicago

Wilson C R M 1987 Hospital-wide quality assurance: models for implementation and development. W B Saunders, Toronto

Centre for Medical Education, Dundee 1995 Moving to audit: an education package for chiropodists, clinical psychologists, dieticians, occupational therapists, physiotherapists, radiographers and speech and language therapists. The Post-Graduate Office, Ninewells Hospital and Medical School, Dundee, Scotland

History

Alper H (ed) 1996 A history of Queen Mary's University Hospital Roehampton. Richmond, Twickenham and Roehampton Healthcare NHS Trust

Therapy

British Association of Chartered Physiotherapists in Amputee Rehabilitation (BACPAR) 1997 Amputation rehabilitation: a guideline for the education of students. The Chartered Society of Physiotherapy, London

Hagedorn R 1992 Occupational therapy: foundations for practice. Models, frames of reference and core skills. Churchill Livingstone, Edinburgh

Goodwill C J, Chamberlain M A, Evans C 1997 Rehabilitation of the physically disabled adult, 2nd edn. Stanley Thomas (Publishers LTD) Cheltenham, UK

Hansen R A, Atchison B 1993 Conditions in occupational therapy: effect on occupational performance. Williams and Wilkins, Baltimore

Maczka K 1990 Assessing physically disabled people at home. Therapy in practice. Chapman and Hall, London

Neistadt M E Bleasedale Crepeau E 1998 Willard and Spackmans Occupational Therapy 9th Edn. J P Lippincott, Philadelphia

Nichols P J R 1980 Rehabilitation medicine: the management of physical disabilities. Butterworth, London

Pedretti L W 1996 Occupational therapy: practice skills for physical dysfunction. 4th edition. Mosby, St Louis

Penso D E 1987 Occupational therapy for children with disabilities. Therapy in practice. Chapman and Hall, London

Reed K L, Nelson Sanderson S 1992 Concepts in occupational therapy, 3rd edn. Williams and Wilkins, Baltimore

Trew M, Everett T 1997 Human movement: an introductory text, 3rd edn. Churchill Livingstone, Edinburgh

Trombly C A 1997 Occupational therapy for physical dysfunction, 4th edn. Williams and Wilkins, Baltimore

Turner A, Foster M, Johnson S E 1996 Occupational therapy and physical dysfunction: principles, skills and practice, 4th edn. Churchill Livingstone, Edinburgh

Young M E, Quinn E 1992 Theories and principles of occupational therapy. Churchill Livingstone, Edinburgh

Van Deusen J, Brunt D 1997 Assessment in occupational therapy and physical therapy. W B Saunders Company, Philadelphia

Prosthetics

American Academy of Orthopaedic Surgeons 1981 Atlas of limb prosthetics: surgical and prosthetic principles. C V Mosbv. St Louis

Day H J B Kulkarni J R Datta D 1993 Prescribing upper limb prostheses. Amputee Medical Rehabilitation Society, London

Department of Health and Social Security 1986 Amputation statistics for England, Wales and N. Ireland for the year 1985. DHSS, Norcross, Blackpool

Klopsteg P E, Wilson P D 1954 Human limbs and their substitutes. McGraw-Hill, New York

Mastro B A 1980 Elected reading: a review of orthotics and prosthetics. American Orthotic and Prosthetic Association, Washington

Murdoch G 1970 Prosthetic and orthotic practice. Edward Arnold, London

Murdoch G, Donovan R G (eds) 1988 Amputation surgery and lower limb prosthetics. Blackwell Scientific, Edinburgh

Phillips G 1990 Best foot forward. Granta Editions, Cambridge

Redhead R G, Day H J B, Marks L J, Lachmann S L 1991 Prescribing lower limb prostheses. Disablement Services Authority (from NHS Supplies Authority, Sheffield)

Royal College of Surgeons of England 1967 Symposium on limb ablation and limb replacement. Annals of the Royal College of Surgeons of England 40(4)

Vitali M, Andrews B G, Robinson K P, Harris E H 1986 Amputations and prostheses. Baillière Tindall, London

Wilson A B 1976 Limb prosthetics, 5th edn. Robert E Krieger, New York

Amputation surgery: vascular disease

Abramson D I, Miller D S 1981 Vascular problems in musculoskeletal disorders of the limbs. Springer-Verlag, New York

Bloom A, Ireland J 1980 A colour atlas of diabetes. Wolfe Medical Publications, London

Burgess E M, Romano R L, Zettl C P 1969 The management of lower extremity amputations: surgery, immediate postsurgical prosthetic fitting, patient care. Veterans Administration, Washington

Faris I 1982 The management of the diabetic foot. Churchill Livingstone, Edinburgh

Gerhardt J J, King P S, Zett J H 1982 Amputations: immediate and early prosthetic management. Hans Huber, Bern

Gillis Leon 1954 Amputations. Heinemann, London

Greenhalgh R M 1985 Diagnostic techniques and assessment procedures in vascular surgery. Grune and Stratton, London

Harris N H, Birch R 1995 Postgraduate textbook of clinical orthopaedics, 2nd edn. Blackwell Science, Oxford

Levy W S 1983 Skin problems of the amputee. Warren H Green, St Louis

Little J M 1975 Major amputations for vascular disease. Churchill Livingstone, Edinburgh

Malt R A 1978 Surgical techniques illustrated 3(3). Amputations of the lower extremity. Little Brown, Boston

Murdoch G, Bennet A, Wilson A 1996 Amputation, surgical practice and patient management. Butterworth Heinemann, London

Saleh M 1993 Amputation surgery. In: Evans D (ed) Techniques in orthopaedic surgery. Blackwell Scientific Publications, Oxford

Siegfried J, Zimmermann M 1981 Phantom and stump pain. Springer-Verlag, Berlin

Walker W F 1980 A colour atlas of peripheral vascular disease. Wolfe Medical Publications, London

Warren R, Record E E 1967 Lower extremity amputation for arterial insufficiency. Little Brown, Boston

Equipment for disabled people and community practice

Bumphrey E E 1995 Community practice: a text for occupational therapists and others involved in community care, 2nd edn. Harvester Wheatsheaf, Hertfordshire

Compton A, Ashwin M 1992 Community care for healthcare professionals. Butterworth Heinemann, London

Dambrough A, Kinrade D 1995 Directory for disabled people, 7th edition. Prentice Hall / Harvester Wheatsheaf, Hertfordshire

Disability Information Trust; Equipment for Disabled People. Mary Marlborough Centre, Nuffield Orthopaedic Centre, Oxford, UK
    Arthritis: an equipment guide 1997
    Children with disabilities 1993
    Communication and access to computer technology 1995
    Employment in the workplace 1994
    Furniture 1997
    Gardening – an equipment guide 1997
    Hoists, lifts, and transfers 1996
    Home management and housing 1995
    Manual wheelchairs – a practical guide 1998
    Outdoor transport 1994
    Personal care 1996
    Powered wheelchairs and scooters – a practical guide 1998
    Sport and leisure 1996
    Walking and standing aids 1997
    Wheelchair accessories 1998

Disabled Living Foundation, London. Choosing an electric wheelchair

Equipment and services for people with disabilities. Health Publications Unit, Department of Health and the Central Office of Information

Goldsmith S 1984 Designing for the disabled, 4th edn. Royal Institute of Architects, London

Ham R, Aldersea P, Porter D 1998 Wheelchair users and postural seating. Churchill Livingstone, Edinburgh

Male J, Massie B 1990 Choosing a wheelchair. The Royal Association for Disability and Rehabilitation (RADAR), London

Mandlestam M 1997 Equipment for older or disabled people and the law. Jessica Kingsley Publishers, London

Mandlestam M 1990 How to get equipment for disability. Disabled Living Foundation. Jessica Kingsley Publishers, London

National Council for Voluntary Organisations 1996 The voluntary agencies directory, 15th edn. NCVO Publications, London

National prosthetic and wheelchair services report 1993–1996 College of Occupational Therapists, London

RADAR 1995 Getting the best from your wheelchair: a guide to using a basic wheelchair. The Royal Association for Disability and Rehabilitation, London

Statham R, Korczak J, Monaghan P 1988 House adaptations for people with physical disabilities. Department of the Environment, HMSO, London

Tuttiet S 1990 Wheelchair cushions summary report, 2nd edn. Department of Health Disability Equipment Assessment Programme

Wheelchair training resource pack 1996 College of Occupational Therapists, London

Other

British Standards, Prosthetics and Orthotics:

Part 1 Section 1.1 Glossary of general terms relating to external limb prostheses and external orthoses BS 7313 ISO 8549–1

Part 1 Section 1.2 Glossary of terms relating to external limb prostheses and wearers of external limb prostheses BS 7313 ISO 8549–2

Part 2 Method of describing limb deficiencies present at birth BS 7313 ISO 8548-1

Part 3 Method of describing lower limb amputation stumps BS 7313 ISO 8548–2

Part 4 Method of describing upper limb amputation stumps BS 7313 ISO 8548–3

Bryceson A, Pfalzgraff R E 1990 Leprosy, 3rd edn. Churchill Livingstone, Edinburgh

Coates T T 1983 Practical orthotics for chiropodists. Actinic Press, London

Coombs R, Friedlander G 1987 Bone tumour management. Butterworth, London

Croucher N 1989 Tales of many mountains. Amanda Press, London

Disabled Drivers' Motor Club Handbook 1985 Ins and outs of car choice: a guide for elderly and disabled people. Department of Transport, London

Hart E 1986 Victoria, my daughter: a true story of courage. Bodley Head, London

Jopling W H 1985 Handbook of leprosy, 3rd edn. Heinemann Medical, London

Klenerman L 1982 The foot and its disorders. Blackwell Scientific, London

Kohner N 1988 Caring at home. National Extension College, Cambridge

Maczka K 1990 Assessing physically disabled people at home. Chapman and Hall, London

Medical Devices Agency Bulletin No. 16. Guidance notes for manufacturers of prosthetic and orthotic devices

Morris J 1993 Pride against prejudice: transforming attitudes to disability. The Women's Press, London

Oliver M 1990 The politics of disablement. Macmillan, London

Shakespeare T, Gillespie-Sells K, Davies D 1996 The sexual politics of disability. Cassell, London

The Children's Act 1989 An introductory guide for the NHS. HMSO, London

Watson J M 1986 Essential action to minimise disability in leprosy patients. The Leprosy Mission, London

Watson J M 1986 Preventing disability in leprosy patients. The Leprosy Mission International, London

Pain management

Caudill A 1994 Managing pain before it manages you. Guildford Press

Broome A, Jellicoe H 1987 Living with your pain. British Psychological Society, Leicester, in association with Methuen and Co. Ltd., London

Gatchell R J, Turk D C 1996 Psychological approaches to pain management. A practitioner's handbook. Guildford Press

Melzack R, Wall P D 1985 The challenge of pain. Penguin, Harmondsworth

Sherman R A, Devor M, Jones C D E, Katz J, Marbach J J 1997 Phantom Pain. Plenum Press, New York

Turk D C, Melzack R 1992 Handbook of Pain Assessment. Guildford Press

Wells P, Frampton V, Bowsher D 1997 Pain management by physiotherapy, 2nd edn. Butterworth Heinemann Ltd, Oxford

Journals

The organisations publishing journals relevant to the rehabilitation of the amputee are listed in Appendix 1.

Index

Page numbers in italics refer to tables and figures.